REOPERATIVE GYNECOLOGIC SURGERY

"A wise and experienced surgeon has said, 'The second most difficult decision to make in surgery is when to operate. The most difficult decision is when to reoperate.' The truth of this aphorism is readily apparent to most clinical surgeons."

Ronald K. Tompkins, M.D., 1988

Reoperative Gynecologic Surgery

DAVID H. NICHOLS, M.D.
Professor of Obstetrics and Gynecology
Brown University Program in Medicine
Director, The Center for Women's Surgery at Brown University and Women and Infants Hospital of Rhode Island
Providence, Rhode Island

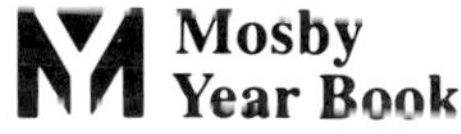

St. Louis Baltimore Boston Chicago London Philadelphia Sydney Toronto

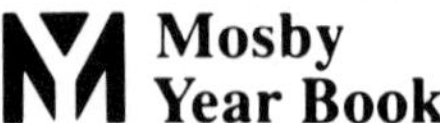

Dedicated to Publishing Excellence

Sponsoring Editor: Stephanie Manning
Assistant Director, Manuscript Services: Frances M. Perveiler
Production Coordinator: Nancy C. Baker
Proofroom Supervisor: Barbara Kelly

Mosby–Year Book, Inc.
11830 Westline Industrial Drive
St. Louis, MO 63146

1 2 3 4 5 6 7 8 9 0 CL/MV 95 94 93 92 91

Library of Congress Cataloging-in-Publication Data
Reoperative gynecologic surgery / [edited by] David H. Nichols.
p. cm.
Includes bibliographical references.
Includes index.
ISBN 0-8151-6383-5
1. Generative organs, Female—Reoperation. 2. Generative organs, Female—surgery—Complications and sequelae. I. Nichols, David H., 1925-
[DNLM: 1. Genitalia, Female—surgery. 2. Postoperative Complications. 3. Surgery, Operative. WP 660 R424]
RG104.2.R46 1991 91-13296
618.1′45—dc20 CIP
DNLM/DLC

To Robert, Landel and David, to carry on further the surgical traditions in which their grandfather so firmly believed.

CONTRIBUTORS

James L. Breen, M.D.
Department of Obstetrics and Gynecology
St. Barnabs Medical Center
Livingston, New Jersey

Steven L. Curry, M.D.
Director, Obstetrics and Gynecology
Hartford Hospital
Hartford, Conneticut

Julian E. De Lia, M.D.
Associate Professor of Obstetrics and Gynecology
University of Utah School of Medicine
Salt Lake City, Utah

Bruce H. Drukker, M.D.
Professor and Chairperson, Department of Obstetrics and Gynecology and Reproductive Biology
Michigan State University
East Lansing, Michigan

Celso-Ramón García, M.D.
Director of Reproductive Surgery
William Schippen, Jr. Professor of Human Reproduction
Department of Obstetrics and Gynecology
University of Pennsylvania
Philadelphia, Pennsylvania

David L. Hemsell, M.D.
Professor of Obstetrics and Gynecology
Director, Division of Gynecology
The University of Texas
Southwestern Medical Center
Dallas, Texas

Jaroslav F. Hulka, M.D.
Professor
Department of Obstetrics and Gynecology
University of North Carolina School of Medicine
Chapel Hill, North Carolina

W. Glenn Hurt, M.D.
Professor
Department of Obstetrics and Gynecology
Medical College of Virginia
Richmond, Virginia

Saul Lerner, M.D.
Professor of Obstetrics and Gynecology
University of Massachusetts Medical School
Worchester, Massachusetts

L. Russel Malinak, M.D.
Professor
Department of Obstetrics and Gynecology
Baylor University
Medical Director
Center for Reproductive Medicine and Surgery
Methodist Hospital
Houston, Texas

Douglas J. Marchant, M.D.
Professor of Obstetrics and Gynecology
Professor of Surgery
Tufts University School of Medicine
New England Medical Center
Boston, Massachusetts

Augustine M. McNamee, M.D.
Clinical Assistant Professor
Department of Anesthesia
Rhode Island Hospital
Brown University School of Medicine
Providence, Rhode Island

Linda Mitchel-Frye
Resident, Obstetrics and Gynecology
Medical College of Georgia
Augusta, Georgia

George S. Mitchell, M.D.
Professor
Department of Obstetrics and Gynecology
The University of Texas Health Science Center
San Antonio, Texas

David H. Nichols, M.D.
Professor of Obstetrics and Gynecology
Brown University Program in Medicine
Director, The Center for Women's Surgery at Brown University and Women and Infants Hospital of Rhode Island
Providence, Rhode Island

Giglia Parker, M.D.
Clinical Assistant Professor
Department of Obstetrics and Gynecology
Brown University Program in Medicine
Providence, Rhode Island

Timothy H. Parmley, M.D.
Professor of Obstetrics and Gynecology
University of Arkansas for Medical Sciences
Little Rock, Arkansas

John D. Thompson, M.D.
Professor, Department of Gynecology and Obstetrics
Emory University School of Medicine
Atlanta, Georgia

James M. Wheeler, M.D., M.P.H.
Assistant Professor
Department of Obstetrics and Gynecology
Director, In Vitro Fertilization
Baylor University School of Medicine
Houston, Texas

Clifford R. Wheeless, M.D.
Associate Professor of Obstetrics and Gynecology
Johns Hopkins University School of Medicine
Chairman, Department of Obstetrics and Gynecology
Union Memorial Hospital
Baltimore, Maryland

Tiffany J. Williams, M.D.
Professor
Department of Obstetrics and Gynecology
Mayo Medical School
Mayo Clinic
Rochester, Minnesota

PREFACE

Throughout the civilized world there are more women living longer. To these women longevity is a poor reward unless accompanied by a meaningful quality of life. When correctable disorders of the urogenital systems subtract from this quality of life, it is the mission of the gynecologic surgeon to address these needs effectively and efficiently. Once thoughtful consideration indicates a surgical remedy, the initial procedure should be selected carefully and performed with greatest precision so that it will provide a permanent solution to the patient's problem. When these efforts, however strongly motivated, have not been successful, the possibility of reoperation must be entertained.

At no time in previous history have the opportunities for preservation or restoration of quality of life been more readily available. At the same time the costs of hospitalization have never been so great. We are in an era when our hospital system can shoulder the expense of surgery for a given condition only once. The luxury of reoperation to say nothing of the repetition of risk, pain, and inconvenience for the patient will not long be tolerated.

When reoperation is necessary through some tragedy of inadequate initial preoperative assessment, a poor choice of technical procedure, improficiency in its performance, the appearance of unforseeable and unpreventable complications, or the cumulative effects of tissue aging, the patient, often an older woman, requires special reassessment and the most careful surgical decision making.

To salvage the situation, the reoperative procedure must be done with greatest precision. The surgeon must take into consideration the often altered physiologic status of the patient as well as the changes and scarring, both psychological and anatomic, brought about by the previous operation.

To address and solve these issues as they affect the female reproductive system is the purpose of this book. The best American authors for each chapter have been carefully selected for their interest and accomplishments in each of the areas addressed. They have generously directed their efforts to emphasize both prevention and salvage.

David H. Nichols, M.D.

PREFACE

ACKNOWLEDGMENTS

The editor acknowledges with pleasure the skillful contributions of illustrations of Melford Diedrick and Allison Boisselle made to illustrate the author's views in various previous publications, especially the monograph, "Vaginal Surgery" published by Williams & Wilkins of Baltimore. The artistic contributions of Robert Hoagland, Nance Place, and Diane Raeke to this book are much appreciated. Dr. Giglia A. Parker provided valuable manuscript suggestions. The conceptual planning of James Ryan, the editorial skills and patience of Nancy Puckett and Stephanie Manning and production skills of Nancy Baker of Mosby–Year Book, Inc., have been invaluable and are sincerely appreciated. The patience and forbearance of my co-workers at Brown University and at the Women & Infants Hospital of Rhode Island have been an indulgence without parallel. The burden of typing and retyping the manuscript has been most ably borne by our secretaries, Kathy Hawes and Donna Coppola.

David H. Nichols, M.D.

CONTENTS

COLOR PLATES

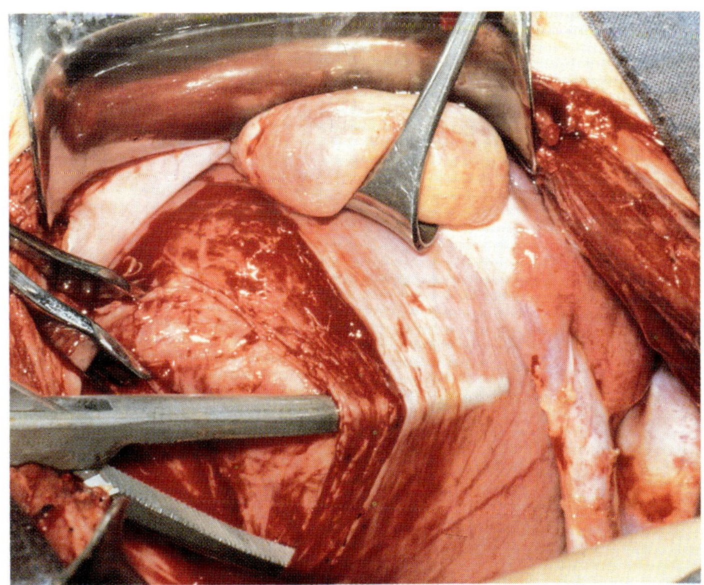

PLATE 1.—One large myoma and numerous small and intermediate-sized myomas are seen in the anterior uterine wall. Because of the distortion, we cannot immediately apply a tourniquet around the lower uterine segment. The large, centrally situated myoma must be enucleated first and is approached through a midline incision. (When the myoma is to be approached more laterally, a transverse incision is made to parallel the blood supply from the uterine vessels to the uterine wall.) The midline incision has been made with a Shaw hemostatic scalpel; the section through the myometrium has been extended to the myoma, and dissection will be continued between the myoma and its capsule as shown. As soon as the surface of the myoma has been exposed, it is grasped by a tenaculum to which traction is applied, reducing blood loss. (Photograph by Lester V. Bergman, courtesy of LTI Medica® and The Upjohn Company. Copyright © 1986 by Learning Technology Incorporated.)

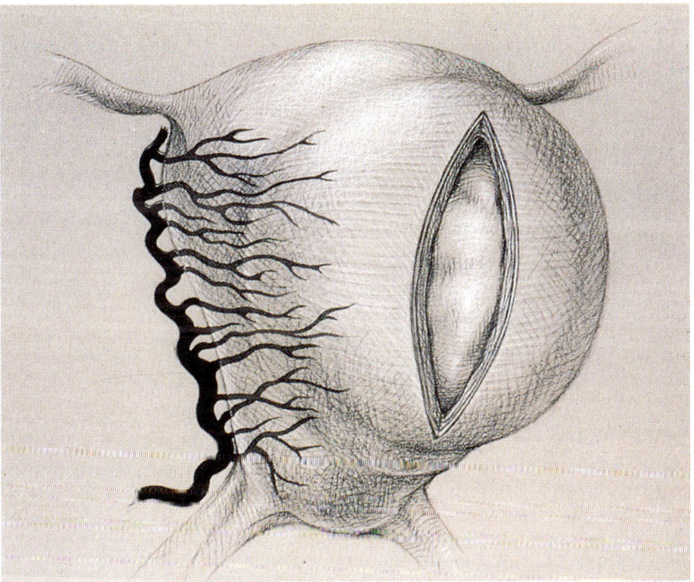

PLATE 2.—The midline incision through the thinnest area over the bulging myoma has been carried to the capsule of the tumor. After further dissection beneath the capsule, the mass is delivered with traction. Notice the branches from the left uterine artery (Drawing by Beverly Kessler, courtesy of LTI Medica® and The Upjohn Company. Copyright © 1986 by Learning Technology Incorporated.)

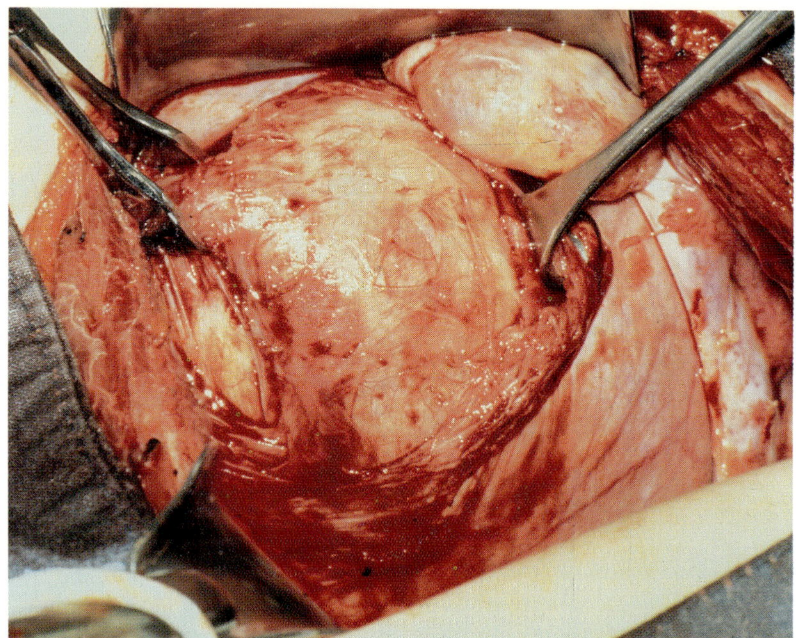

PLATE 3.—The myoma is delivered from the uterine bed while continued traction on the myoma reduces the bleeding. (Photograph by Lester V. Bergman, courtesy of LTI Medica® and The Upjohn Company. Copyright © 1986 by Learning Technology Incorporated.)

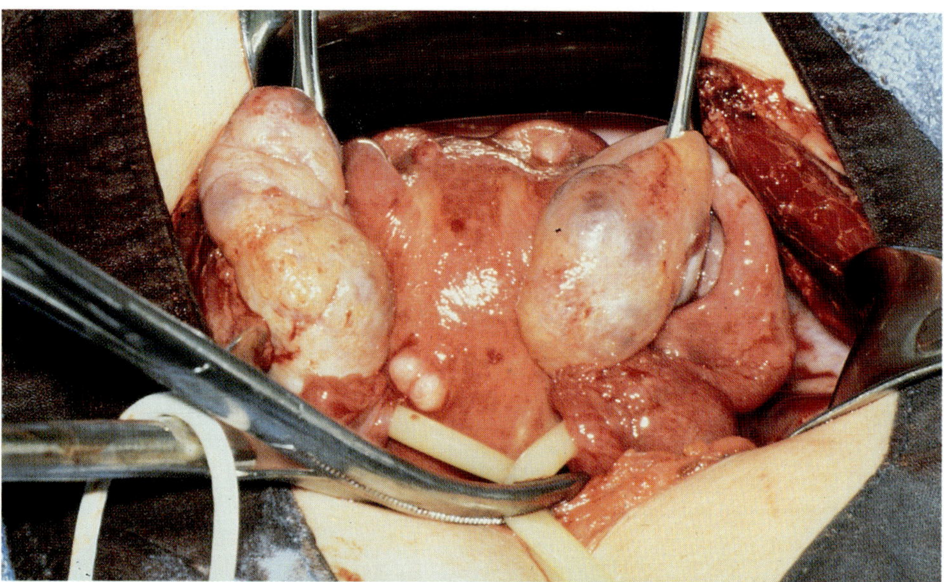

PLATE 4.—The uterus has been elevated with clamps on the utero-ovarian ligaments, and a section of latex tubing has been placed around the entire uterine body, encompassing both the fallopian tubes and ovaries to compress the infundibulopelvic and uterine vessels. Traction on a Kelly clamp applied posteriorly makes the tubing a tourniquet, and a second Kelly will be applied for stepwise tightening of the tubing. This technique produces considerable hemostasis. (Photograph by Lester V. Bergman, courtesy of LTI Medica® and The Upjohn Company. Copyright © 1986 by Learning Technology Incorporated.)

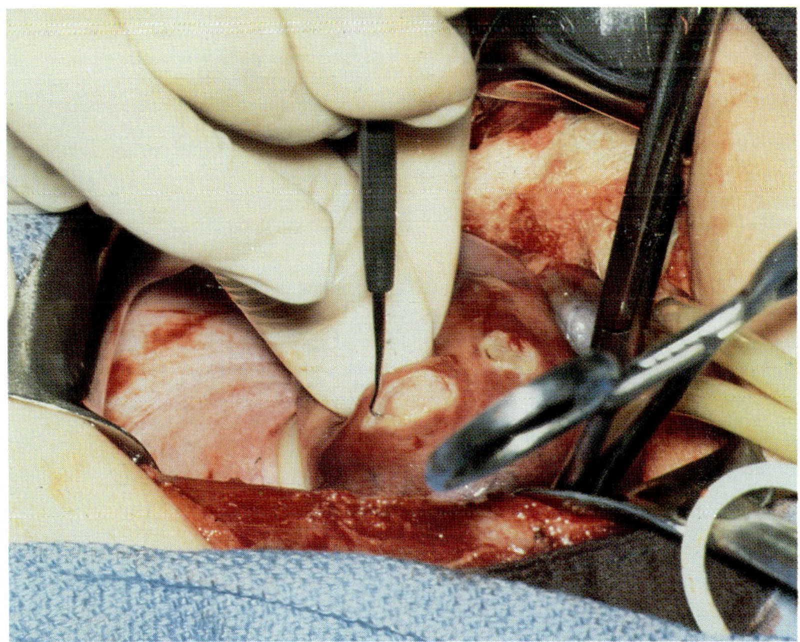

PLATE 5.—The capsule of a smaller leiomyoma has been incised and the tumor elevated by a skin hook to which traction has been applied. (Photograph by Lester V. Bergman, courtesy of LTI Medica® and The Upjohn Company. Copyright © 1986 by Learning Technology Incorporated.)

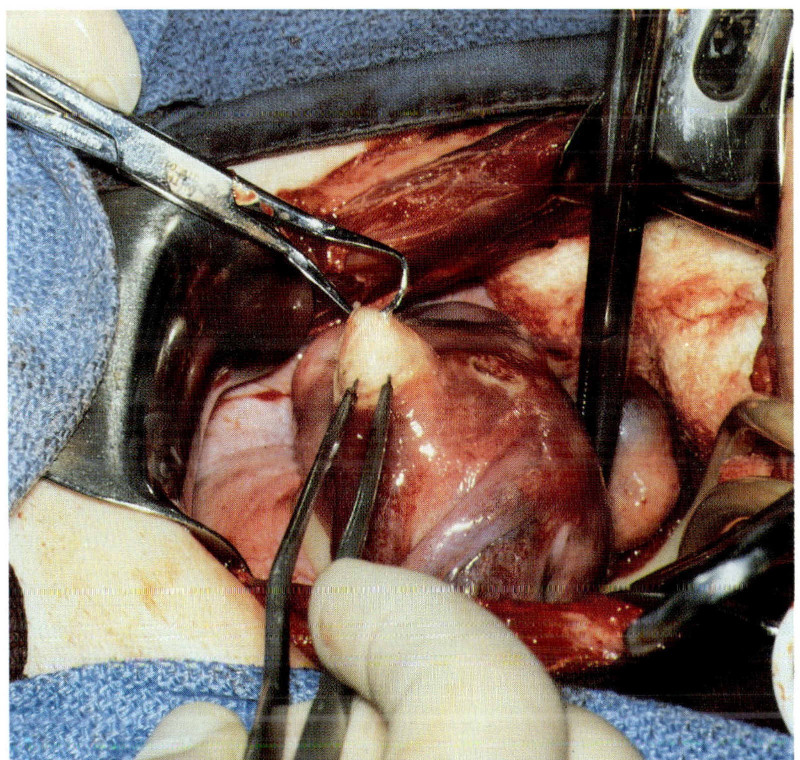

PLATE 6.—The skin hook is replaced by a towel clip, and the myoma is shelled out from its bed within its capsule. Bipolar microforceps may aid in the dissection. (Photograph by Lester V. Bergman, courtesy of LTI Medica® and The Upjohn Company. Copyright © 1986 by Learning Technology Incorporated.)

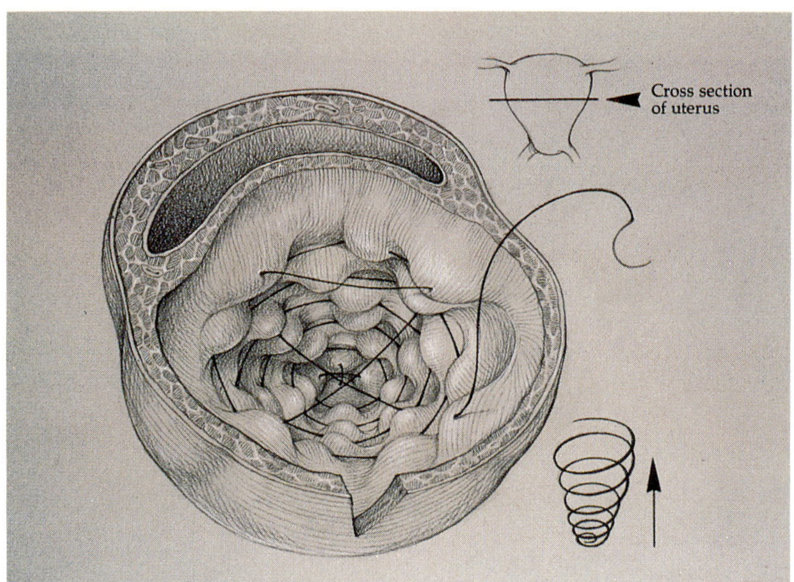

PLATE 7.—The defect in the myometrium following myomectomy is closed with a continuous circumferential approximating suture, and crisscross mattress sutures are used as needed to further obliterate the dead space. Two more sutures were placed after the deep one, shown in the depths of the wound. Additional crisscross mattress sutures will be placed. A centrally situated submucous myoma may not be demonstrated by palpation, and hysterotomy may occasionally be necessary to locate and remove the elusive tumor. Meticulous technique of repair is important to avoid occlusion of the uterine tubes in the cornual area. Size 4-0 polyglycolic acid–type suture is used (Drawing by Beverly Kessler, courtesy of LTI Medica® and The Upjohn Company. Copyright © 1986 by Learning Technology Incorporated.)

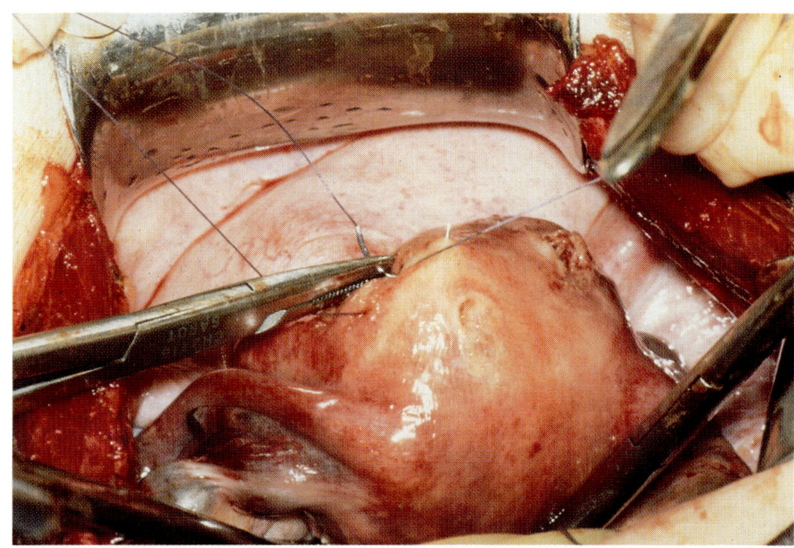

PLATE 8.—After the deeper layers have been circumferentially ligated, a running no. 4-0 polyglycolic acid–type suture is placed in the subperitoneal myometrium. Oozing around the edges may require coagulation with the bipolar current. The tourniquet is removed. If the operation has extended beyond 2 hours, the existing crop of ovarian follicles will probably die, and the menstrual flow will be delayed until the maturation of a new crop of follicles from the more resistant primordial germ cells 2 or 3 weeks postoperatively. (Photograph by Lester V. Bergman, courtesy of LTI Medica® and The Upjohn Company. Copyright © 1986 by Learning Technology Incorporated.)

Chapter 1

General Considerations

David H. Nichols, M.D.

The goals of reoperative gynecologic surgery are the same as those of primary gynecologic surgery: the relief of symptoms, the restoration of useful function, and the reestablishment of anatomic relationships. A decision for reoperation requires some assumptions concerning the causes of failure of the original surgery. Understanding of the etiology of the failure may evolve from the surgeon's consideration of the following issues: Is it clear that the original surgery was the best solution to relieve the patient's symptoms? If so, was the best of several possible operations selected for this particular patient? Was the procedure performed expertly by an experienced surgeon? Was the quality of postoperative care appropriate to the needs of this particular patient?

Some introspective soul searching is required if the original operation was performed by oneself. Reviewing objectively one's personal record of success and noting the long-term result after prolonged longitudinal postoperative follow-up of one's patients is an essential habit all gynecologic surgeons should develop.

Any operative exercise must have realistic goals to be achieved. The surgeon must faithfully determine postoperatively whether or not these expectations have been realized and, if not, why not. If results are less than ideal, one must develop a plan to prevent these problems among future patients.

Once again, the surgeon should take a detailed history from the patient emphasizing subtle clues concerning the onset and progression of the patient's disability or of its persistence since the previous surgery. It is helpful to ask and understand the patient's perception of her problem.

Copies of previous surgical dictations, pathology reports, and discharge summaries should be obtained, whenever possible, and studied. One should ask the patient's permission to contact the original surgeon when this might seem likely to produce candid answers not evident in the signed dictations.

Having considered what steps have already been taken to relieve her suffering, one should note whether the latter were even partially effective.

A careful and unhurried physical examination seeking mechanical clues that might explain the operative failure should be performed. The surgeon should endeavor to correlate the patient's symptoms with positive findings, and these observations should be promptly recorded. For those suspected conditions likely made worse by the pull of gravity, pelvic examination should be conducted with the patient in the standing as well as lithotomy position, first while she is at rest and then while she is bearing down.

Positive findings relevant to the patient's problem must be summarized.

A firm and definitive preoperative diagnosis should be made and recorded. There must be careful correlation between symptoms and findings with realistic assessment of both patient and physician expectations of the results of surgery. The surgeon must be convinced that a new surgical plan is likely, though not guaranteed, to provide relief for the patient. If there is any doubt as to the appropriateness of a surgical remedy, the opinion and consultation of a more experienced colleague should be obtained.

All of these conclusions should be reviewed for the surgeon's memory refreshment immediately before reoperation.

Unproved or novel procedures should be considered only with great caution in the patient for whom reoperation is a consideration; however, when there are no obvious surgical alternatives, the patient must be clearly informed of the risks involved and the likelihood of success of the procedure. If the surgeon's optimism is unsubstantiated by a record of success, corroboration by consultation with a more experienced colleague should be sought, particularly if there is any doubt within the surgeon's mind as to the efficacy of the surgical plan. Nevertheless, as Zollinger says, "There must be only one 'captain of the ship,' and one surgeon alone must coordinate all diagnostic procedures, consultations, and treatments. There is no place for fragmentation of responsibility in any part of the preoperative, operative, or postoperative care of the patient who requires reoperative surgery."[1]

PREOPERATIVE CARE

A recommendation and decision for reoperation should be implemented only after meticulous assessment of the patient's history and correlation with the objective findings of physical examination. The surgeon should be familiar with all recent relevant surgical advances and described techniques that are likely to be applicable to this particular clinical problem.

There should be careful psychologic assessment of the patient's expectation of the results of the surgery, balanced with those of the surgeon. It is imperative that the surgeon's expectations be based on fact and experience and not on wishful thinking.

When indicated, appropriate preoperative recognition, evaluation, and treatment of coincident medical disorders that are likely to affect the risk and outcome of surgery should be undertaken. The patient's status with respect to problems such as heart disease, pulmonary disease, obesity, diabetes, and hypoestrogenism should be thoughtfully considered before the final presentation to the patient of the problem and its proposed solution. All necessary or desirable laboratory work should be completed and evaluated. When medical consultation will effectively provide an unprejudiced risk-benefit assessment, it should be obtained, recorded, and followed. The proposed length of hospitalization and the need and place for appropriate postoperative convalescence should be carefully outlined. Necessary alterations in lifestyle should be discussed with the patient.

The timing of reoperative surgery should be optimized. It is important that physiologic homeostasis after the previous surgery has been obtained and that edema and wound healing have stabilized. An operative time that will provide unhurried surgical intervention into the patient's condition is selected. The surgeon should be unencumbered by pressures of surgical overcommittment or by the patient's unresolved physiologic or psychologic adjustment.

INTRAOPERATIVE CARE

Morning surgery is best for reoperation when the minds and bodies of the surgeon and surgical team are alert and unfatigued. The surgeon should have arranged for the best qualified assistants available. An adequate length of time for surgery will have been booked. An appropriate anesthetic will be planned following preoperative evaluation by a skilled anesthetist.

Thoughtful consideration will have been given to include patient positioning, choice of incision, choice of suture material, and availability of special instruments that may be required. Antibiotics will not displace adequate surgical asepsis, nor will drains replace adequate and effective hemostasis. The surgeon should dictate the operative report promptly and thoroughly while the details are still freshly in mind.

POSTOPERATIVE CARE

Postoperative care begins the minute the patient enters the recovery room. The patient's loved ones should be promptly informed of the details of surgery and told when it is likely that they may see the patient and what they may expect.

The surgeon should make daily unhurried postoperative hospital visits to the patient with assessment of her responses to healing and therapy. Recognizing and responding to her psychologic concerns is important. With the implementation of discharge planning, the patient must be given information as to the surgeon's availability postoperatively for advice, counsel, and concern. She must be told in detail of changes such as unexpected pain, bleeding, or fever that should be brought to the surgeon's attention. Her convalescence should be outlined, questions solicited, and a plan made for postoperative examination. Verbal instructions are so often misinterpreted or forgotten that brief, written instructions are desirable and valuable.

Each surgeon should develop a plan for long-term follow-up and analysis of patients both as individuals and within series of cases so that the end results and effectiveness in reaching the surgical goals may be correlated with the techniques performed. Thus, the need for future modifications will become obvious and can be implemented, underlining the dynamic and evolutionary character of our surgical discipline.

REFERENCE

1. Zollinger RM: Some principles of reoperative surgery, in Tompkins RK: *Reoperative Surgery*. Philadelphia, JB Lippincott Co, 1988, pp 1–7.

Chapter 2

Evisceration

Clifford R. Wheeless, Jr., M.D.

Evisceration may be vaginal or abdominal. Fortunately, this complication is rare. Both vaginal and abdominal evisceration are preceeded by disruption of the vaginal or abdominal wound. Wound disruption, or dehiscence, generally refers to a separation of the abdominal wound involving the anterior fascia sheath and peritoneum. Vaginal evisceration has been reported without pelvic surgery following the spontaneous rupture of a large enterocele.

Both vaginal and abdominal evisceration are associated with high mortality. Although one recent series reported a mortality of 34% in patients who had operative closure of an abdominal wound evisceration, most authorities report that operative mortality has been reduced to less than 1% in recent years. Few operative complications in modern gynecology have this range of mortality associated with a surgical procedure.

ABDOMINAL EVISCERATION

The frequency of abdominal wound disruption averages 2.6% when all abdominal operations are considered collectively, but the literature ranges from 0.5% to 3%. The etiology of this phenomenon is secondary to systemic as well as local factors.

Systemic factors associated with wound separation and evisceration include age, obesity, atelectasis, coughing, retching, hiccuping, cancer, jaundice, malnutrition, corticosteroids, and immunosuppressive drugs. The most common systemic factor associated with wound separation are those pathophysiological phenomenon associated with increased intraabdominal pressure such as atelectasis with its associated coughing, nausea and vomiting, all of which increase the intraabdominal pressure and put a strain on the suture line in the abdominal wall. Systemic factors that are associated with decreased properties of wound healing play roles in the reduction and alteration of collagen synthesis, collagen reorganization, and influence the effectiveness of the phases of wound healing such as inflammatory, contraction, and epithelialization.

Local Risk Factors

The most important local factors predisposing to abdominal wound separation and evisceration are inadequate closure, inadequate suture material, hemorrhage, and wound infection. The most frequent local factor in wound dehiscence and evisceration is inadequacy of surgical technique. Occasionally the first sign of wound dehiscence manifests when the skin sutures are removed and either intestinal or omental evisceration of intraperitoneal contents occurs (Fig 2–1) Closing the midline abdominal wall incision in layers with fine absorbable suture approximating the peritoneum and the edges of the fascia with permanent suture material have generally been replaced with the mass closure techniques. Mass closure techniques involve placing sutures 2 to 3 cm from the fascia edge and including all layers of the abdominal wall, fascia, muscle, and peritoneum. It was generally believed that interrupted mass closure sutures would have a greater success rate than running mass closure sutures. A recent multicenter prospective, randomized trial compared continuous vs. interrupted sutures in midline abdominal incisions. The overall dehiscence rate was 1.6% in patients with continuous sutures vs. 2% in patients with interrupted sutures.

Many believe that the type of abdominal incision contributes to the incidence of dehiscence and evisceration. With the exception of long paramedian incisions that denervate much of the rectoabdominal wall, there is no evidence that that kind of incision is related to the incidence or frequency of wound dehiscence or evisceration. Exteriorization of drains or stomas through the midline incision rather than through separate stab wound incisions is another factor that may contribute to wound disruption and evisceration.

Wound infection can be associated with a higher incidence of wound disruption and evisceration, particularly if one has used catgut sutures. The process of absorption of catgut sutures in wounds through phagocytosis reduces suture tensile strength. The role of catgut sutures in modern gynecologic surgery is limited, and

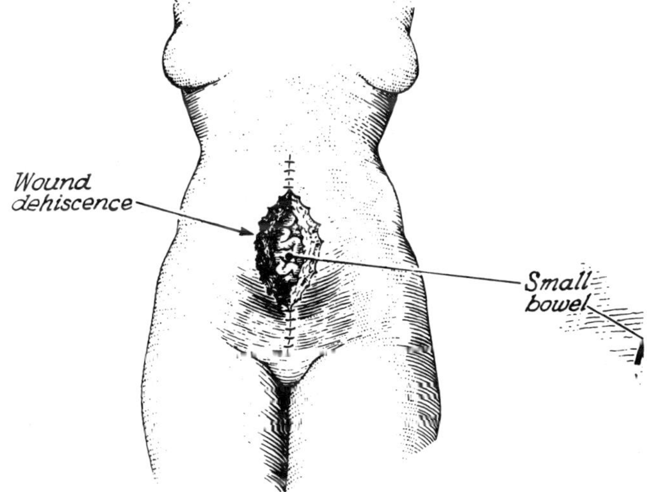

FIG 2–1.
Abdominal wound separation with dehiscence of small bowel through the wound. (From Wheeless CR Jr: Abdominal wound dehiscence, in *Atlas of Pelvic Surgery,* ed 2. Philadelphia, Lea & Febiger, 1988, p 375. Used by permission.)

they should be replaced with modern synthetic absorbable, delayed absorbable, or permanent suture.

The dehiscence rate in interrupted suture lines was significantly higher than in the continuous suture line group when wounds were contaminated. Several well-controlled series have shown no significant differences in the type of synthetic absorbable suture used, for example, polyglycolic acid vs. polyglactin 910.

Diagnosis and Management

The drainage of serosanguineous fluid after 24 hours from an abdominal incision is virtually pathogneumonic of wound separation and impending evisceration. The patient often describes a popping sensation associated with severe coughing or retching.

The mortality associated with wound disruption and evisceration can be dramatically influenced by modern surgical techniques. The patient should be returned to bed immediately, the abdominal viscera covered by moist, sterile towels, and the patient taken promptly to the operating room. The cough reflex should be immediately suppressed by the intravenous (IV) or intramuscular injection of opiates that block the cough center. After general anesthesia, the abdominal contents should be copiously washed using saline or Ringer's lactate solution. All necrotic tissue needs to be excised and all suture removed (Fig 2–2). The intestines should be thoroughly inspected from the ligament of Treitz to the rectosigmoid colon. Any devitalized intestine should be resected and reanastomosis performed (see Fig

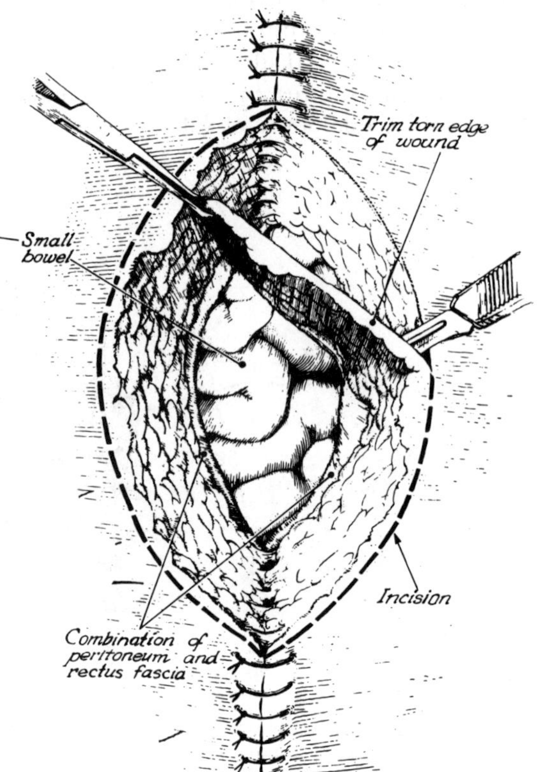

FIG 2–2.
All necrotic tissue, including skin, rectus fascia muscle and peritoneum, should be excised. Necrotic sutures should be removed. (From Wheeless CR Jr: Abdominal wound dehiscence, in *Atlas of Pelvic Surgery,* ed 2. Philadelphia, Lea & Febiger, 1988, p 375. Used by permission.)

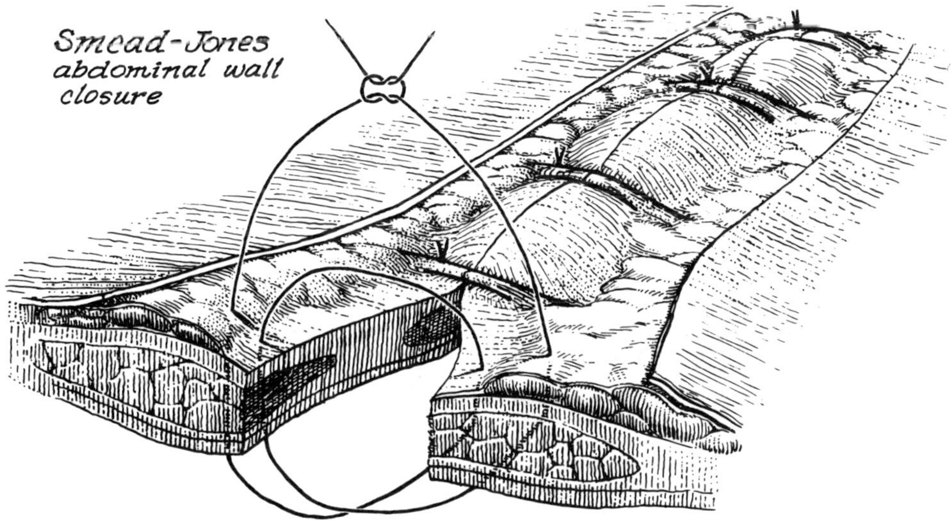

FIG 2–3.
Smead-Jones abdominal wall closure using far-near-near-far sutures.

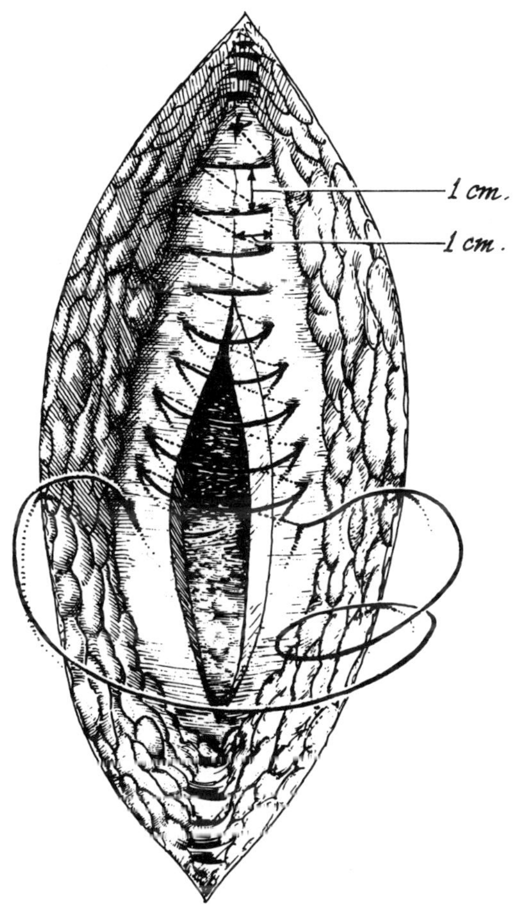

FIG 2–4.
Through-and-through technique of mass closure with running technique placing sutures 1 cm apart.

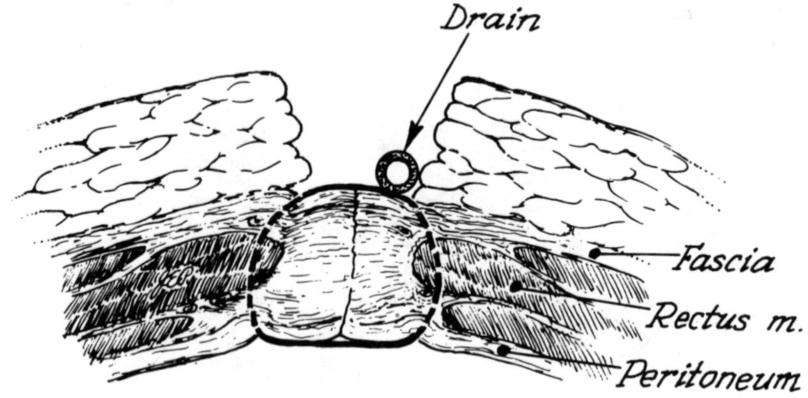

FIG 2–5.
Cross section of the mass closure including all layers, fascia, muscle, and peritoneum. If the subcutaneous tissue and skin are to be closed, a closed suction drain is placed over the fascia and brought out through a separate stab wound.

2–9). The wound should be closed in a mass closure technique using the Smead-Jones far-near-near-far technique (Fig 2–3) or the mass closure running technique (Fig 2–4). Either technique should be performed with large synthetic permanent suture (e.g., polypropylene [Prolene] or nylon). Through-and-through sutures of the entire abdominal from the skin to the peritoneum using large-gauge wire have generally been replaced with buried synthetic permanent sutures such as nylon or Prolene. If the wound is not infected or surgical debridement of necrotic tissue has been adequate (see Fig 2–2), an alternative to open or delayed wound closure may be considered and a closed suction drain placed over the fascia and under the skin and subcutaneous tissue (Fig 2–5). Intravenous antibiotics are used initially in most cases but can be tailored according to cultures taken at the time of operation and the patients' postoperative clinical course. In obese patients, the use of a surgical binder may relieve stress on the wound from the large fat pad and panniculus.

Recurrence of evisceration after reclosure of a dehisced wound is rare, although incisional hernias are later found in approximately 20% of such patients, usually in those with wound infection in addition to dehiscence.

VAGINAL EVISCERATION

Fortunately, vaginal evisceration of the intestine is rare (Fig 2–6). The literature consists of individual case presentations with an occasional review article; less than 40 cases have been reported.

Evisceration occasionally follows vaginal hysterectomy, usually within the immediate postoperative period. However, cases have been reported years later. It has been reported after abdominal hysterectomy and as a spontaneous sequela of rupture of large enteroceles with and without previous hysterectomy.

A contemporary source of vaginal eviscerations has been the suction curettage for termination of pregnancy during which the small intestine is sucked into the eye of a vacuum curette that has perforated the uterine wall (Fig 2–7) and pulled through the perforation in the uterus and out into the vagina (Fig 2–8).

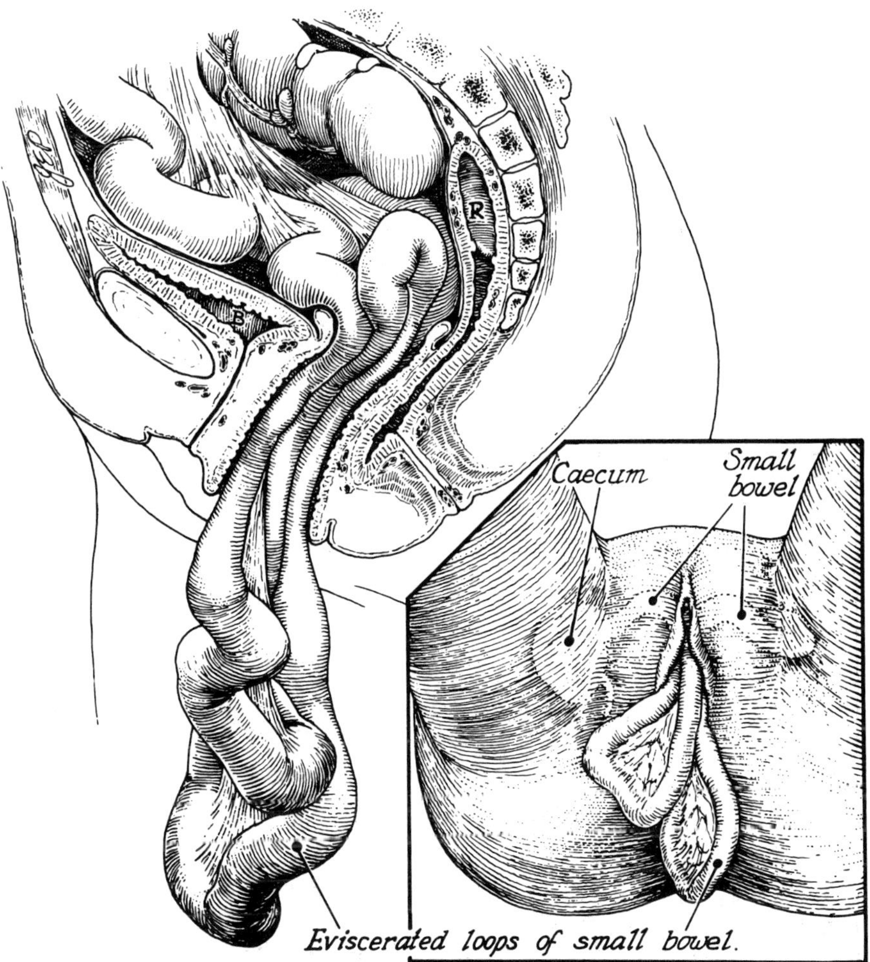

FIG 2–6.
Sagittal view of the lower abdomen and pelvis plus a perineal view *(inset)* with the patient in the lithotomy position show the vaginal evisceration. The sagittal view in particular emphasizes the point that for complete vaginal evisceration to occur, there must be some technique of mobilization of the small bowel mesentery. Otherwise, the length of small bowel mesentery is generally insufficient for the evisceration to occur. (Redrawn from Wheeless CR Jr: Vaginal evisceration following pelvic surgery, in Nichols DH [ed]: *Clinical Problems, Injuries, and Complications of Gynecologic Surgery,* ed 2. Baltimore, Williams & Wilkins Co, 1988, pp 120–129.)

The etiology of vaginal evisceration, except for that associated with suction termination of pregnancy, is confusing. No specific pattern of events can be related in a cause and effect manner.

The anatomy of the small bowel and its mesentery should make vaginal evisceration difficult. Most anatomists describe the mesentery of the small bowel as being 15 to 20 cm long. This distance is insufficient to allow the terminal ileum or jejunum to exit the peritoneal cavity through the vaginal cuff or a uterine perforation and eviscerate. There appear to be two possibilities: (1) certain individuals could have a longer mesentery than the 15- to 20-cm average, or (2) the process involved in evisceration may lengthen the small intestine mesentery by mobilizing it second-

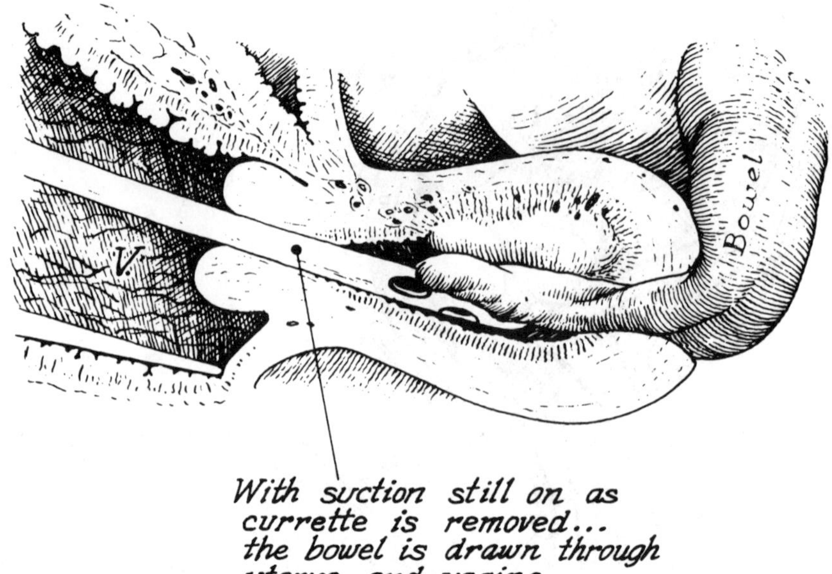

FIG 2–7.
Sagittal view showing the suction curette with attached bowel being pulled through the perforated uterus during a termination of pregnancy. The gestational contents have not been removed. *V*, vagina. (From Wheeless CR Jr: Vaginal evisceration following pelvic surgery, in Nichols DH [ed]: *Clinical Problems, Injuries, and Complications of Gynecologic Surgery,* ed 2. Baltimore, Williams & Wilkins Co, 1988, pp 120–129. Used by permission.)

ary to laceration in the mesentery at the root of its origin (Fig 2–9,A) It is likely that both phenomena occur. Laceration of the small bowel mesentery threatens the continuity of the blood supply to the intestine. However, the laceration could occur in such a location as to spare specific vascular arcades within the small bowel mesentery. This may explain why there are successful reports of simply replacing the

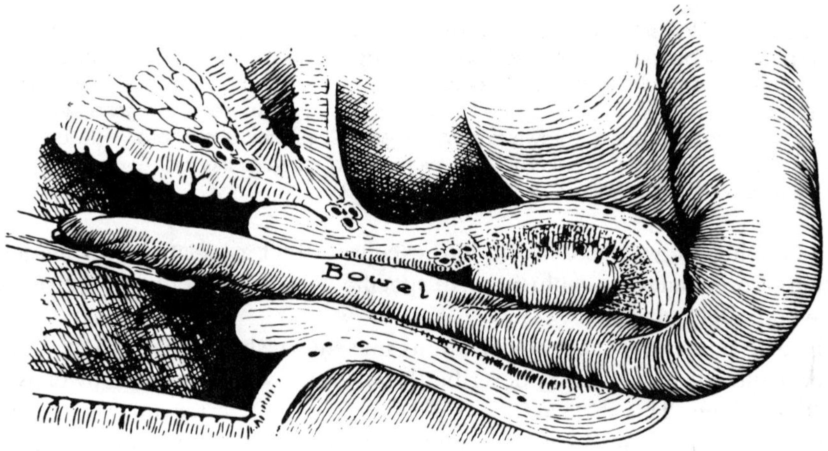

FIG 2–8.
The intestine is eviscerated through the cervix out into the vagina. It is at this point that the intestine is most likely to be injured by confusing it with fetal parts. (From Wheeless CR Jr: Vaginal evisceration following pelvic surgery, in Nichols DH [ed]: *Clinical Problems, Injuries, and Complications of Gynecologic Surgery,* ed 2. Baltimore, Williams & Wilkins Co, 1988, pp 120–129. Used by permission.)

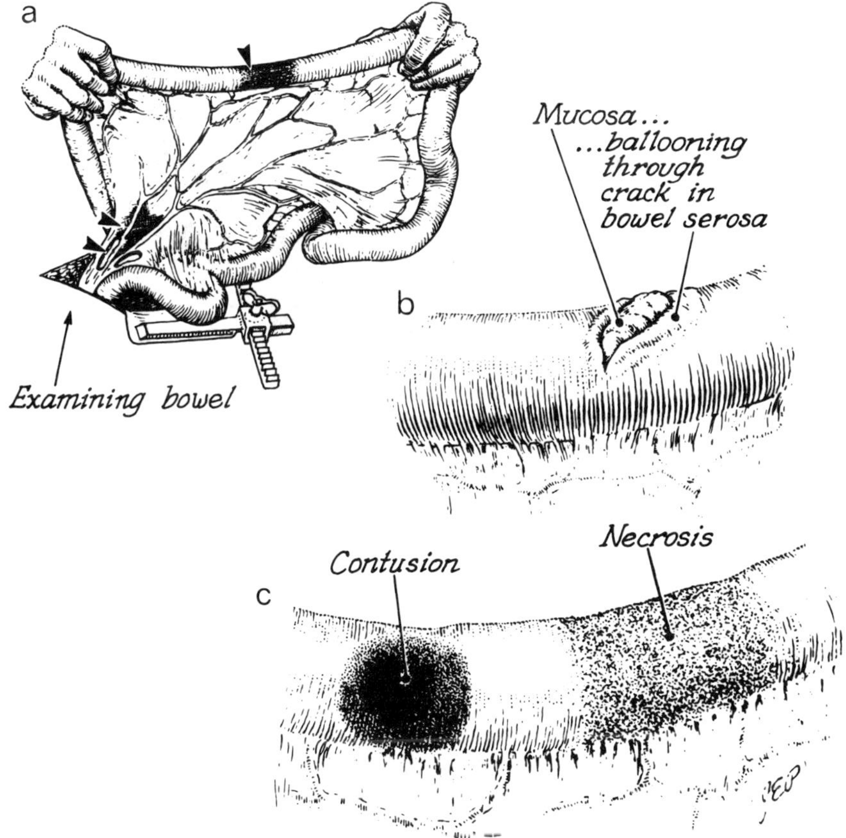

FIG 2–9.
a, this drawing demonstrates the need for complete examination of the intestine from the ligament of Treitz to the cecum. Specific areas of laceration within the mesentery should be searched for and the relationship between the laceration and the vascular integrity of the bowel should be confirmed. **b,** intestinal enterotomies or tears should be searched for and appropriately repaired. **c,** areas of contusion and necrosis should be identified. (From Wheeless CR Jr: Vaginal evisceration following pelvic surgery, in Nichols DH [ed]: *Clinical Problems, Injuries, and Complications of Gynecologic Surgery,* ed 2. Baltimore, Williams & Wilkins Co, 1988, pp 120–129. Used by permission.)

small bowel into the peritoneal cavity via the vaginal route without performing a laparotomy and the patient recovering without incident. However, such a procedure as replacement of the intestine through the vaginal opening without laparotomy could be perilous. The overall mortality from vaginal evisceration has been reported at approximately 10%. From a review of the literature, it appears that much of this mortality is secondary to peritonitis, possibly related to intestinal necrosis. On the other hand, the morbidity from laparotomy in a modern hospital is minimal. Via laparotomy the intestine can be thoroughly inspected and suspicious areas of compromised intestine resected with primary reanastomosis. (Figs 2–9,B and C and 2–10)

Prevention

Prevention of vaginal evisceration following hysterectomy has several possibilities. Collective series of a significant number of patients for statistically valid results

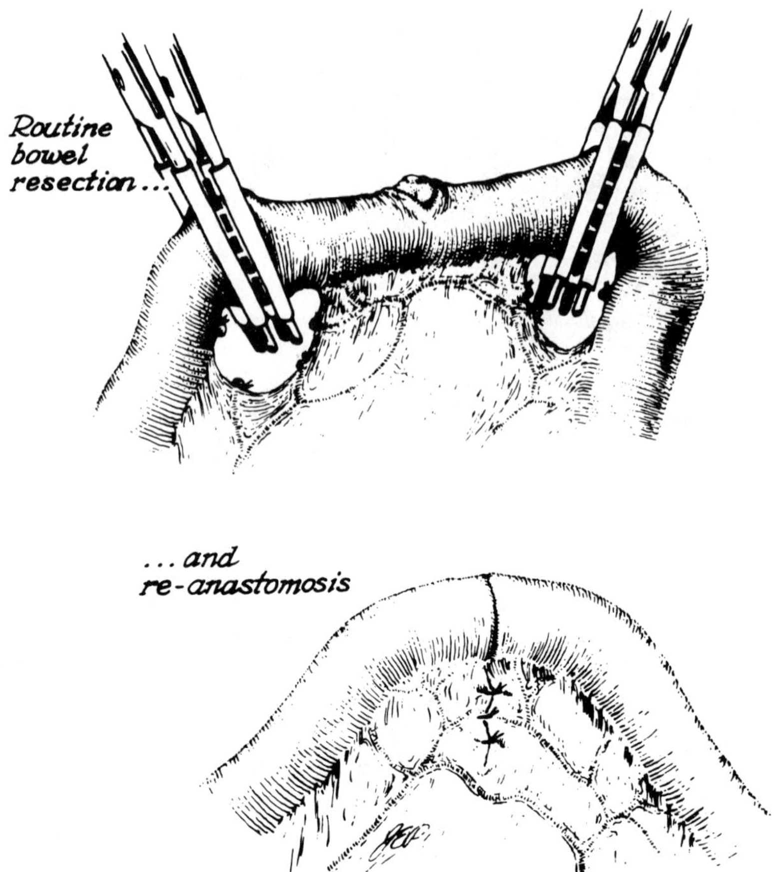

FIG 2–10.
Areas of severe intestinal damage and vascular necrosis should be surgically resected and reanastomosis performed. (From Wheeless CR Jr: Vaginal evisceration following pelvic surgery, in Nichols DH [ed]: *Clinical Problems, Injuries, and Complications of Gynecologic Surgery,* ed 2. Baltimore, Williams & Wilkins Co, 1988, pp 120–129. Used by permission.)

is unavailable. Therefore, the precise etiology of this problem in most cases remains unknown, except for those cases that occurred during termination of pregnancy in which the intestine was pulled through a perforation in the uterine wall. Possibilities for prevention that require discussion include (1) failure to repair enteroceles and cytoceles present at the time of hysterectomy, (2) the pros and cons of leaving the vaginal vault open at the time of hysterectomy, (3) choice and size of suture material used in closure of the vaginal vault, and (4) particularly the technique of anastomosis of the stumps of the supporting ligaments of the pelvis to the angles of the vagina.

Although vaginal eviscerations have occurred from a variety of clinical and anatomic situations, the majority have occurred in association with poor support of the vaginal cuff, posterior fornix, and cul-de-sac after vaginal hysterectomy.

The open vaginal vault is an attractive and tempting possibility for the etiology of vaginal evisceration. However, the open vaginal vault is the technique of many gynecologists, and thousands of hysterectomies have been performed leaving the vaginal vault open with no postoperative vaginal evisceration. When the vaginal vault is left open, its edge is usually sutured with a running locked synthetic absorbable suture referred to as "reefing" the margin of the vaginal cuff. At the vaginal angles, this reefing suture usually includes the stumps of the uterosacral and cardinal ligaments and anastomoses them to the angle of the vagina for additional support. In addition, most surgeons (but not all) peritonealize the pelvis by approximating the anterior and posterior peritoneal surfaces. This covers the open vaginal cuff. However, if one returns to the classic anatomic situation where the average length of the mesentery of the small bowel is 15 to 20 cm, evisceration would be virtually impossible unless an additional event occurred to excessively mobilize the intestine to produce sufficient length to push it through an opening in the vaginal cuff. Therefore, open vaginal cuffs alone are generally insufficient to be the etiology of all vaginal eviscerations. In addition, most vaginal eviscerations reported have occurred after the vaginal cuff has been surgically closed with interrupted sutures.

Choice of suture material may be a factor in the occurrence of vaginal evisceration, but like the open vaginal cuff, an additional factor is usually required to mobilize sufficient intestine to eviscerate out the vagina. If fine synthetic absorbable suture material is used (size 3-0 or less), there is the attractive thesis that the anastomosis of the stumps of the cardinal and uterosacral ligaments could break down and set up the anatomic situation for evisceration. In addition, if enough pressure were acutely exerted on the mesentery of the small bowel via a large Valsalva maneuver to lacerate the mesentery and thereby mobilize the intestine, evisceration could occur. However, insufficient evidence exists for placing the etiology of vaginal evisceration on choice of suture material. I believe synthetic absorbable suture in sizes of 2-0 represents the ideal suture material for closure of the vagina and reanastomosis of the stumps of the uterosacral and cardinal ligaments to the angle of vaginal cuff. Permanent suture used in this area would not eliminate eviscerations but would add morbidity from suture abscesses.

The method of closure of the vagina could also represent a potential threat for vaginal evisceration. All too often the vaginal cuff is closed with figure-of-eight sutures. A figure-of-eight suture, especially if tied tightly, promotes necrosis and healing by second intention. This is not the purpose of the suture in the vaginal cuff. Single sutures tied gently enough to approximate the tissue and prevent hemorrhage are sufficient.

In addition, it is important to plicate the uterosacral ligaments behind the vaginal vault to reduce the cul-de-sac and reduce the tendency toward enterocele formation. I do not believe that the complete classic McCall's plication of the uterosacral ligament is necessary in all hysterectomies and, in fact, represents a threat of suture ligation of the ureter if the uterosacral ligaments are plicated for a distance of more than 4 cm. Although these factors may be a part of this problem, most vaginal eviscerations are associated predominately with large Valsalva's maneuvers, namely, vomiting, coughing, and lifting heavy objects. Severe vomiting and coughing have been reported in most cases in which evisceration has occurred after hysterectomy. Therefore, prevention must include containing these factors within moderation by eliminating overzealous oral feeding and excessive induction of postoperative coughing. Prevention of evisceration at suction abortion must include the safe utilization of techniques for performing the operation, that is, careful dilation of the cervix and repeated sounding of the uterine cavity.

Diagnosis and Management

The key to the reduction of the severe morbidity and mortality associated with evisceration must be early recognition. Most eviscerations through the vagina are associated with lacerations of the mesentery of the small bowel, and the vascular integrity of the small bowel is at stake (see Fig 2–9). When evisceration is caused by suction abortion, the additional factor of trauma by the suction curette to the surface of the bowel makes early recognition extremely important (see Fig 2–8). Early recognition would allow surgical intervention before intestinal necrosis and leakage of intestinal contents into the peritoneal cavity.

Treatment for any evisceration through the vagina should start with pelvic laparotomy. Initial first aid on discovery of the evisceration should be the physiologic protection of the eviscerated loop of intestine by wrapping it in sterile saline-soaked gauze or a sterile moist towel. An exploratory laparotomy through a midline incision should be performed immediately. I emphasize a midline incision; I do not believe that the mesentery of the intestine can be inspected adequately through a Pfannenstiel incision. The intestine is carefully withdrawn through the defect whether it is the perforated uterus or the vaginal cuff (Fig 2–11) A complete inspection of the entire intestine and its mesentery from the ligament of Treitz to the

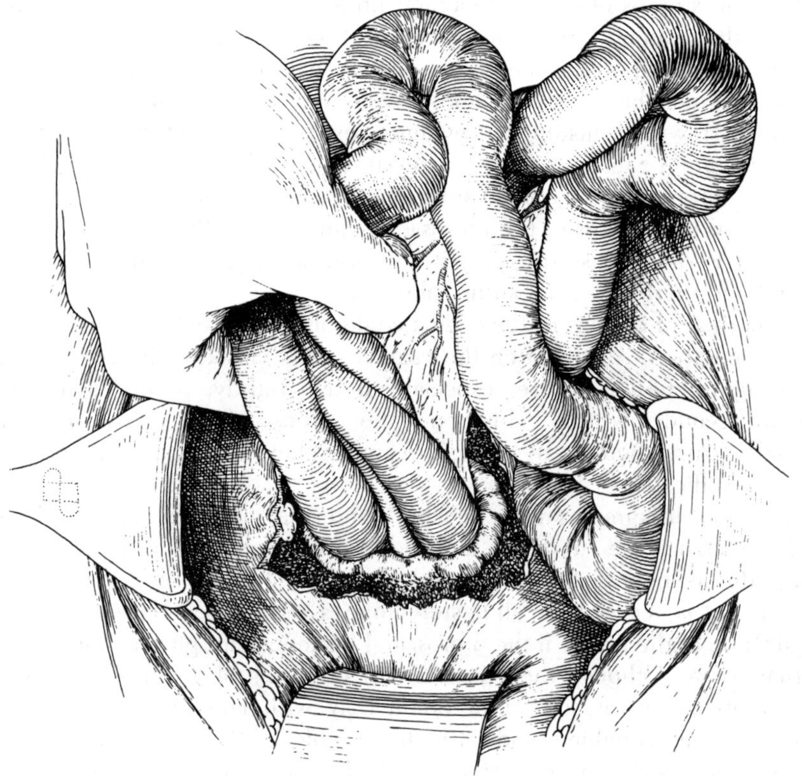

FIG 2–11.
Pelvic laparotomy showing the replacement of the intestine back into the peritoneal cavity through the ruptured vaginal cuff surrounded by the torn peritoneal margins. (From Wheeless CR Jr: Vaginal evisceration following pelvic surgery, in Nichols DH [ed]: *Clinical Problems, Injuries, and Complications of Gynecologic Surgery,* ed 2. Baltimore, Williams & Wilkins Co, 1988, pp 120–129. Used by permission.)

cecum is indicated (see Fig 2–9). The mesentery should be carefully inspected for lacerations and vascular injuries and hemostasis. Suspicious areas of intestine should be resected and reanastomosis performed (see Fig 2–10). I believe there is no role for transvaginal replacement of the intestine into the abdominal cavity without laparotomy because of the possibility of lacerations in the mesentery and undetected injury to the small bowel, especially when evisceration has occurred through the perforated uterus during the performance of a suction abortion. The suction curette could have damaged several pieces of small intestine other than the piece eviscerated through the uterine perforation. After the intestine has been appropriately replaced into the abdominal cavity, inspected carefully, and damaged areas resected, the entire peritoneal cavity is copiously lavaged with normal saline. A Salem sump nasogastric tube is inserted into the stomach and left in place until the patient passes flatus or has a bowel movement. All patients who have sustained enterotomies, and probably the entire group of vaginal eviscerations, should be covered with broad-spectrum antibiotics. Antimicrobial therapy should be guided by appropriate cultures taken at the time of laparotomy, but therapy should be directed toward the anaerobic organisms.

In those cases of evisceration associated with termination of pregnancy, it is vital to complete the termination of pregnancy as part of the repair procedure. All too often in the panic of this unexpected and severe complication, attention is directed toward the intestinal problem and away from the potential severe complication of

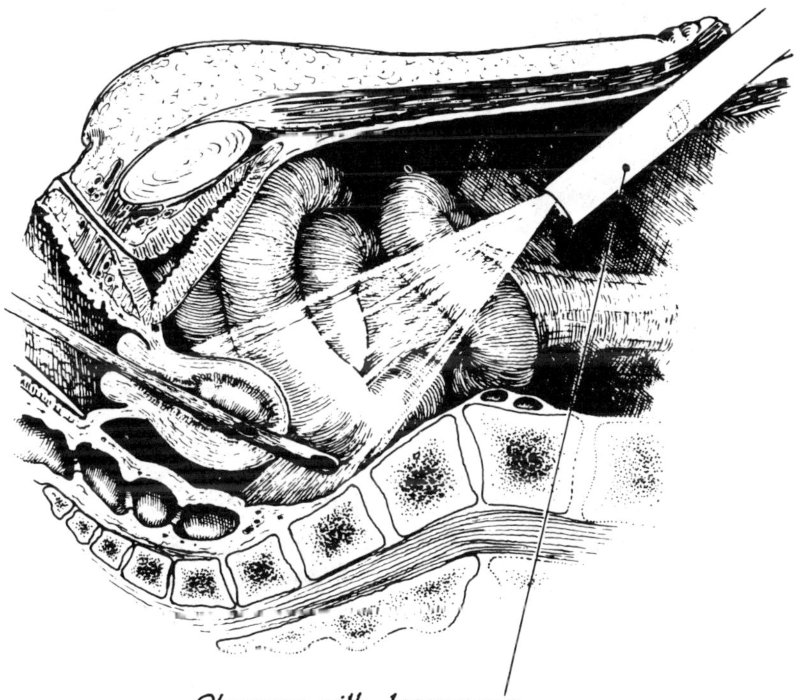

FIG 2–12.
Sagittal view demonstrating the prevention of intestinal evisceration and so forth. (From Wheeless CR Jr: Vaginal evisceration following pelvic surgery, in Nichols DH [ed]: *Clinical Problems, Injuries, and Complications of Gynecologic Surgery,* ed 2. Baltimore, Williams & Wilkins Co, 1988, pp 120–129. Used by permission.)

incomplete abortion with retained gestational contents. One solution to this problem is to have a second surgeon immediately perform laparoscopy through the umbilicus and guide the withdrawl of the suction cannula out of the peritoneal cavity and back into the endometrial cavity (Fig 2–12) where the suction can be resumed and the termination of pregnancy completed (Fig 2–13). Failure to do this leaves products of gestation within the endometrial cavity and creates the potential for the sequelae of incomplete abortion (i.e., infection and hemorrhage).

Repair of the ruptured vagina or perforated uterus differs. The perforation site in the uterus can be closed with simple through-and-through sutures of absorbable material. However, in the case of the ruptured vagina, careful closure with a well-designed plan of ligament suspension and obliteration of the cul-de-sac should be made (Fig 2–14). The suture material should be absorbable, and care should be

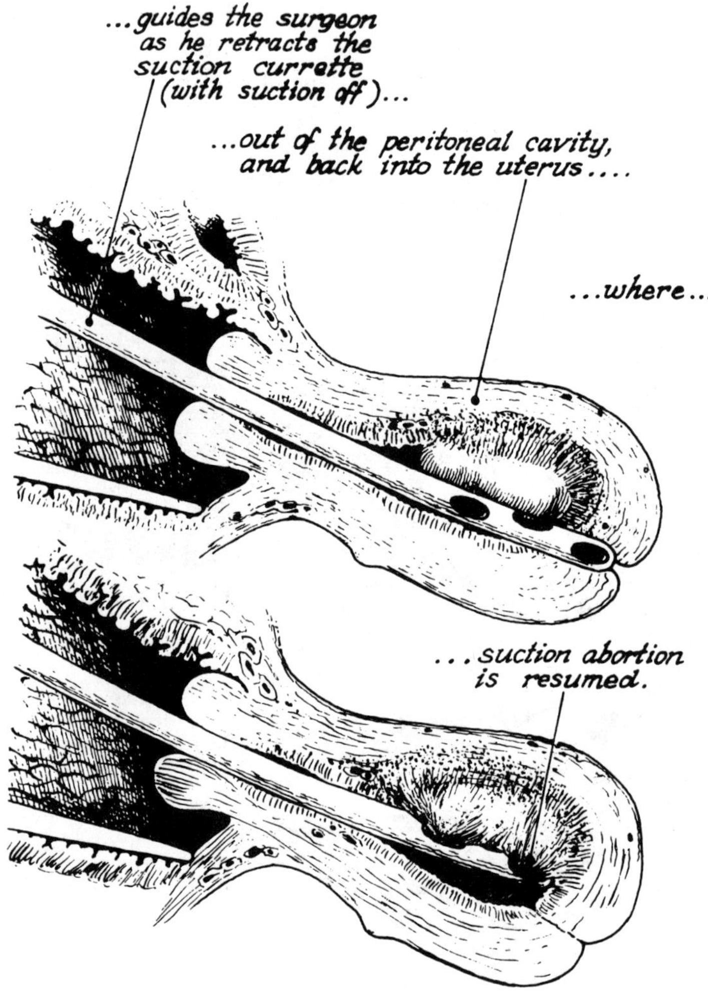

FIG 2–13.
Sagittal drawing showing suction cannula withdrawn into endometrial cavity and so forth. (From Wheeless CR Jr: Vaginal evisceration following pelvic surgery, in Nichols DH [ed]: *Clinical Problems, Injuries, and Complications of Gynecologic Surgery*, ed 2. Baltimore, Williams & Wilkins Co, 1988, pp 120–129. Used by permission.)

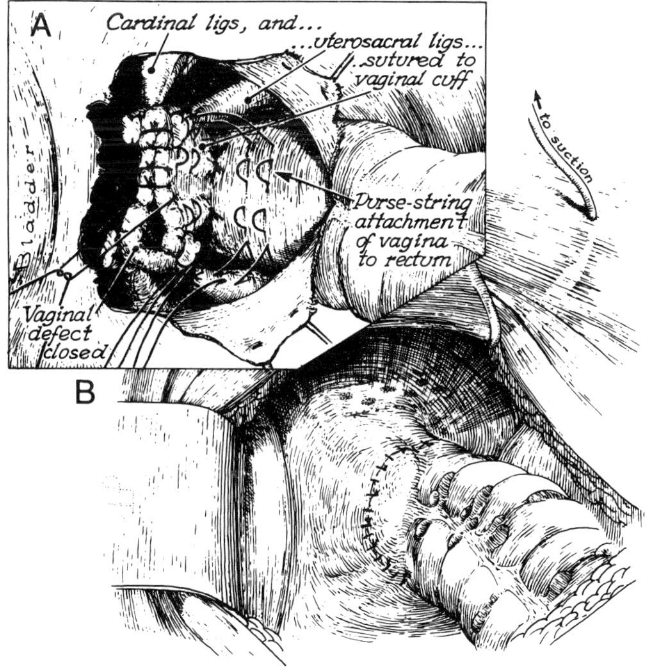

FIG 2–14.
Repair of ruptured vagina and suture of rectosigmoid colon to posterior vaginal cuff **(A).** Reperitonealization of pelvis **(B).** (From Wheeless CR Jr: Vaginal evisceration following pelvic surgery, in Nichols DH [ed]: *Clinical Problems, Injuries, and Complications of Gynecologic Surgery,* ed 2. Baltimore, Williams & Wilkins Co, 1988, pp 120–129. Used by permission.)

taken to reduce areas of necrosis to a minimum. The opening in the vagina should be excised back to fresh, healthy tissue. Closure with interrupted absorbable suture is preferable. A separate step to locate and suture the stumps of the uterosacral and cardinal ligaments to the angles of the vagina should be made (see Figure 2–14,A). In addition, the anterior surface of the rectosigmoid colon should be sutured to the posterior vaginal cuff to obliterate the cul-de-sac (see Fig 2–14,B) Complete resection of all necrotic tissue along the vaginal cuff and stumps of the supporting ligaments is necessary. This is a particularly important step if fecal material has spilled into the peritoneal cavity. One should not be surprised at the development of a postoperative pelvic abscess if necrotic tissue that has been bathed in the intestinal contents is left within the pelvis postoperatively. Antibiotic therapy will not be sufficient to override this breach in surgical technique. I advocate placing all of these patients on the intermittent pneumatic pressure cuffs to the legs for 5 days. Those patients who do not have return of intestinal function within 3 to 4 days postoperatively should be given IV hyperalimentation (total parenteral nutrition). Many of the series in the literature have reported prolonged ileus following vaginal evisceration. If the entire intestine has been completely explored and the surgeon is comfortable as to the vascular integrity of the intestine, prolonged ileus should be treated conservatively with nasogastric drainage and IV hyperalimentation. However, if the intestine has been replaced vaginally and there has not been adequate exploration of the intestine, the question of vascular integrity and necrosis of the bowel should be considered. Repeat, or second-look, laparotomy should be considered, and the vascular integrity of the bowel should be ensured.

Although evisceration of the small intestine through the vagina is an extremely serious event, patients have an excellent chance for recovery if intestinal necrosis and peritonitis have not occurred. Moreover, if proper closure of the vaginal vault with elimination of the cul-de-sac and careful approximation of the supporting ligaments to the angles of the vagina is made during the repair process, the likelihood of recurrence is small.

A gynecologist may be in practice for a lifetime and never encounter a case of vaginal evisceration. Because of its rarity, it has been difficult for any one clinic to gain a large volume of experience in treating this phenomenon. Nevertheless, it seems logical to treat vaginal evisceration as one would treat abdominal evisceration following dehiscence of a postoperative abdominal incision. In treating evisceration of the abdominal wall, the surgeon would never consider replacing the intestine through the traumatic abdominal opening or dehiscent wound without a thorough inspection of the peritoneal cavity. This same principle should be observed in vaginal evisceration.

BIBLIOGRAPHY

Alexander HC, Prudden J: The causes of abdominal wound dehisced disruption. *Surg Gynecol Obstet* 1966; 122:1223.

Banerjee SR, Daudi I, et al: Abdominal wound evisceration. *Curr Surg* 1983; 40:432.

Fagniez JL, Hay JM, et al: Abdominal midline incision closure. *Arch Surg* 1985; 120:1351.

Fox PF, Kowalczyk AS: Ruptured enterocele. *Am J Obstet Gynecol* 1971; 111:592.

Fox WP: Vaginal evisceration. *Obstet Gynecol* 1977; 50:223.

Gammelgaard N, Jensen J: Wound complications after closure of abdominal incisions with Dexon or Vicryl. *Acta Chir Scand* 1983; 149:505.

Goligher JC, Irvin TT, et al: A controlled clinical trial of three methods of closure of laparotomy wounds. *Br J Surg* 1975; 62:823.

Gray H, The digestive system, in Goss CM (ed): *Anatomy of the Human Body,* ed 29. Philadelphia, Lea & Febiger, 1973, p 1230.

Greenburg AG, Saik RP, Peskin GW: Wound dehiscence. *Arch Surg* 1979; 114:143.

Halasz NA: Dehiscence of laparotomy wounds. *Am J Surg* 1968; 116:210.

Hall BS, Phelan JP, Pruyn SC, et al: Vaginal evisceration during coitus. *Am J Obstet Gynecol* 1978; 131:115.

Hunt TK: Disorders of repair and their management, in Hunt TK, Dumphy JE (eds): *Fundamentals of Wound Management.* New York, Appleton-Century-Crofts, 1979, pp 68–69.

McNellis D, Torkelson L, McElin TW: Late postoperative vaginal vault disruption. *Am J Obstet Gynecol* 1966; 94:543.

Nichols DH, Randall CL: Complications of surgery, in *Vaginal Surgery,* ed 3. Baltimore, Williams & Wilkins Co, 1989, p 441.

Pemberton LB, Manax WG: Complications after vertical and transverse incisions for cholecystectomy. *Surg Gynecol Obstet* 1971; 132:892.

Penninck FM, et al: Abdominal wound dehiscence in gastroenterological surgery. *Ann Surg* 1979; 189:342.

Powell JL: Vaginal evisceration following vaginal hysterectomy. *Am J Obstet Gynecol* 1973; 115:276.

Rolf BB: Vaginal evisceration. *Am J Obstet Gynecol* 1970; 107:369.

Sanders RJ, DiClementi D: Principles of abdominal wound closure: Prevention of wound dehiscence. *Arch Surg* 1977; 112:118.

Wheeless CR Jr: Abdominal wound dehiscence, in Wheeless CR Jr (ed): *Atlas of Pelvic Surgery,* ed 2. Philadelphia, Lea & Febiger, 1988, p 374.

Wheeless CR Jr: Vaginal evisceration following pelvic surgery, in Nichols DH (ed): *Clinical Problems, Injuries, and Complications of Gynecologic Surgery,* ed 2. Baltimore, Williams & Wilkins Co, 1988, pp 120–129.

Chapter 3

Incisional Hernia

George W. Mitchell, M.D.

PREDISPOSING FACTORS

If all gynecologic operations were performed on young healthy individuals, there would be few incisional, or ventral, hernias, but this is not the group most liable to surgery and its consequences. Factors predisposing to the development of ventral hernia are listed in Table 3–1. In life-threatening situations requiring surgical intervention, all of these factors must be ignored, but in the decision to perform elective surgery, herniation is one of the possible complications that must be taken into account. Adverse predisposing factors of a general systemic type are for the most part self-evident, but even in a healthy person a well-healed wound leaves the abdominal wall weaker than it was before, and additional incisions through the same site weaken it still further.

INCISIONS

The surgeon has some control over operative factors, but this control is not absolute. For instance, if the same area must be reentered a few hours or even a few weeks after a preceding operation, the surgeon is well advised to reopen the original incision, since a new parallel or perpendicular incision may further compromise the regenerating blood and nerve supply of the area. The most commonly used incisions for gynecologic operations are shown in Figure 3–1; of these, the lower midline is certainly the most popular. For cesarean sections, the transverse modified Pfannenstiel incision is replacing the vertical incision, probably because of the marked diastasis of the rectus muscles produced by pregnancy and the easy access to the lower uterine segment. Transverse muscle cutting incisions, the Maylard (Fig 3–2) and the Czerny (Fig 3–3), provide excellent exposure for retropubic operations, such as those performed by gynecologic urologists, and for the resection of the lymph nodes of the lateral pelvic walls. Transverse skin incisions leave a cosmetic scar and are more in demand by patients. Some statistics suggest that transverse incisions undergo fewer dehiscences than vertical incisions and give rise to

TABLE 3–1.
Factors Predisposing to Wound Disruption

1. Preoperative
   - Age
   - Systemic disease
     - Diabetes, cancer, anemia, pulmonary
   - Nutrition
     - Obesity, hypoproteinemia
   - Previous surgery
   - Irradiation
   - Drugs
     - Chemotherapy, steroids
2. Operative
   - Type and length of incision
   - Length of operation
   - Poor hemostasis
   - Necrotic tissue
   - Type of closure
   - Suture material
3. Postoperative
   - Wound infection
     - Hematomas, seromas
   - Distention
     - Ileus, ascites
   - Exertion
     - Coughing, vomiting, hiccups

fewer postoperative hernias, but the tension on both types of incision is equal, as is the quality of the tissue, and it is possible that the reported differences may be due to other variables such as the suture material used and the type of closure. Transverse incisions can be an embarrassment if the focus of the operation proves to be higher in the abdomen.

Rather than seriously damage the rectus muscle in a frustrating attempt to find the midline after previous surgery, it is sometimes advisable to do a muscle-splitting incision directly through the sheath of the rectus itself. This incision offers exposure just as good as a midline incision and can be extended above the umbilicus without difficulty but has the disadvantage that more bleeding may be encountered as a result of vessels perforating the sheath from the inferior epigastric artery. Incisions close to or along the semilunar line at the junction of the transversalis and oblique muscles (pararectus) are sometimes used for retroperitoneal operations involving the ureter, pelvic lymph nodes, or localized infections, but the resulting scar is relatively weak. The healing process is also affected by the length of the incision despite the much quoted apocryphal statement that incisions heal from side to side and not from top to bottom. The tension on the closure of a midline incision is proportional to the square of the length of the incision, which means that the longer the incision, the more likely it is to pull apart.

Closure of Incisions

Hemostasis should be 100% complete when the incision is closed. Seromas and hematomas accumulating in the subcutaneous space or deep to the fascia give rise

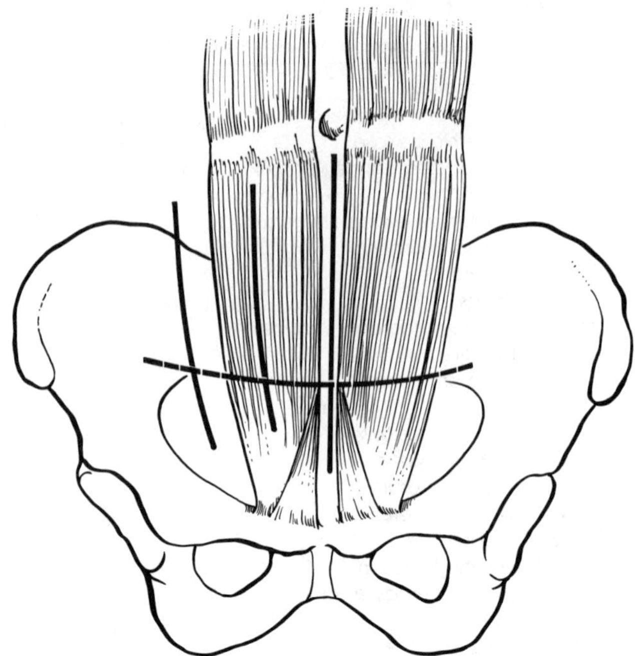

FIG 3–1.
Placement of midline, muscle-splitting, pararectal, and low transverse incisions.

to infection and may even burst open the incision by the pressure of their accumulation. The cautery is a valuable tool in this process, since it is both effective and expeditious, but the overuse of the cautery causes necrosis and gives rise to infection. When the subcutaneous tissues have been widely undercut during the closure or there is likely to be a considerable dead space left behind, drainage is desirable, and this should be done by suction drains brought out through a stab wound at least 5 cm away from the incision. In operations involving gross infection or fecal contamination, the skin should be left open and closed several days later.

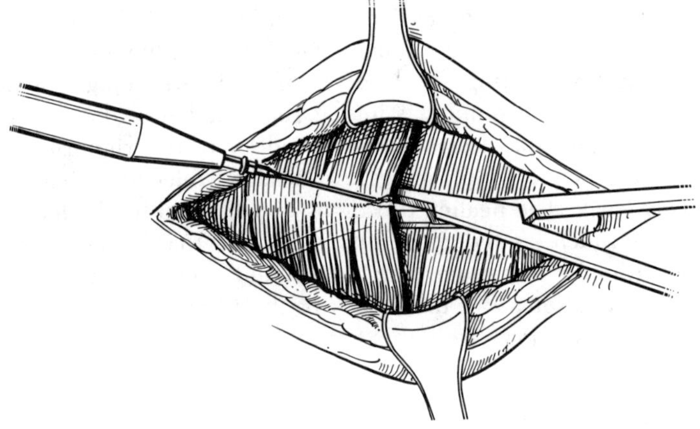

FIG 3–2.
Maylard incision. A long Kelly clamp is thrust under the rectus muscle, and the muscle is transected with the Bovie cautery, taking care not to damage the inferior epigastric vessels.

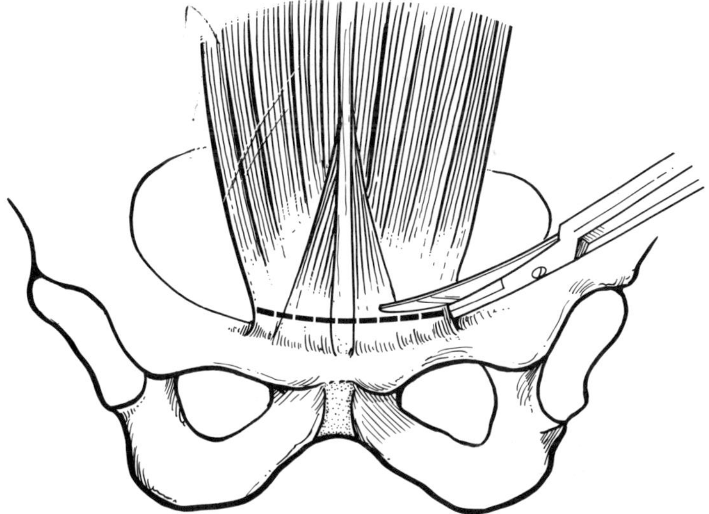

FIG 3–3.
Czerny incision. The tendinous insertion of the rectus muscles and the origin of the pyramidal muscles are cut away from the pubis and reflected upward.

Wound dehiscence through one or more layers of the abdominal wall is a complication of gynecologic surgery that occurs in between 0.3% and 3% of cases. When only the skin opens in isolated areas postoperatively, it is of no great significance, but the more common separation of the skin and subcutaneous tissues down to the fascia, usually caused by infection, prolongs hospitalization and requires either reclosure after the wound is clean and granulating or a protracted period of healing by second intention. If the fascia is involved in the infection or gives way as a result of tension, the situation is more serious and subsequent herniation more likely. Complete dehiscence, for which the term evisceration is frequently used, implies the extrusion of abdominal contents through the incision and requires immediate surgical intervention. The mortality rate from this complication remains high, and in those who survive, the possibility of hernia formation is great.

Suture Materials

All experts agree that the type of closure of the incision has an important bearing on the likelihood of dehiscence and the possibility of the future development of hernia, but there is little agreement regarding what the exact nature of that closure should be. There is a similar lack of consensus regarding appropriate suture material. From the beginning of the 20th century, general surgeons preferred to close their patients' wounds in layers with nonabsorbable suture material, usually silk, although cotton and linen were also used. Metallic sutures have been available for more than 100 years, and monofilament steel wire remains to this day the preference in some quarters. Gynecologists often followed suit, but with the development of chromicized catgut in the 1920s, most turned to that type of suture material. During this era, statistics were adduced to show that closures with catgut were as strong as those with nonabsorbable material and that the incidence of dehiscence and herniation was not increased.

The development of longer lasting synthetic absorbable suture material and relatively inert nonabsorbable suture material in the 1960s again radically altered the

TABLE 3–2.
Nonabsorbable Sutures

Type	Generic Name	Ethicon, Inc.† Trade Name	Davis & Geck‡ Trade Name	Deknatel, Inc.§ Trade Name
Synthetic braided	Uncoated polyester	Mersilene	Dacron	Cottony Dacron
	Polybutilate-coated polyester	Ethibond		
	Silicone-coated polyester		Ti-cron	
	Polytetrafluoro-ethylene-coated polyester			Polydek
	Polytetrafluoro-ethylene-coated polyester			Tevdek
	Uncoated nylon	Nurolon		
	Uncoated nylon with tubing fluid	Pliabilized Nylon		Braided Nylon
	Nylon-coated with silicone		Surgilon	
Synthetic monofilament	Monofilament nylon	Ethilon	Dermalon	Monofilament Nylon
	Monofilament nylon with tubing fluid	Pliabilized Nylon		
	Polybutester		Novafil	
	Polyethylene		Dermalene	
	Polypropylene	Prolene	Surgilene	Deklene
Metallic				
	Stainless steel (316L)			
	Monofilament	Monofilament Stainless Steel	Monofilament Stainless Steel	Monofilament Stainless Steel
	Twisted	Twisted Stainless Steel	Flexon	
	Braided	Braided Stainless Steel		
Natural fiber				
	Uncoated twisted silk	Virgin Silk	Virgin Silk	
	Twisted silk coated with silicone		Twisted Silk Coated with Silicone	
	Uncoated braided silk	Perma-Hand		
	Braided silk coated with silicone	Perma-Hand	Braided Silk Coated with Silicone	
	Twisted cotton	Surgical Cotton	Surgical Cotton	

*From Edlich RF, Rodeheaver GT, Thacker JG: *J Urol* 1987; 137:373–379. Used by permission.
†Somerville, NJ.
‡Danbury, Conn.
§Queens Village, NY.

pattern of usage. The commercial market for products of this kind is now exploding, and as each new product comes on the market, it quickly develops a coterie of adherents. Nevertheless, those who were trained with the more old-fashioned materials may continue to adhere doggedly to them and claim their superiority. The wide range of choices is shown in Tables 3–2 and 3–3. Even though the surgeon's preference has a major role in determining what is to be used, the following objective points can be made:

1. Nonabsorbable sutures are strong and last a lifetime, but they are foreign bodies that may serve as niduses for infection.
2. Silk is facile to use but reactive in tissue, cotton is obsolescent, and linen is obsolete.
3. Wire is relatively inert but hard to handle.
4. Nylon and polyester are more flexible than wire but require five throws per knot.
5. Braided sutures are more likely to promote infection than monofilament sutures.
6. The tensile strength of absorbable sutures lasts from 10 (catgut) to 40 days (synthetic).
7. Synthetic nonabsorbable sutures are stiff, tend to come untied, and require five throws per knot.

TABLE 3–3.
Absorbable Sutures

Type	Generic Name	Ethicon, Inc. Trade Name	Davis & Geck Trade Name	Deknatel, Inc. Trade Name
Synthetic braided	Coated polyglactin 910	Vicryl		
	Uncoated polyglycolic acid		Dexon "S"	
	Coated polyglycolic acid		Dexon Plus	
Synthetic monofilament	Polyglyconate		Maxon	
	Polydioxanone	PDS		
Natural fiber	Plain gut with tubing fluid	Plain Gut	Plain Gut	Plain Gut
	Chromic gut with tubing fluid	Chromic Gut	Chromic Gut	Chromic Gut
	Plain gut impregnated with glycerin		Soft Gut	
	Chromic gut impregnated with glycerin		Soft Gut	
	Reconstituted plain collagen	Plain Collagen		
	Reconstituted chromic collagen	Chromic Collagen		

*From Edlich RF, Rodeheaver GT, Thacker TG: *J Urol* 1987; 137:373–379. Used by permission.

8. Catgut sutures are more difficult to standardize for quality, give way early, but require only three throws per knot.
9. Synthetic absorbable suture material lasts long enough for complete wound healing.

A sensible middle-of-the-road position based on the facts would suggest that silk and catgut should not be used as the principal suture in fascial closure, that long-lasting synthetic absorbable sutures are satisfactory in most instances, and that relatively inert synthetic nonabsorbable material is advantageous in difficult cases and in hernia repair.

Suturing Techniques

As has been noted, a variety of different techniques of closure have evolved, which have been shown by various authors to be successful in reducing the incidence of postoperative dehiscence. The only conclusion to be reached is that there is no universal method that can be acclaimed supremely successful. One important variable other than the technique may explain the discrepancy in statistics; in many centers that accumulate large volumes of cases, the incisions are closed by personnel low on the hierarchical totem pole, often without supervision. This is particularly true of cesarean sections, and the results of these closures are bound to reflect the inexperience. On the other hand, future authors interested in compiling data to support their particular method are more likely to remain in attendance and either perform or supervise the closure.

The peritoneum is usually closed with a running absorbable suture. Since this mesothelial layer ordinarily regenerates spontaneously within 24 hours, some surgeons believe that it is unnecessary to close it, but common sense suggests that an additional layer might be helpful in some instances in preventing total extrusion of the intestines after fascial separation. The fascia may be closed with straight inter-

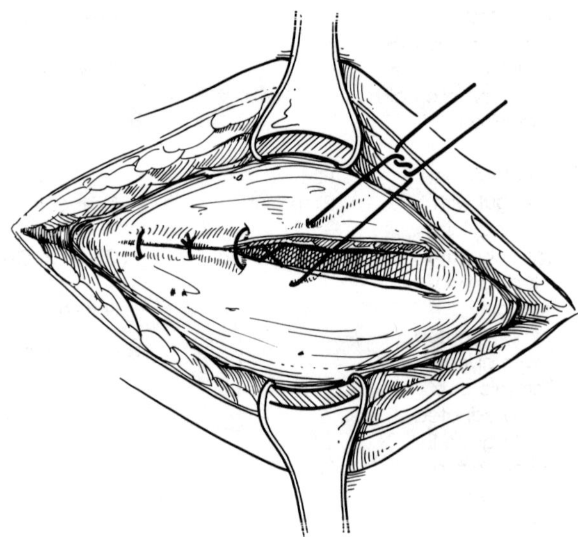

FIG 3–4.
Closure of the Maylard incision with interrupted figure-of-eight sutures incorporating the severed ends of the rectus muscles.

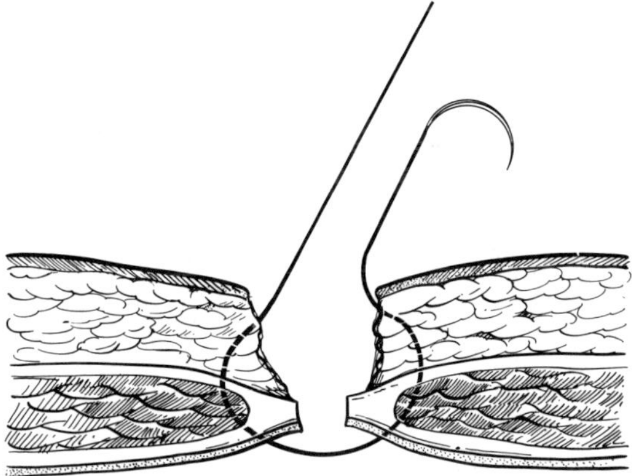

FIG 3–5.
The continuous closure with nonabsorbable suture includes all layers.

rupted sutures (see Fig 3–12), with figure-of-eight sutures (Fig 3–4), or with a running suture (Fig 3–5). The first takes more time but has the advantage that if one goes, all of them do not go. The second is less likely to pull out but bunches up tissue, making it more likely to undergo necrosis. The third is faster and probably satisfactory if the suture material can be depended on. Possibly influenced by tradition, my preference is for the first. Important principles in all of these techniques are white fascia to white fascia apposition, the placement of sutures at least 1 cm from the fascial edge, the ability to tie securely but not to maximum constriction, and closure without tension. The anesthesiologist can be of great help in the latter respect. Closure of transverse incisions is very similar except at the lateral margins where the fascia of the internal oblique must be united with that of the external oblique on each side of the incision. An attempt should be made to incorporate the rectus muscle in the fascial suture in the midportion of the incision when a Maylard incision (see Fig 3–4) has been made or to pull the tendons of the rectus muscle under the distal fascial edge in the case of the Czerny incision (Fig 3–6). Failure to do so does not necessarily initiate hernia formation but may cause an unsightly subfascial muscle bulge that subsequently can be seen and felt by the patient.

The Smead-Jones closure, far-near-near-far and its modification (Fig 3–7), has

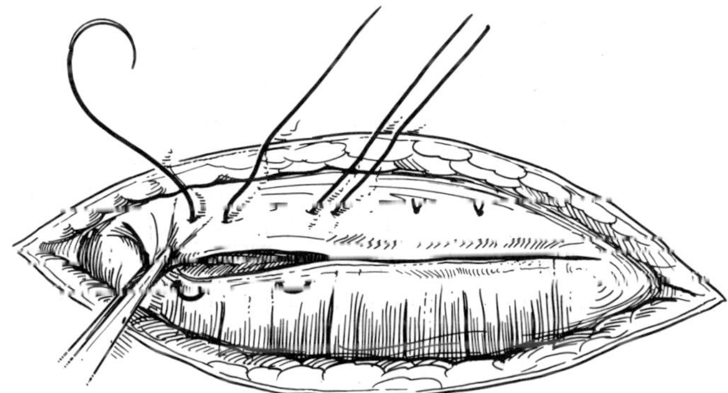

FIG 3–6.
Closure of the Czerny incision using interrupted pulley sutures to draw the tendinous insertions of the rectus muscles beneath the distal fascia.

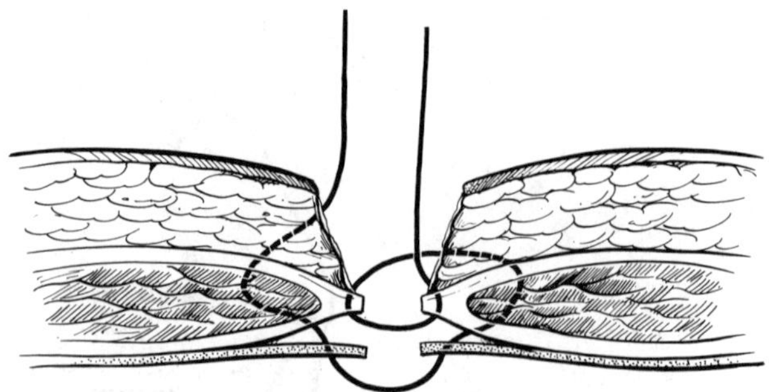

FIG 3–7.
The modified Smead-Jones far-far-near-near closure includes all layers except the skin.

achieved great popularity in recent years and is often used in what the surgeon believes to be difficult cases. I have always believed that what is good for difficult cases might also be appropriate for simple cases, but this philosophy does not seem to be widespread. The data indicate that this is an excellent type of closure in that dehiscenses are rare.

Even more recently, many general surgeons have adopted a form of mass closure using a nonabsorbable running suture to unite all layers of the abdominal wall except the skin (see Fig 3–5). This has been advocated by Gallup for gynecologic surgery, including prolonged difficult oncologic operations. The apparent effectiveness of this method makes it another option for those seeking a rapid simple technique with which to conclude surgery. The results match those of other types of closure.

The use of through-and-through stay sutures, either of wire, nylon, or polyester, to add support to layer for layer closures has been advocated for many years. Like adding a belt to suspenders to hold up the trousers, this double harness would seem to be superior to either method alone, but statistics on dehiscence do not support that concept.

HERNIAS

Incisional hernias occur when the fascial margins and adjacent muscles separate, leaving a defect through which peritoneal pouches containing abdominal contents protrude. More often than not the poor protoplasm of the patient is responsible, but additional factors include infection, defective suture material, and tension on the closure from abdominal distention or any type of unusual exertion (see Table 3–1). In a lower abdominal vertical incision, this is more likely to happen in the lower pole of the incision because of the weakness of the posterior sheath of the rectus muscle below the semicircular line, where only the transversalis fascia is present. The rate of occurrence of ventral hernias varies according to the population at risk but is reported to occur following approximately 1% of all gynecologic surgery. The incidence increases after superficial wound infection and even more drastically after dehiscence and reclosure. The size of the fascial defect may have no bearing on the volume of the hernia, since escaping loops of bowel and omentum may quickly undermine the superficial subcutaneous tissues and skin and spread out over much of the abdominal wall. Of course, the smaller the fascial defect, the greater the likelihood of incarceration of the intestine with possible constriction of blood supply and infarction. The fascial ring is usually quite large in ventral hernias, however, and vascular impairment of the bowel is rare compared with inguinal hernias.

Diagnosis

The diagnosis of incisional hernia is usually made by the patient, who feels lower abdominal pressure and discomfort and occasionally can observe peristalsis of the intestine beneath the skin. She may also note that the lump becomes worse with straining, coughing, or even standing and recedes when she lies down. Occasionally she will have the impression that something is giving way and will note that the hernia becomes larger over a period of time, especially when her lifestyle requires considerable exertion. The patient's story is not absolutely pathognomonic of the presence of hernia but is very close to being so; objective evidence is provided by palpation of the edge of the fascial ring, sometimes very difficult in the obese patient. Additional evidence can often be obtained by ultrasound cuts through the abdominal wall, which, in the hands of an expert, can demonstrate even very small protrusions. Mistakes are also made with this technique. Of the triad of history, physical examination, and ultrasound, it is well to have at least two of the three positive before proceeding with surgical treatment.

Some hernias are extremely large, making it seem as if the entire abdominal contents are within the hernia sac, and some such patients are very old, very sick, or morbidly obese. The likelihood of failure of surgical correction under these circumstances is high, and, since the operation is always lengthy, the patient may die due to anesthesia or postoperative complications. The failure rate also increases with the number of previous unsuccessful attempts at repair. Under any of these circumstances, decision analysis requires the careful balancing of the pros and cons of surgery with the possibility of managing the patient with abdominal binders and an adjusted lifestyle. Large hernias of long standing may be well tolerated by some individuals, and medical supply houses offer a variety of adjustable garments that can be made to fit almost any abdominal distortion.

Surgical Repair

Once surgery has been elected, a well-planned preoperative regimen should be initiated (Table 3–4).

TABLE 3–4.
Treatment Before Hernia Surgery

1. Shave, shower, and cleanse abdomen 1 hr before
2. Nasogastric tube
3. Foley catheter
4. Bowel prep
   - Cathartics, enemas
   - Neomycin, 1 gm four times in 24 hr
   - Erythromycin, 1 gm four times in 24 hr
5. Prophylactic antibiotics intravenously

The patient should be admitted the day before surgery so that appropriate measures to cleanse the bowel and reduce the bacterial content can be initiated. These measures are necessary because the bowel is frequently adherent in the peritoneal sac, and dissection of adhesions may cause bowel perforation at a time when it is least expected. Proper preoperative preparation reduces the morbidity following such an accident. A nasogastric tube should be placed the night before surgery so that the intestine can be completely decompressed, and the skin should be cleansed well before the patient's call to the operating room. Shaving is usually unnecessary for vertical incisions and should be kept to a minimum for all types because of increased bacterial contamination of the skin. If it is necessary, it should be done close to the time of surgery.

The basic principles of hernia repair have been sacred since the days of Halsted: dissection and excision of the peritoneal sac, high ligation of the peritoneal defect, fascia to fascia closure without tension, and absolute hemostasis. In addition, it is desirable to excise excess skin and subcutaneous tissue in amounts appropriate for a cosmetic superficial closure. A broad-spectrum antibiotic should be given intravenously before the skin incision is made.

The previous scar is resected along with a margin of normal skin (Fig 3–8), and the subcutaneous tissues are sharply dissected from the surface of the hernial sac (Fig 3–9). When the sac is exposed, I prefer to open it, being careful not to injure adherent underlying structures, and with a finger inside as a guide, to continue the dissection of subcutaneous tissue and muscle down to the point of protrusion above the fascia (Fig 3–10). The sac may now be more fully opened and its edges grasped with Kocher clamps to provide counter traction while the surgeon mobilizes bowel and omentum away from the peritoneal surface by cutting adhesions (Fig 3–11). Metzenbaum scissors are ideal for this purpose, and the dissection continues until all abdominal contents are free of the sac and returned to the abdominal cavity. Before the omentum and intestines are abandoned, a sharp search for possible bleed-

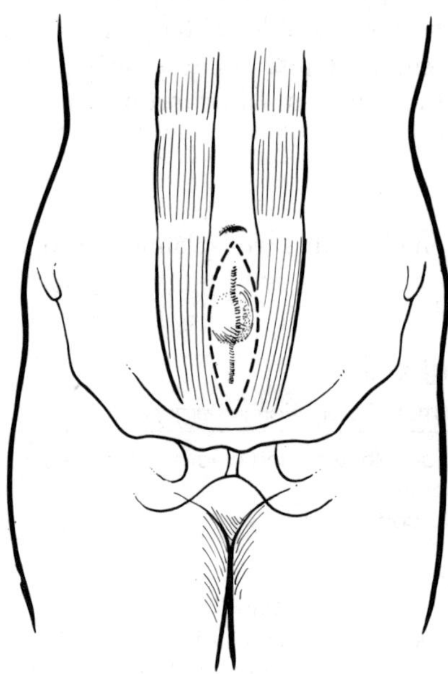

FIG 3–8.
Elliptical incision to excise previous scar and redundant skin over the hernia.

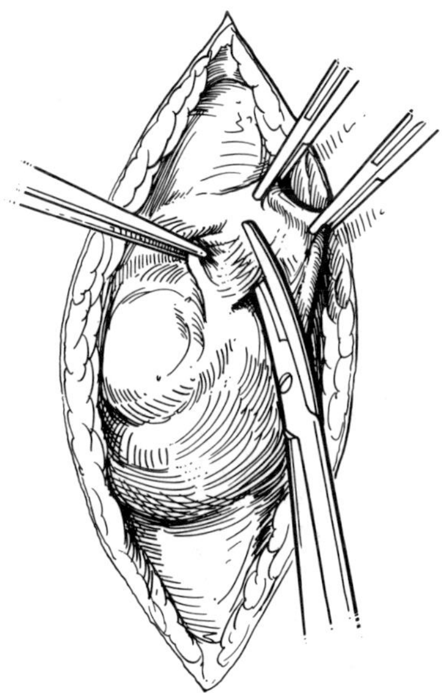

FIG 3–9.
While traction is maintained on the fascial edge, the peritoneal covering of the hernia sac is cut away from its undersurface.

ing points is imperative. The redundant peritoneum is then excised; often at the fascial level the peritoneum and rectus sheath are fused, and the fascial edges are attenuated and ragged. When this is the case, it is essential to resect the combined fascia and peritoneum ruthlessly, mobilizing the rectus muscles as necessary in the process, until a level where the fascia is healthy and strong is reached. Attempts to retain and use fascia of obviously poor quality in the repair are certain to increase the likelihood of failure.

Before the repair is begun, each fascial edge is grasped with an Allis clamp, and the two edges are drawn together to see whether there will be tension on the closure. In the event that there is no tension and the underlying peritoneum is not fused to the fascia, the peritoneum is closed separately with a running suture, and the fascia is closed with interrupted synthetic, monofilament, nonabsorbable material, placing the sutures at least 1 cm from the edge and 1 cm apart (Fig 3–12). The overlapping double-layer imbrication of the fascia has not been shown to have any advantage over a simple side-to-side technique.

When traction on the fascial edges indicates that the incision cannot be closed without undue tension, the problem may be solved by extensive mobilization of the anterior rectus fascia, cutting back the subcutaneous tissue from the surface as far as is necessary to permit the fascial edge to be pulled to the midline (Fig 3–13). It is usually also necessary to separate the rectus muscle from its fascial attachments and to mobilize the posterior sheath as well. This maneuver is often successful in allowing closure without tension, and since the peritoneum is often fused with the fascia, as previously noted, both layers may be united at the same time with interrupted sutures. Further mobilization of the rectus fascia can also be achieved by relaxing incisions close to the semilunar line, where the transversalis muscle joins the oblique musculature, but this weakens the abdominal wall in that area and has been superseded by the use of prostheses.

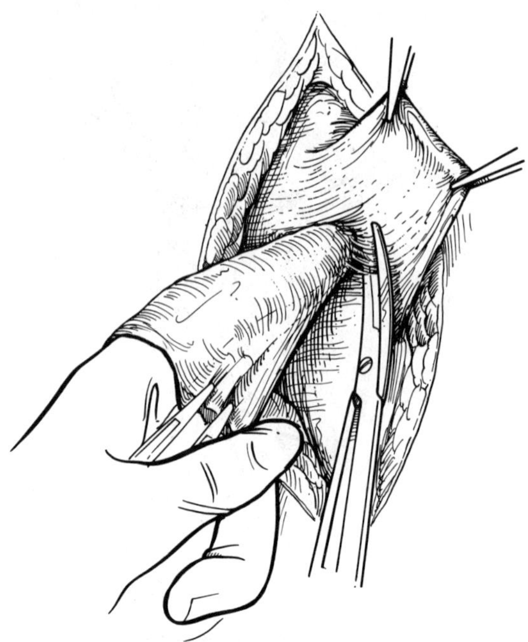

FIG 3–10.
The hernia sac is opened and kept on traction while a finger inside guides the dissection downward to the origin of the hernia.

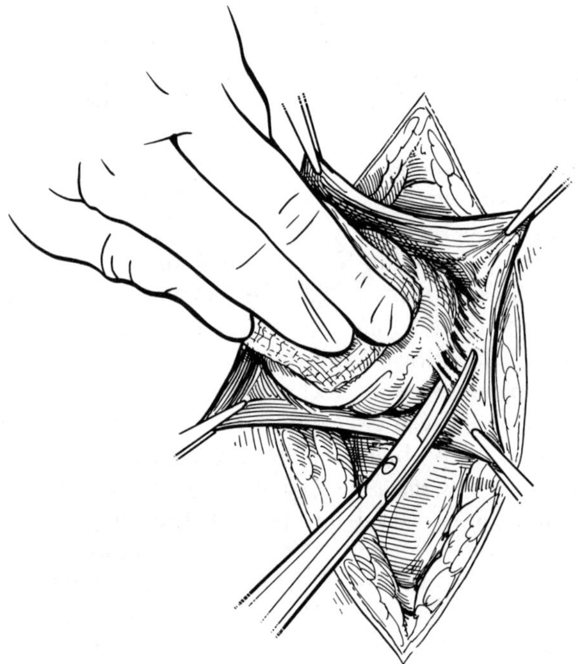

FIG 3–11.
Traction is maintained on the peritoneum and counter traction on the contents of the hernia while internal adhesions are lysed to permit return of the intestines and omentum to the general abdominal cavity.

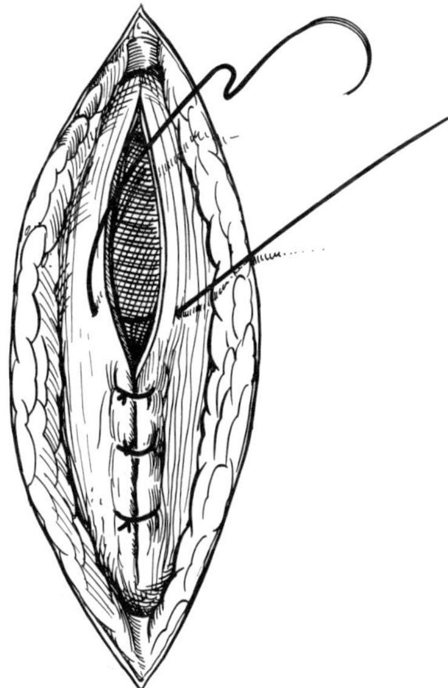

FIG 3–12.
The fascia is being closed over the mesh with interrupted nonabsorbable sutures.

When a large amount of fascia has been resected to obtain a substantial layer for closure or the hernia defect is unusually wide, it may be impossible to bring the fascial edges together. This absolute tissue deficiency may be compensated by the use of prostheses, a bewildering variety of which have been promoted over the past 100 years. In the 19th century, animal tendons, skin and fascia, and metal filigrees, particularly silver, were tried with little success. Early in this century the patient's own transplanted fascia and skin were used with some successes but a high morbid-

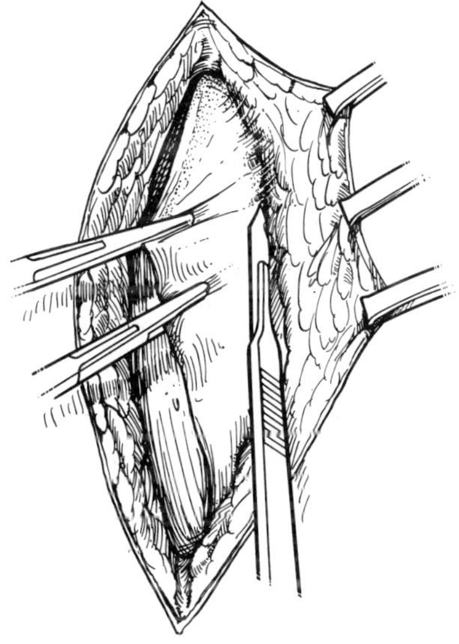

FIG 3–13.
The subcutaneous tissues are mobilized from the superior surface of the fascia so that it can be resected as necessary and closed without tension.

ity. In the 1920s, preserved ox fascia seemed to hold promise because of its successful use in dogs, but it was not well tolerated in humans. During the following decade, tantalum mesh was introduced and was not only well tolerated but could be placed directly in contact with the underlying intestine without causing complications. Over the years it underwent work fracture, but by then the mesh was extensively replaced by the ingrowth of connective tissue. Although tantalum and steel mesh are still available for this purpose, more flexible and durable synthetic materials have been developed, of which polyethylene and polypropylene are the most frequently selected. These are inserted in the wound in the form of a fine, gauzelike mesh. When the peritoneum and fascial edges cannot be approximated, the mesh is tailored with scissors to the size of the defect and sutured to the retracted fascial margins around its perimeter (Fig 3–14). The edge of the mesh is doubled over for about 1 cm so that the sutures can be placed through a double layer to avoid their pulling out. The mesh thus lies directly over and in contact with the intestine, and the subcutaneous tissues and skin are closed over it.

When all of the fascia is unduly attenuated and the closure is considered insecure, the repair can be reinforced with mesh placed either beneath or above the fascial closure. It is technically easier to place it above the fascia, but in this position it is more likely to give rise to infection in the subcutaneous tissues, since the mesh is a major foreign body lying in a large dead space where fluid collection is certain. The mesh is in a relatively protected position below the fascial closure, but it is more difficult and time consuming to suture it in this location (Fig 3–15). Non-

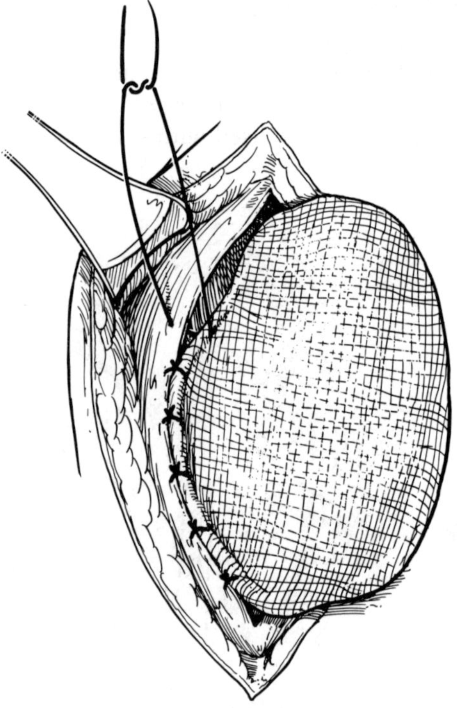

FIG 3–14.
Because of an absolute deficiency of fascia and peritoneum, the folded edge of the mesh is sutured to the retracted fascial edge. It lies in contact with the intestines below and the subcutaneous tissues above.

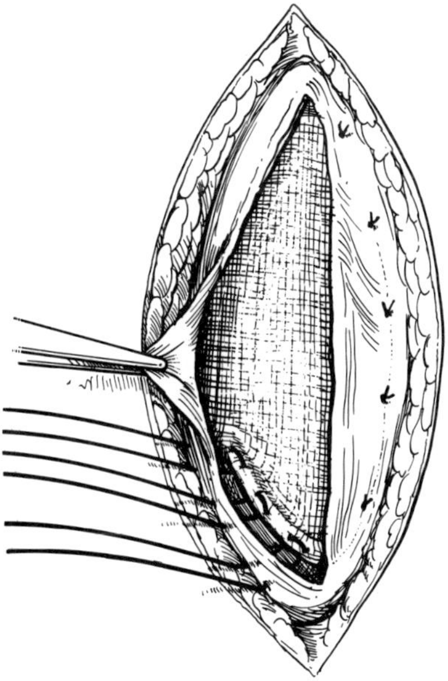

FIG 3–15.
The synthetic mesh has been tailored and placed beneath the fascia to support the closure. The folded edge of the mesh is being drawn beneath the fascia with pulley sutures placed well back from the edge.

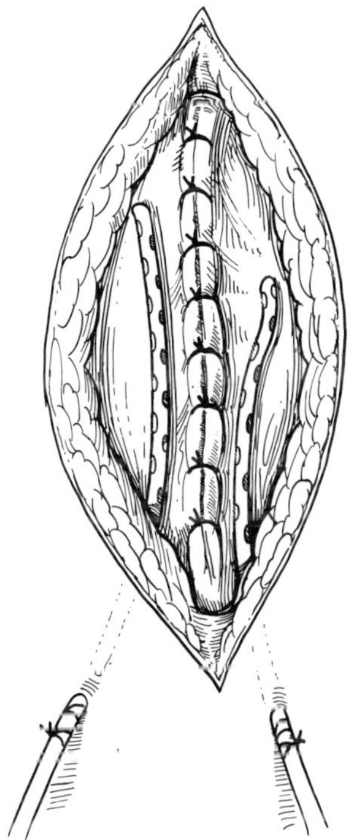

FIG 3–16.
Suction drains are inserted through separate stab wounds in the dead space left by undercutting the subcutaneous tissues and are sutured at the skin level.

absorbable sutures are desirable. When the repair is successful, the mesh is eventually completely replaced by connective tissue.

The essential feature of hernia repair is the fascial closure, with or without the addition of a prosthesis, but careful attention must be paid to the subcutaneous tissues and the skin. Because they have often been extensively undercut, these structures must be examined for bleeding points, however minute, and patches of redundant fat likely to become necrotic must be excised. The skin that has been mobilized by undercutting should be resected enough to provide a firm but not taut closure and joined by clips or sutures according to the surgeon's preference. Before the skin is closed, one or two suction drains, depending on the amount of dead space beneath the skin, are inserted through separate stab wounds and sutured at the skin level (Fig 3–16). A tight dressing is applied for 24 hours, and the patient is taken to the recovery room.

Postoperative Care

Postoperatively, the patient's nasogastric tube is kept in place until she begins to pass gas per rectum. Until that time she is fed intravenously, beginning a liquid diet at the onset of bowel function and progressing to a soft and then regular diet. Early removal of the tube and oral feeding are likely to cause abdominal distention that may jeopardize the repair. Early ambulation is advisable, supporting the abdominal wall with some type of soft binder. Prophylactic antibiotics are not continued for more than 24 hours. Smoking is discouraged, and every attempt is made to alleviate coughing, vomiting, and hiccups. The dressing is removed in 24 hours and the wound inspected. After that a light dressing may be applied or the wound left open to the air, and inspections are carried out at least once daily. The drain or drains are removed within 48 hours unless the volume of drainage remains high (100 mL or more daily). At the time of discharge, the patient is instructed to reduce physical activities for at least 1 month and cautioned about the possibility of superficial fluid collection, especially when a prosthesis has been used. When such collections occur, they must either be aspirated or, if chronic, again placed on constant suction drainage. Infections are treated as in any other wound, but occasionally removal of a prosthesis may be necessary for healing. Since no two hernias are alike, success rates are difficult to determine.

BIBLIOGRAPHY

Baggish MS, Lee WK: Abdominal wound disruption. *Obstet Gynecol* 1975; 46:530.

Bucknall TE, Teare L, Ellis H: The choice of a suture to close abdominal incisions. *Eur Surg Res* 1983; 15:59.

Chan STF, Esufali ST: Extended indications for polypropylene mesh closure of the abdominal wall. *Br J Surg* 1986; 73:3.

Edlich RF, Hodeheaver GT, Thacker JG: Considerations in the choice of sutures for wound closure of the genitourinary tract. *J Urol* 1987; 137:373.

Gallup DG, Talledo OE, King LA: Primary mass closure of midline incisions with a continuous running monofilament suture in gynecologic patients. *Obstet Gynecol* 1989; 73:675.

George CD, Ellis H: The results of incisional hernia repair: A twelve year review. *Ann R Coll Surg Engl* 1986; 68:185.

Gilsdorf RB, Shea MM: Repair of massive septic abdominal wall defects with Marlex mesh. *Am J Surg* 1975; 130:634.

Halevy A, Oland Y, Adam YG: Stainless steel wire for closure of abdominal operative wounds. *Am Surg* 1978; 44:342.

Helmkamp BF: Abdominal wound dehiscence. *Am J Obstet Gynecol* 1977; 128:803.

Jenkins SD, Klamer TW, Parteka JJ: A comparison of prosthetic materials used to repair abdominal wall defects. *Surgery* 1983; 94:392.

Katz S, Izhar M, Mirelman D: Bacterial adherence to surgical sutures: A possible factor in suture induced infection. *Ann Surg* 1981; 194:35.

Kenady DE: Management of abdominal wounds. *Surg Clin North Am* 1984; 64:803.

Kon ND, Meredith JW, Poole GV Jr, et al: Abdominal wound closure: A comparison of polydioxanone, polypropylene, and Teflon-coated Dacron sutures. *Am Surg* 1984; 50:549.

Koontz AR: Preliminary report on the use of tantalum mesh in the repair of ventral hernias. *Ann Surg* 1948; 127:1079.

Koontz AR, Shackelford RT: Tissue reaction to ribbon catgut and preserved ox fascia lata strips. *Ann Surg* 1942; 115:1186.

Lewis RT: Knitted polypropylene (Marlex) mesh in the repair of incisional hernias. *Can J Surg* 1984; 27:155.

Mattingly RF, Thompson JD: *TeLinde's Operative Gynecology*, ed 6. Philadelphia, JB Lippincott Co, 1985.

Mead PB, Pories SE, Hall P, et al: Decreasing the incidence of surgical wound infections. *Arch Surg* 1986; 121:458.

Murray DW Jr, Blaisdell FW: Use of synthetic absorbable sutures for abdominal and chest wound closure. *Arch Surg* 1978; 113:477.

Nehme AE: Repair of large incisional hernias with Marlex mesh. *Int Surg* 1982; 67:398.

Nichols RE: Postoperative wound infection. *N Engl J Med* 1982; 307:1701.

Rubin LK, Maplesden DC: Suturing with stainless steel wire. *Vet Med* September 1977, p 1431.

Rubio PA: New technique for repairing large ventral incisional hernias with Marlex mesh. *Surg Gynecol Obstet* 1986; 162:275.

Skandalakis JE, Gray SW, Mansberger AR Jr, et al: *Hernia: Surgical Anatomy and Technique.* New York, McGraw-Hill Book Co, 1989.

Sloop RD: Running synthetic absorbable suture in abdominal wound closure. *Am J Surg* 1981; 141:572.

Sowa DE, Masterson BJ, Nealon N, et al: Effects of thermal knives on wound healing. *Obstet Gynecol* 1985; 66:436.

Stillman RM, Marino CA, Seligman SJ: Skin staples in potentially contaminated wounds. *Arch Surg* 1984; 119:821.

Varma S, Johnson LW, Ferguson HL, et al: Tissue reaction to suture materials in infected surgical wounds—a histopathologic evaluation. *Am J Vet Res* 1981; 42:563.

Wallace D, Hernandez W, Schlaerth JB, et al: Prevention of abdominal wound disruption utilizing the Smead-Jones closure technique. *Obstet Gynecol* 1980; 45:226.

Chapter 4

"Recurrent" Stress Urinary Incontinence

W. Glenn Hurt, M.D.

Stress urinary incontinence (SUI) is the involuntary loss of urine that occurs as a direct result of sudden, stress-induced increases in intra-abdominal pressure. Characteristically, the loss of urine occurs coincident with the acme of the stress. Stress urinary incontinence becomes clinically significant when it is an embarrassing social and hygienic problem.

"Recurrent" SUI is used in the generic sense to refer to all cases of SUI, both persistent and recurrent, which may follow an operation undertaken to cure the condition. It is necessary to consider other types of urinary incontinence in the diagnosis and management of patients with "recurrent" SUI.

INCIDENCE

Urinary continence in women is not always absolute. At least 50% of young adult nulliparous women admit to some leakage of urine when coughing or sneezing or as a result of some other forms of physical exertion. Usually their leakage is not so severe or so frequent as to be a social or hygienic problem and is of little clinical consequence.

It is estimated that at least 10% of women 20 to 60 years of age and 30% of women more than 60 years of age have significant urinary incontinence.[1] The majority of these women have SUI. One half of all women with SUI will have "pure" SUI; the other half will have SUI in combination with some other form of urinary incontinence.

More than 125 surgical procedures have been recommended for the treatment of SUI. This large number of procedures attests to the fact that no one operation can cure all patients. Patient, diagnostic, operative, and assessment variables make it difficult to review the surgical literature and predict the cure rates of various surgical procedures. Studies that have attempted the objective assessment of the results of SUI surgery report anterior vaginal repair cure rates of 36% to 60% and abdominal retropubic colpopexy (i.e., Burch) cure rates of 80% to 90%.[2] Following primary surgical procedures, 15% to 20% of the patients will have recurrent SUI, and an additional 15% to 20% will have urge incontinence or some other type of lower urinary tract dysfunction that causes them to be dissatisfied with the results of their surgical procedure. All such cases are, in a sense, therapeutic failures.

It is important that every effort be made to ensure the success of the first operative procedure undertaken as treatment of SUI. This is especially true since it is the first operative procedure that is most likely to cure a patient's SUI. Subsequent procedures have failure rates that increase in proportion to their number.

To improve the chances for cure, I will review the preoperative, operative, and postoperative factors that are thought to contribute to surgical failure. I will discuss the evaluation of patients with recurrent SUI and will make recommendations regarding the treatment of patients with recurrent SUI.

PREOPERATIVE FACTORS

There are many different causes of urinary incontinence (Table 4–1). The treatment of each is vastly different. Therefore, it is the physician's responsibility to evaluate each patient in a manner that will precisely diagnose the cause of her urinary incontinence. Preoperative diagnostic errors can result in failure to recognize the cause or causes of a patient's urinary incontinence and, therefore, be a major contributor to the failure of the operation.

Many patients have had surgery for SUI when their preoperative diagnosis was based solely on their history of urine leakage. Although the clinical history is valuable in documenting urinary symptomatology and its onset and severity, it cannot be depended on to accurately diagnose the specific cause of a patient's urinary incontinence. A recent study undertaken to determine the ability of the urologic history to predict urodynamically proved SUI concluded that the symptom of stress incontinence is highly sensitive (93%) with respect to the final diagnosis, but when taken alone, it has such low specificity (19%) that it is of little diagnostic value.[3]

TABLE 4–1.
Causes of Urinary Incontinence

Causes of Urinary Incontinence
Stress urinary incontinence
Urge incontinence
Detrusor instability
Irritative conditions
Neuropathic incontinence
Overflow incontinence
Psychogenic incontinence
Miscellaneous causes
Urethral diverticulum
Drug induced
Congenital incontinence
Urethral hypospadias
Ectopic ureter
Bladder exstrophy
Genitourinary fistula
Ureteral
Vesical
Urethral

The physical examination should be used to evaluate the patient's mental attitude, her overall state of health, and the current status of all medical conditions that might be related to her urinary incontinence. Chronic respiratory diseases, neurologic disorders, and hormonal deficiencies should receive special attention. They may be a cause of or contribute to a patient's urinary incontinence.

The pelvic examination of patients who complain of urinary incontinence should be more than an attempt to demonstrate pelvic relaxation. It is a common mistake for clinicians to use evidence of anterior vaginal relaxation to confirm the diagnosis of SUI. The two should not be equated. Stress urinary incontinence is frequently seen in patients with little or no pelvic relaxation. At the other extreme, some patients with marked degrees of pelvic organ prolapse will find themselves unable to pass urine unless they manually reduce the prolapse. When the symptom of stress incontinence is combined with evidence of anterior vaginal wall relaxation in an effort to predict urodynamically proved genuine SUI, the positive predictive value of pure SUI is 60% and the false positive diagnosis rate is 40%.[3]

The pelvic examination should be used not only to look for weaknesses within the pelvic support system but to determine the condition of all pelvic tissues and to demonstrate the patient's urinary incontinence. Stress testing is the most reliable method of diagnosing SUI. It has the highest predictive values, both positive and negative, of all tests. Unfortunately, it cannot be used to distinguish pure SUI from those mixed forms of incontinence of which SUI may be only one component. Stress testing should be performed when the patient has a full bladder. If stressful maneuvers do not demonstrate a patient's incontinence when she is in the lithotomy position, she should be allowed to assume the erect position for additional attempts at demonstrating her incontinence. The diagnosis of urinary incontinence should not be made unless the incontinence is objectively demonstrable. A patient whose SUI cannot be demonstrated should not be considered a candidate for SUI surgery.

Patients who complain of urinary incontinence should have their urine tested to rule out the possibility of a urinary tract infection. Such infections can cause lower urinary tract dysfunction and result in urinary incontinence. The eradication of a urinary tract infection will often relieve the patient's symptoms and preclude the need for further diagnostic procedures. Sterile urine should be a prerequisite for urodynamic testing. Invasive testing in patients with infected urine places them at risk for developing an acute urinary tract infection and casts doubt on the reliability of all urodynamic studies.

No urinary incontinence evaluation is complete unless cystometry has been performed. Cystometry is the primary method of detecting detrusor instability, which is the cause of at least 10% to 15% of all female urinary incontinence. It is also a frequent finding in those patients who have mixed forms of urinary incontinence. One third to one half of all patients with SUI have some evidence of detrusor instability. The treatment of detrusor instability is primarily medical; the treatment of SUI is primarily surgical. Patients who have SUI and detrusor instability should be told of the significance of the coexistence of the two types of urinary incontinence. Detrusor instability should be aggressively treated before any attempt is made to surgically correct SUI. If a patient's preoperative detrusor instability cannot be corrected and persists after surgery, or if it occurs for the first time after surgery, it may be a cause of urgency, frequency, and urge incontinence. The patient with postoperative urinary incontinence due to detrusor instability will consider surgery undertaken to correct her condition a failure, even though she may have been cured of her coexistent SUI.

In the treatment of SUI, surgical failure predisposes the patient to subsequent surgical failure. This fact emphasizes the need for the careful selection and performance of each continence procedure. Historically, anterior vaginal repairs have been considered the operation of choice for all cases of SUI. There is the dictum, "Do the first operation from below, and if it fails, then go above." This dictum has been sighted as the reason for many cases of recurrent SUI. It is now apparent, by objective assessment, that the cure rates of SUI treated by a retropubic procedure are consistently better than the cure rates of SUI treated by an anterior vaginal repair. Consequently, it makes little sense to routinely perform an anterior vaginal repair as treatment for SUI. The routine anterior vaginal repair, as performed by most surgeons, is not a procedure designed primarily for the cure of SUI. It is an operation designed for the correction of pelvic relaxation; it is limited in the extent to which it can elevate and stabilize the urethrovesical junction. Even its most ardent proponents do not recommend it for the treatment of patients with recurrent SUI.

OPERATIVE FACTORS

The primary aim of the majority of SUI procedures is to elevate the urethrovesical junction to a high retropubic position within the abdominal zone of pressure and to maintain its position during sudden increases in intra-abdominal pressure. To be most effective, the operation must preserve posterior rotational descent of the bladder, the compressibility of the urethra, and the integrity of the internal urethral sphincter mechanism.

Failure to accomplish the goals of a particular SUI procedure may be due to lack of knowledge of the technical aspects of the procedure or to lack of experience in performing it. Unfortunately, training programs are limited in the experience that they can provide in the performance and follow-up of procedures to correct incontinence. As a result, the gynecologic surgeon who does not become proficient in several different types of SUI procedures will be limited in the ability to successfully perform surgery for incontinence when intraoperative findings dictate the need to modify the proposed procedure.

Incontinence may be the result of previous surgery that has resulted in the fibrosis and fixation of the pelvic tissues. Such scarring can adversely affect the continence mechanism by distorting the anatomic relationship between the urethra and bladder that favors continence, by interfering with posterior rotational descent of the bladder during stress, damaging the urethra's internal and external sphincteric mechanisms and its overall compressibility, or both. All pelvic operations should avoid direct and indirect injuries to the urethra. Laceration, devascularization, or denervation of the urethra may cause it to lose its sphincteric capability and become a functionless drainpipe. It also may cause urinary incontinence as a result of lower urinary tract dysfunction or the formation of a genitourinary fistula.

The results of incontinence procedures depend on the integrity of the tissues that are used to support the urethrovesical junction. Since injury, attenuation, and atrophy of the tissues that normally support the proximal urethra and the urethrovesical junction contribute to the development of SUI, it is important to prepare all pelvic tissues for surgery and to use the tissues to provide permanent support for the proximal urethra and the urethrovesical junction. When the patient's tissues are inadequate for this purpose, it may be necessary to consider the use of fascial or synthetic straps for a more durable repair.

Suture material and suture placement are critical to the success of continence surgery. Catgut is a poor choice for repair and suspension operations. It causes an intense inflammatory response, promotes fibrosis, has poor tensile strength, and is rapidly absorbed. The newer delayed absorbable and permanent suture materials are recommended because of their low reactivity, their higher tensile strength, and their slower rate of absorption. The critical sutures in needle retropubic and abdominal colposuspension procedures are the ones that are placed in tissues on either side of the urethrovesical junction. These sutures are used to elevate and maintain the urethrovesical junction within the retropubic space (of Retzius). It is recommended that permanent suture be used for such suspensions and that it be tied in a manner that will not result in necrosis or release. Furthermore, it is important that the primary suspending sutures be placed on either side of the urethrovesical junction, which is normally about 4 cm from the external urethral meatus. If these sutures are placed below the urethrovesical junction, they fail to restore it to a high retropubic position. If they are placed above the urethrovesical junction, they tend to "urethralize" the trigone and interfere with the posterior rotational descent of the bladder.

It is important in incontinence surgery to detect and correct all weaknesses within the pelvic support system. To concentrate on the elevation and stabilization of the urethrovesical junction and to neglect other evidence of pelvic organ prolapse predisposes the operation to failure. The function of the urinary continence mechanism depends on the relationship of the urethra and bladder, but this relationship can be influenced by the presence of a cystocele, enterocele, rectocele, or prolapsed uterus. Suspension of the urethrovesical junction and failure to correct other evidence of pelvic organ prolapse are likely to accentuate weaknesses within the pelvic support system and require the patient to have additional surgery.

POSTOPERATIVE FACTORS

During the immediate postoperative period, hematomas, infections, and overdistention of the bladder can cause recurrent incontinence through damage to the suspending sutures and tissues, the bladder, or the urethra. It is recommended that all patients who have operations for pelvic support defects observe a period of physical restraint to permit adequate healing. Patients should be advised that excessive coughing, straining, or lifting during the healing phase can cause recurrent incontinence and pelvic organ prolapse. An increasing number of patients are involved in strenuous occupational and recreational activities. If such activities are likely to contribute to recurrent incontinence or prolapse, they should be reduced or eliminated.

Estrogen prevents weakening and atrophy of the pelvic support system, enhances the function of the internal urethral sphincter mechanism, and preserves the pliability of the soft tissues of the pelvis. Menopausal patients need long-term estrogen replacement therapy. If they quit taking estrogen, they may see a gradual deterioration in the efficiency of their continence mechanism.

Chronic respiratory diseases that cause sudden increases in intra-abdominal pressure may contribute to the failure of surgery for incontinence. The repetitive stress of a chronic cough may be more than tissues can bear. Smokers who undergo incontinence surgery should be advised to quit smoking or risk the return of urinary incontinence.

A number of postoperative complications may result from incontinence surgery and cause urinary leakage. Detrusor and urethral instability may cause urge incontinence, bladder neck obstruction may cause overflow incontinence, and genitourinary fistula may cause continuous leakage.

EVALUATION

Patients who have "recurrent" SUI should have a complete urogynecologic evaluation with urodynamic studies (Table 4–2). Every effort should be made to determine why the operative procedure or procedures failed, the anatomic, physiologic, and pathologic changes that are present, and the current cause or causes of urinary incontinence.

The patient should be asked to keep a urinary diary for at least 3 consecutive days as she goes about her daily routine. She should record the time and amount of fluid intake and urinary output. Also, she should record all episodes of urgency and incontinence and make some comment regarding the circumstances associated with each. The urinary diary provides objective evidence of the patient's symptomatology. It is also a valuable means of assessing the results of therapy.

The patient's general history should be supplemented by an incisive urologic history that documents the urinary symptoms and their onset and severity. Incontinence questionnaires have proved helpful in assuring completeness of the urologic history. It is also useful for the questionnaire to include a space for the patient to

TABLE 4–2.
Evaluation of Patients With Recurrent SUI

Urinary diary
History and physical examination
Q-tip quantification of urethral mobility
Urinary residual measurement
Urine culture
Stress testing to demonstrate incontinence
Uroflowmetry
Multichannel urethrocystometry
Urethral pressure profilometry
Voiding cystourethrography
Periurethral electromyography
Urethrocystoscopy
Optional studies
Bead chain urethrocystocolpography
Voiding cystourethrography
Intravenous urography
Videocystourethrography
Consultation

list significant medical illnesses, previous surgical procedures, allergies, and all recent and current medications.

The general physical examination should detail the patient's body habitus, the condition of her respiratory system, and any findings that are the result of chronic illnesses or previous surgery. The neurologic examination should be focused to detect central, spinal, and peripheral nervous system disorders that might affect the lower urinary tract. Attention should be given to the evaluation of sacral nerves 2, 3, and 4 that provide the principal motor supply for the detrusor and for the periurethral striated muscle. A detailed pelvic examination should be performed to ascertain the condition of the tissues, to determine the size, shape, position, and mobility of the pelvic organs, and to detect all weaknesses within the pelvic organ support system.

Every effort should be made to demonstrate the patient's urinary incontinence. If the patient comes to the examining room with a full bladder, she may be asked to cough while in the lithotomy and erect positions, to heel bounce, and to listen to the flow of running water to see if leakage will occur. After the patient has emptied her bladder, she should be catheterized for measurement of residual urine. The specimen should be tested for evidence of a urinary tract infection or sent for bacteriologic culture. At this time, a Q-tip test may be performed to quantify the mobility of the urethrovesical junction. If the patient did not demonstrate her incontinence when previously stress tested, a straight catheter should be used to slowly fill the bladder with sterile room temperature saline. An effort is made to determine the bladder volume when she feels the first urge to void and when she is at maximum capacity. When the bladder is full, the catheter is removed and stress testing is repeated with the patient in the erect position. It is important to actually observe the patient's leakage in an effort to determine its timing in relationship to stress and to document the characteristics of urine leakage.

Uroflowmetry may be performed following initial stress testing, before instrumentation of the lower urinary tract, when the patient is asked to empty her bladder. It is a study that should be repeated to verify its results.

Cystometry should be performed in all patients who are being evaluated for urinary incontinence. It is the primary method of assessing detrusor activity, bladder sensation, and bladder capacity. Multichannel urethrocystometry is recommended for those with recurrent SUI. It should simultaneously measure bladder, urethral, and abdominal (vaginal or rectal) pressure. Subtracted measurements may be used to calculate detrusor pressure and urethral closure pressure. During the filling of the bladder, it is important to note the first sensation of filling, the first desire to void, and the maximum cystometric capacity. Passive and dynamic urethral pressure profilometry may be performed as part of the urethrocystometric examination. This provides a urethral pressure profile and permits calculation of the maximum urethral closure pressure, the functional profile length, pressure transmission ratios, and so forth. When the bladder is full, the patient should be stress tested in the erect position to detect detrusor instability and to demonstrate urinary incontinence. Voiding cystometry may be performed to evaluate the contractile function of the detrusor. Electromyography of the periurethral striated muscle is useful in detecting vesicourethral sphincter dyssynergia.

Urethrocystoscopy is performed to detect mucosal lesions, growths, diverticula, and so on within the bladder and urethra. It is important to observe the reaction of the detrusor and urethra during filling and to observe the base of the bladder, the urethrovesical junction, and the proximal urethra when the patient is asked to squeeze as if voluntarily interrupting her urinary stream and to bear down as if she were trying to have a bowel movement. Dynamic urethrocystoscopy is used to confirm the findings of the Q-tip test in determining the mobility of the urethrovesical junction and of the pelvic examination in determining the presence or absence of a cystocele or cystourethrocele.

A number of imaging techniques are available for documenting the anatomic relationships of the pelvic organs, for detecting urethral diverticulum, and for visualizing the function of the lower urinary tract. Bead chain urethrocystocolpography is useful in documenting the anatomic relationships of the urethra, bladder, and vagina and the location of each with respect to recognizable bony landmarks within the pelvis. It is recognized as the gold standard for determining the anatomic changes wrought by surgical procedures. Intravenous urography, voiding cystourethrograms, and other tests may be indicated to determine the condition of the urinary tract, to detect genitourinary fistulas, to demonstrate a diverticulum, and so forth. Such tests should be freely utilized.

Many urologic laboratories use ultrasound and videocystourethrography in diagnosing lower urinary tract disorders. The latter, combined with urethrocystometry, gives a comprehensive evaluation of the anatomic and physiologic functions of the lower urinary tract.

In the evaluation of a patient with recurrent SUI it is important to know when consultation or referral is in order. Urodynamic testing and surgery for recurrent SUI is most beneficial when undertaken by physicians who have a special interest in urogynecology.

THERAPY

Detrusor instability can be a cause of urgency, frequency, and urge incontinence in persons who have had continence surgery. It is helpful to know if this problem was a preoperative finding that persists, if it developed for the first time during the immediate postoperative period, or if it was a delayed complication. Detrusor instability that develops during the immediate postoperative period is often due to a lower urinary tract infection or to bladder trauma. It usually resolves promptly following the eradication of the infection and completion of the healing process. Preoperative detrusor instability that persists into the postoperative period or that occurs as a delayed complication of incontinence surgery is much more refractory to bladder retraining and pharmacologic therapy.

As a result of a suspension procedure, patients with a weak detrusor may have their postoperative course complicated by voiding dysfunction or urinary retention. They may benefit by pressure-flow studies and electromyography of their periurethral striated muscle to define the status of their voiding mechanism. Some will learn to void efficiently using alternative voiding techniques. Pharmacologic therapy may be used to reduce outlet resistance. Intermittent self-catheterization is recommended to prevent overdistention of the bladder.

Bladder neck obstruction may cause detrusor instability or retention and overflow incontinence. If there is significant obstruction of the bladder neck, release of the suspending sutures may be necessary. Before reoperation to release the sus-

TABLE 4–3.
Recurrent SUI: Procedures and Their Indications

Retropubic colposuspension
Adequate vagina with mobile walls
Bladder neck descent
Depressed pressure transmission
Suburethral sling urethropexy
Inadequate vagina with immobile walls
Open bladder neck
Low urethral closure pressure
Periurethral polytef injections
Good anatomic relationships
Good pressure transmission
Low urethral closure pressure
Artificial sphincter
Intractable incontinence

pending sutures, it is important to define the patient's detrusor function because she may decide that self-catheterization is preferable to urinary incontinence.

Therapy for recurrent SUI will, of course, be dictated by the patient's current type of incontinence, its severity, and her physical condition and findings. Mild recurrent SUI may be managed by perineal pads, pelvic muscle exercises, and pharmacologic therapy. Estrogen augments the internal urethral sphincter mechanism by its action on the mucosa, the vascular plexus, the connective tissue, and the smooth muscle. It also contributes to the pliability of the pelvic tissues and the integrity of the pelvic support system. α-Adrenergic agonist therapy, such as imipramine, may be used to strengthen the internal urethral sphincter mechanism.

After a complete evaluation of their condition, patients with moderate or severe recurrent SUI should be considered candidates for repeat continence surgery. There is general agreement that surgery for recurrent SUI should consist of some type of retropubic urethral suspension. The standard anterior colporrhaphy has no place in the treatment of recurrent SUI.

The procedures that I currently recommend as treatment for recurrent SUI and indications for each are listed in Table 4–3. Most recurrent SUI can be cured by an abdominal retropubic colposuspension or a suburethral sling urethropexy. There are a few older patients who are at increased risk for major surgical procedures and whose incontinence can be improved by periurethral polytef injections. These three procedures will be described. The artificial sphincter is being recommended for patients with intractable incontinence. At this time, I believe that the placement of an artificial sphincter should remain in the hands of those who are investigating its use.

Retropubic (Modified Burch) Colposuspension

The patient is placed on the operating table, and anesthesia is administered. The patient's heels are strapped in stirrups (Allen Universal), and she is placed in a modified lithotomy position with hips slightly flexed and the lower extremities slightly abducted. The foot of the operating table is dropped from under the lower extremities. The abdomen, inner thighs, perineum, and vagina are prepared and draped to allow simultaneous abdominal and vaginal access. A sterile Foley catheter is placed transurethrally into the bladder and connected to straight drainage.

A lower abdominal incision is made into the peritoneal cavity. If a hysterectomy or salpingo-oophorectomy is indicated, it is performed, and the pelvis is reperitonealized. A Moschcowitz or Halban closure of the cul-de-sac (of Douglas) is completed using permanent suture. The anterior parietal peritoneum is approximated.

The patient is placed in a slight reverse Trendelenburg position. A small retractor (Balfour) is used to retract the lower medial margins of the rectus muscles. Moist laparotomy packs are used to dissect the retropubic space (of Retzius). If the patient has had a previous retropubic procedure, an extraperitoneal cystotomy should be performed and the bladder separated from the pubis and pubic symphysis under direct vision using sharp dissection. Once the depths of the retropubic space have been dissected bilaterally, the operating surgeon should place a sterile sleeve and glove onto the nondominant arm and hand. Approximately 50 mL of indigo carmine–colored sterile saline is instilled into the bladder via the Foley catheter's drainage system, and the catheter is clamped to prevent the escape of the colored solution from the bladder.

The first and second fingers of the surgeon's nondominant hand are placed into the vagina so the tips of the fingers will straddle the urethrovesical junction as identified by the Foley balloon. The urethrovesical junction should be about 4 cm from the external urethral meatus. The tip of one of the vaginal fingers is used to elevate the vaginal wall that overlies it into the retropubic space. A sponge stick or Kelly dissector is used to move the lateral aspect of the urethrovesical junction from over the elevated vaginal wall. When the overlying tissues have been removed, the fibromuscular wall of the vagina appears glistening white, and on palpation, the vaginal wall will be all that is felt between the tips of the vaginal and abdominal fingers.

A no. 0 or 00 permanent suture is threaded onto a needle (Mayo, no. 5) and passed twice through the entire thickness of the anterior vaginal wall at a point 1.5 to 2 cm lateral to the urethrovesical junction. A second suture of similar material is placed in a similar manner 1 to 1.5 cm lateral and superior to the first (Fig 4–1). The long arms of both sutures are clamped with different small clamps so as to distinguish the medial from the lateral suture. The vaginal wall on the opposite side of the urethrovesical junction is elevated, and the overlying tissues are moved medially. Identical suture placement is undertaken, and the long arms of each suture are clamped with the same small clamp sequence to differentiate the medial from the lateral suture. The sutures are elevated to judge their potential for suspending the urethrovesical junction. If it is satisfactory, a needle is threaded sequentially onto one arm of each suture, and that arm of the suture is passed through Cooper's ligament at a point above its location in the anterior vaginal wall. One arm of each suture is placed before any of the suspending sutures are tied (Fig 4–2).

The elevation of the urethrovesical junction may be determined by elevation of the tips of the surgeon's vaginal fingers, observation of the urethrovesical junction via a cystoscope, Q-tip deflection of approximately −20 degrees with respect to the horizontal, or observation of the bladder neck via the suprapubic cystotomy. The extent of elevation of the urethrovesical junction is determined more by experience than by scientific measurement. Once the surgeon feels that the urethrovesical junction is in proper position, the suspending sutures are tied to elevate and main-

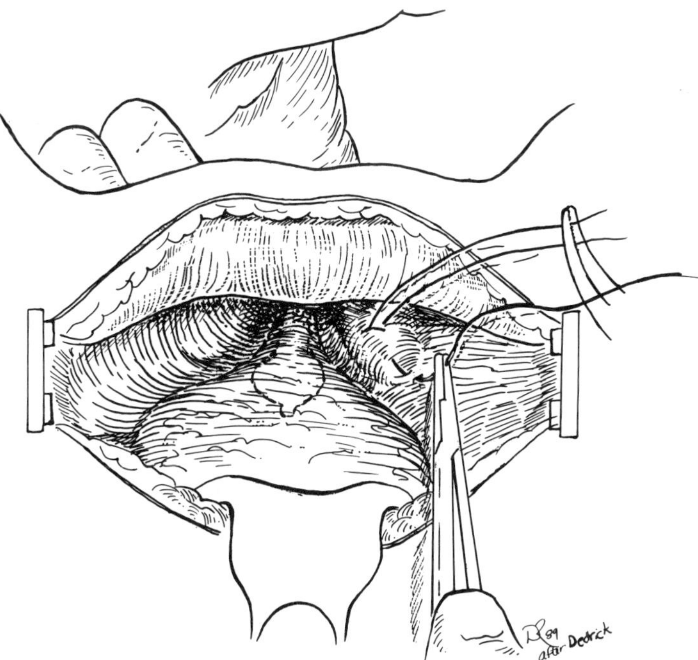

FIG 4–1.
Retropubic colposuspension. A vaginal finger elevates the anterior vaginal wall into the retropubic space for placement of the second suture to the right of the urethrovesical junction.

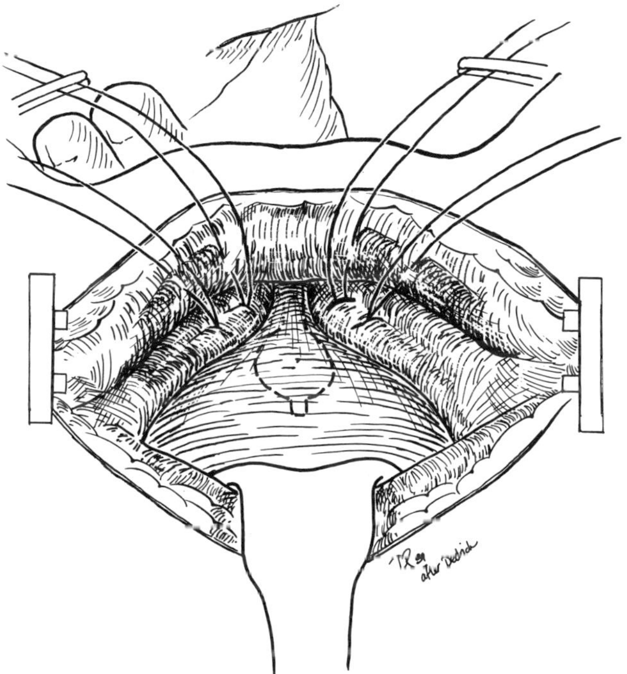

FIG 4–2.
Retropubic colposuspension. The four suspending sutures have been placed through Cooper's ligament.

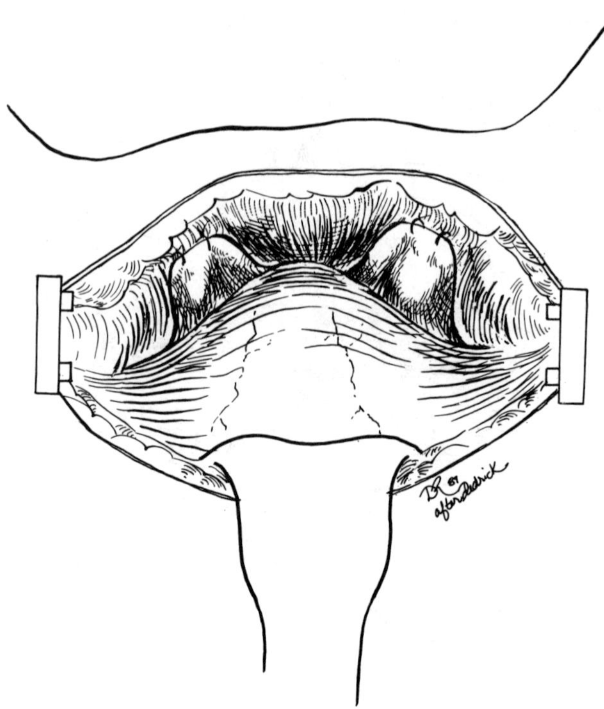

FIG 4–3.
Retropubic colposuspension. The four suspending sutures have been tied.

tain the urethrovesical junction within the retropubic space (Fig 4–3). Care should be taken to be sure that the urethra is not compressed against the symphysis pubis or otherwise unduly obstructed. If there has been excessive bleeding within the retropubic space, suction drains (Jackson-Pratt) may be placed and brought out through separate stab incisions in the lower abdomen.

The medial margins of the rectus muscles are loosely approximated along the midline to prevent ventral herniation of the dome of the bladder. The anterior abdominal incision is closed in the routine manner. A suprapubic catheter is preferred for postoperative bladder drainage. Following its placement, the transurethral Foley catheter is removed, and the patient is sent to the recovery room.

The suprapubic catheter is clamped on the third or fourth postoperative day to permit voiding trials. It is not removed until the postvoid residual urine is consistently less than 80 to 90 mL.

The most frequent complications of a retropubic colposuspension are delayed voiding, urinary tract infection, pyrexia, lower urinary tract injury, and wound infection. The expected cure rate of recurrent SUI with a retropubic colposuspension should be 90%.

Suburethral Sling Urethropexy

The patient is placed on the operating table and anesthesia is administered. If a strip of the patient's fascia lata is to be used for the sling, the patient is placed on her side, with thighs and legs parallel, slightly flexed, and with a pillow between them. The upper part of the thigh is prepared and draped. A transverse 4-cm incision is made through the skin above the inferior condyle and just above the superior margin of the patella. The subcutaneous tissues are retracted to expose the fascia lata. Two parallel incisions are made 1.5 to 2 cm apart and in line with the fibers of the fascia lata. Another incision in the fascia joins the distal ends of the two parallel incisions. The flap of fascia lata is lifted and threaded into a fascial stripper (Masson or Wilson) (Fig 4–4). The fascia lata is stripped for a distance of at least 18 cm. The strip is removed by cutting the superior end of the fascial strip. The exposed fascial incisions are approximated with delayed absorbable or permanent suture, the skin incision is closed, and bandages are applied. This fascia is laid aside in a moistened sterile towel until it is needed.

If a synthetic strap is to be used for the suspension of the urethra, a strap that measures 2 by 20 cm is cut from a sheet of sterile polytetrafluoroethylene (Gore-Tex*) 1 mm thick.

The patient's heels are strapped in stirrups (Allen Universal), and she is placed in a modified lithotomy position with hips moderately flexed and the lower extremities slightly abducted. The foot of the operating table is dropped from under the lower extremities. The abdomen, inner thighs, perineum and vagina are prepared and draped to allow simultaneous abdominal and vaginal surgery preferably by two surgical teams. A sterile Foley catheter is placed transurethrally into the bladder and connected to straight drainage. Indigo carmine–colored saline is instilled into the bladder, and the Foley catheter clamped so as to retain the colored saline within the bladder. Subsequent leakage of the blue dye into the operative field should alert the surgeons to the possibility of bladder injury.

The abdominal surgical team makes a transverse curvilinear 8- to 10-cm incision in the lower abdomen approximately 3 cm above the symphysis and exposes the anterior abdominal aponeurosis. The vaginal surgical team incises the full thickness of the anterior vaginal wall in the midline from within 1 cm of the external urethral meatus to the vaginal apex. The vesicovaginal space is widely dissected bilaterally to the pubic rami. The vaginal surgeon uses the index finger to pierce the endopelvic fascia laterally and dissect the retropubic space (of Retzius) the full depth of the symphysis on either side of the urethrovesical junction. The pubocervical fascia is plicated beneath the urethrovesical junction. This fascia will act as a cushion between the urethra and the fascial sling.

The abdominal surgical team should make bilateral 2-cm incisions through the abdominal aponeurosis at the lateral margins of the rectus muscles or 3 to 4 cm from the midline. A long uterine packing forcep or a suture ligature carrier (Pereyra type) is passed through one incision in the anterior abdominal aponeurosis into the retropubic space so that it comes into direct contact with the vaginal surgeon's index finger. The forcep or ligature carrier is guided down through the retropubic space and out of the vaginal port on the corresponding side of the urethra. The end of the fascial or synthetic strap is picked up by the uterine packing forcep or sutures in the end of the strap are threaded into the ligature carrier. The retrieving instrument is drawn up through the retropubic space bringing the end of the strap through the incision in the abdominal aponeurosis. The same procedure for the retrieval of the opposite end of the strap is performed on the opposite side (Fig 4–5). Care is taken to keep the strap flat throughout its course.

One end of the strap is sewn to the superior surface of the anterior abdominal

*Gore-Tex, W.L. Gore & Assoc., Inc., Flagstaff, AZ.

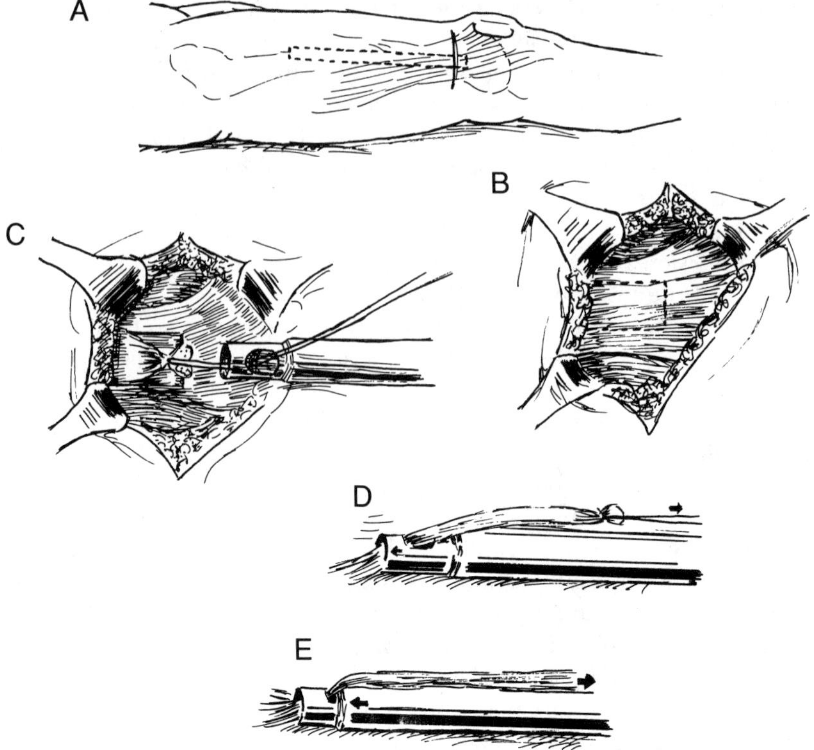

FIG 4–4.
Suburethral sling urethropexy. The thigh is prepared and draped, and the incisions have been made for obtaining the fascia lata strap **(A)**. The fascia is incised as indicated by the *dashed line* **(B)**. The incised fascia is threaded into the fascia stripper **(C)**, and the stripper advanced subcutaneously **(D)** as far as it will go, while traction to the free end of the strip is maintained in the opposite direction, as shown by the *small arrow*. When the stripper can be advanced no further, the outer sleeve is unscrewed and slid distally as a guillotine over the opening in the central barrel **(E)**, transecting the fascia. The fascial strap and the stripper are removed, and the visible fascial defect closed with a few interrupted sutures, as in the skin incision. (Redrawn from Nichols DH: The sling operation, in Cantor EB [ed]: *Female Urinary Stress Incontinence.* Springfield, Ill, Charles C Thomas, Publisher, 1979, p. 254. Used by permission.)

aponeurosis with permanent suture in a manner that will secure it and at the same time close the fascial defect within the aponeurosis. The opposite end of the strap is then drawn up through the anterior abdominal aponeurosis so that the suburethral portion of the strap barely supports the urethrovesical junction. Interrupted permanent sutures are used to attach the suburethral portion of the strap to those tissues on either side of the urethrovesical junction to help hold the strap in place. The unsecured end of the strap is then sewn to the superior surface of the anterior abdominal aponeurosis with permanent suture in a manner that will secure it and also close the fascial defect. The medial edges of the anterior vaginal wall are trimmed and approximated with interrupted delayed absorbable suture. The anterior abdominal wall is closed in a routine manner. A suprapubic catheter is preferred for postoperative bladder drainage. After it is placed, the transurethral Foley catheter is removed.

When voiding trials are to be undertaken, the suprapubic catheter is clamped.

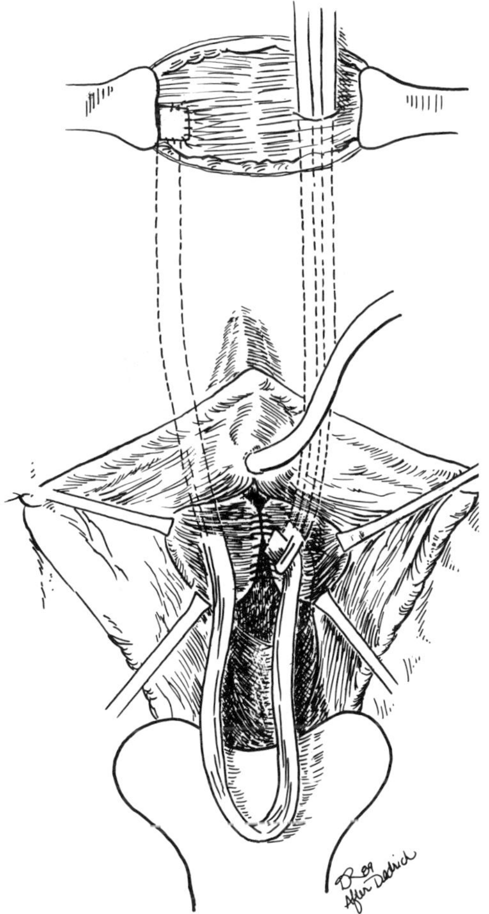

FIG 4–5.
Suburethral sling urethropexy. The fascia lata strap is in place on the right side of the urethra and is being retrieved on the left side of the urethra.

The suprapubic catheter is not removed until the postvoid residual urine is consistently less than 90 mL.

The most frequent complications of the suburethral sling procedures include delayed voiding, urinary tract infection, pyrexia, hematuria, seroma, lower urinary tract injury, wound infection, and urinary fistula. Parker and colleagues[4] report a cure rate of 84%, and Beck and colleagues[5] report a cure rate of 98% when a suburethral fascia lata sling is used as treatment for recurrent SUI.

Periurethral Polytef Injections

The patient is placed on the operating table, and anesthesia is administered. The patient is placed in a modified lithotomy position, and the vulva is prepared and draped to permit vaginal access. Urethrocystoscopy is performed. Simultaneously, a long 16-gauge needle and Lewy syringe, both loaded with polytef paste, are inserted at the 3 o'clock position alongside the urethra so that the tip of the needle reaches to the urethrovesical junction. With the tip of the needle against the

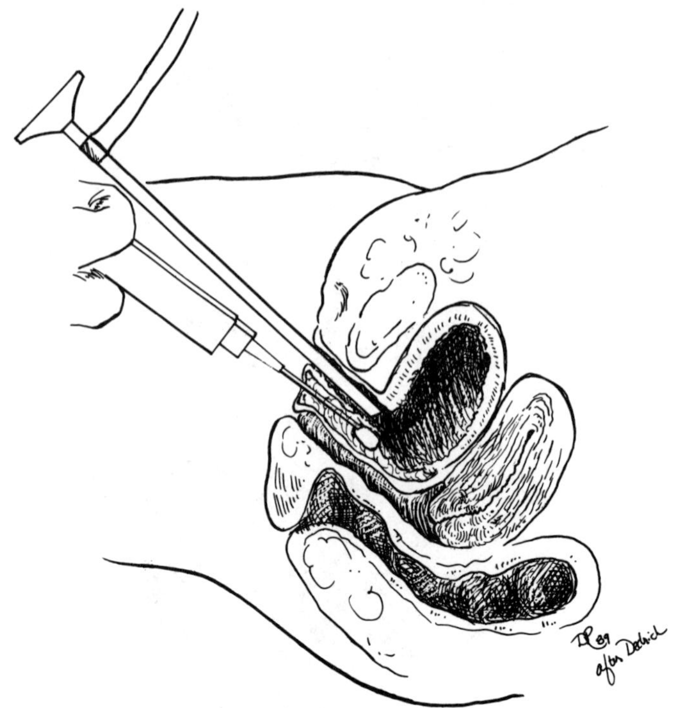

FIG 4–6.
Polytef paste is being injected about the urethra.

wall of the urethra, 3 to 4 mL of polytef is injected (Fig 4–6). The 6 and 9 o'clock positions are subsequently injected in an effort to distribute a total of 10 to 15 mL of polytef about the sides and lower portion of the urethrovesical junction. The injection of the polytef paste should reduce the caliber and increase the resistance of the proximal urethra.

Urethral pressure profiles before, during, and after this procedure are helpful in determining the effects of the procedure. It may be necessary to repeat the procedure in 3 to 4 months to achieve maximum benefit. Periurethral polytef injections do not preclude performance of subsequent continence procedures.

Carrion and Politano, in a series of 51 females with urinary incontinence of various causes, report that polytef injections restored continence in 51%, markedly reduced urinary leakage in 20%, and resulted in little or no improvement in 29%.[6] They note that 8 of the 15 patients with little or no improvement in their incontinence received only one series of polytef injections.

REFERENCES

1. Urinary incontinence in adults. *Natl Inst Health Consensus Dev Conf Statement* 1988; 7:1.
2. Hilton P: Urinary incontinence in women. *Br Med J (Clin Res)* 1987; 195:426–432.
3. Walters MD, Shields LE: The diagnostic value of history, physical examination, and the Q-tip cotton swab test in women with urinary incontinence. *Am J Obstet Gynecol* 1988; 159:145–149.

4. Parker RT, Addison WA, Wilson CJ: Fascia lata urethrovesical suspension for recurrent stress urinary incontinence. *Am J Obstet Gynecol* 1979; 135:843–852.
5. Beck RP, McCormick S, Nordstrom L: The fascia lata sling procedure for treating recurrent genuine stress incontinence of urine. *Obstet Gynecol* 1988; 72:699–703.
6. Carrion HM, Politano VA: Periurethral polytef (Teflon) injection for urinary incontinence, in Raz S (ed): *Female Urology*. Philadelphia, WB Saunders Co, 1983, pp 293–298.

BIBLIOGRAPHY

Burch JC: Urethrovaginal fixation to Cooper's ligament for correction of stress incontinence, cystocele, and prolapse. *Am J Obstet Gynecol* 1961; 81:281–290.

Burch JC: Cooper's ligament urethrovesical suspension for stress incontinence. *Am J Obstet Gynecol* 1968; 100:764–774.

Diokno AC, Hollander JB, Alderson TP: Artificial urinary sphincter for recurrent female urinary incontinence: Indications and results. *J Urol* 1987; 138:778–780.

Furlow WL: Artificial sphincter, in Stanton SL, Tanagho EA (eds): *Surgery of Female Incontinence*, ed 2. New York, Springer-Verlag New York, 1986, pp 155–173.

Chapter 5

Eversion of the Vagina

David H. Nichols, M.D.

Although uncommon, recurrent massive eversion of the vagina is not rare. It may be of various degree, with or without recurrence of the other forms of genital prolapse such as enterocele, cystocele, and rectocele. It involves a significant redescent of the vaginal vault, at first a partial eversion (Fig 5–1), which, if unattended, proceeds to a complete eversion of the vagina (with the uterus if it is present). Descent of the uterus is a passive accompaniment of the vaginal vault prolapse and is, therefore, the result and not the cause of genital prolapse. Hysterectomy, though usually desirable, is but one feature of surgical pelvic reconstruction. The essential steps toward successful pelvic reconstruction lie within the choice of appropriate procedure, the techniques of the repair itself, and the precision and proficiency of the surgeon.

Usually there is a history of preceding hysterectomy, either transabdominal or transvaginal. Often there was a particular weakness in the support of the vaginal vault, which may or may not have been recognized and effectively addressed by the initial surgeon (Fig 5–2). The onset of recurrent massive eversion of the vagina is sometimes insidious. At other times it follows directly some sudden increase in intra-abdominal pressure as from a fit of coughing or vomiting or having lifted something heavy, such as a piece of furniture. The patient, often older and frequently dehydrated, may be given to a chronic habit of straining at stool. She may become aware of a sudden sensation of something having given way within the pelvis, with an accompanying backache and feeling of fullness, which is worse in the erect position. An obvious and externally visible bulge in the vagina may become evident. It enlarges over a period of time but invariably recedes when the patient lies down when gravity pulls her genital parts in another direction.

The sole exception to this situation is the patient with an incarcerated procidentia, in which the amount of tissue edema becomes so severe that spontaneous or induced manual reduction within the pelvis is no longer possible. Such incarceration constitutes a surgical emergency, because ureteral obstruction, necrosis, and gangrene of the tissues may supervene if the condition is not relieved. For the patient with an incarcerated prolapse, the immediate treatment is strict bed rest. The prolapsed parts should be wrapped in soaks of hypertonic saline to reduce the edema. Manual reposition within the pelvis may be tried two or three times daily as the edema subsides, the tenderness abates, and reduction once again becomes possible. The reposited prolapse should be held in place with an intravaginal pes-

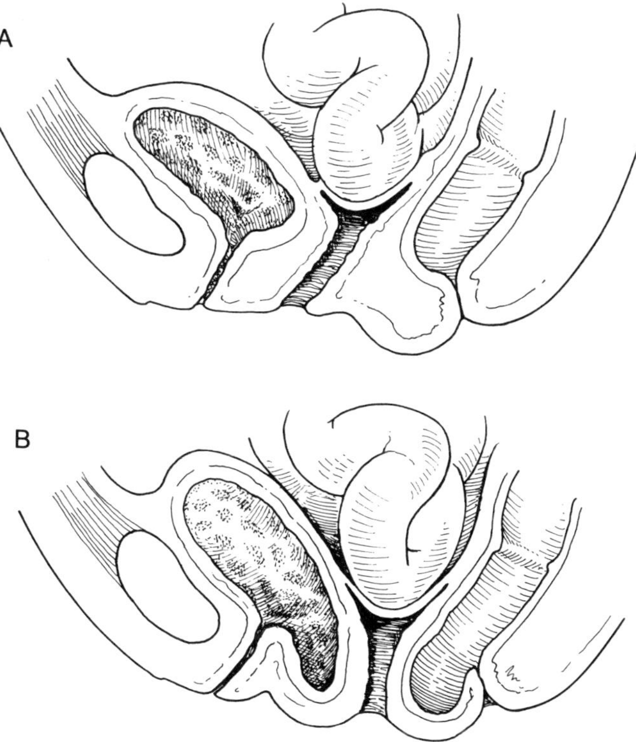

FIG 5–1.
Partial posthysterectomy eversion of the vagina without cystocele and rectocele is shown in **A.** Partial posthysterectomy eversion of the vaginal vault with obvious cystocele and rectocele are shown in **B.** (Redrawn from Nichols DH, Randall CL: *Vaginal Surgery,* ed 3. Baltimore, Williams & Wilkins Co, 1989, p 331.)

sary until appropriate reconstructive surgery can be performed. If irreducible after 2 or 3 days of therapy, surgery should be performed.

The patient often describes the bulge of recurrent prolapse as a "bubble" involving the bladder. When it begins to interfere with the wearing of her clothing or the comfort of sitting down, she will request relief. There is a surprising lack of initial urinary symptoms or incontinence, although later digital elevation of the bladder may be required for urination. Symptoms of rectal dysfunction or pain are uncommon.

The patient with recurrent massive eversion of the vagina is usually, though not invariably, postmenopausal and parous. There may be a family history of severe genital prolapse. Recent weight loss may precipitate aggravation of the prolapse by removing ischiorectal fat from its supporting position beneath the pelvic diaphragm (Fig 5–3). The presence of wide abdominal striae strongly suggests an underlying elastic tissue defect.

PATHOGENESIS

Initially, there is eversion of a poorly supported vaginal vault, with coexistent enterocele in 60% to 70% of patients. At first one may note only a small displace-

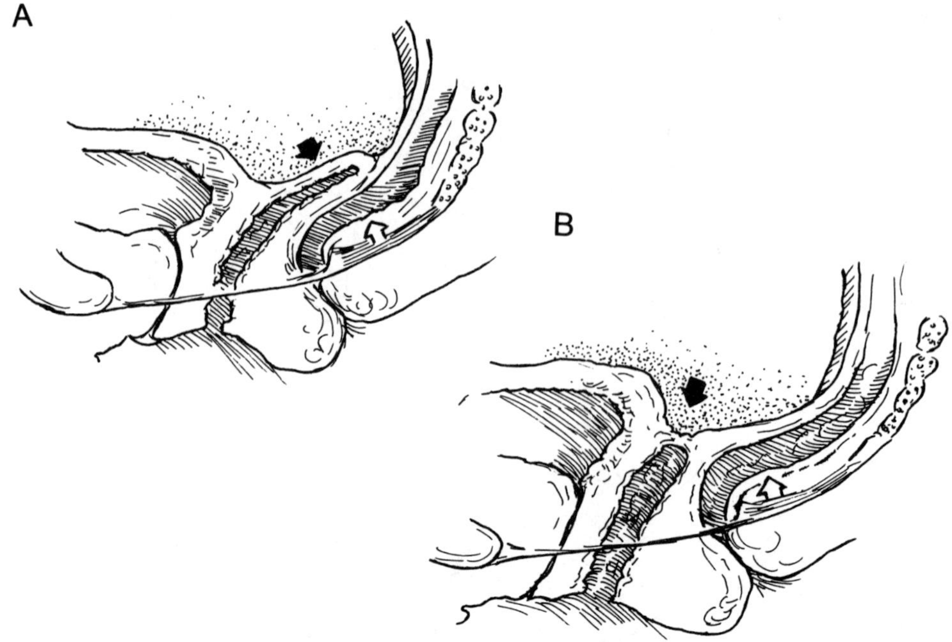

FIG 5–2.
The long posthysterectomy vagina in which the vaginal vault is supported above the intact levator plate *(white arrow)* and posterior to its anterior margin is shown in **A.** Increases in intra-abdominal pressure *(black arrow)* tend to squeeze the vagina against the intact levator plate. In **B,** however, the vault of a shorter posthysterectomy vagina ends anterior to the intact levator plate *(white arrow),* and increases in intra-abdominal pressure *(black arrow)* are exerted in the axis of the vagina, tending to cause it to telescope and to become even shorter. (Redrawn from Amreich J: *Wien Klin Wochenschr* 1951; 63:74–77.)

ment type of cystocele, which will often disappear with replacement of the vault. There is usually an abnormally inclined, vertically oriented vaginal axis, signifying some disturbance in the integrity of the levator plate. When this is severe, there may be some flattening of the anorectal angle. The patient may admit on questioning a minor degree of loss of confidence in her rectal continence.

As the vault descends further, it brings with it more of the bladder as a larger cystocele. Later, the lower supports of the vagina are compromised. As the urogenital diaphragm becomes stretched, there is a degree of rotational descent of the bladder neck. Since the posterior portion of the bladder has come down first, there is usually with its unimpeded descent some expected persistence and even increase in the cystourethral angle with preservation or return of urinary continence. As the prolapse progresses to total vaginal eversion, the dilating wedgelike effect of the prolapse on the levator ani increases the width of the genital hiatus and accentuates the defect in the integrity of the pelvic diaphragm and then of the perineal body. Coincident full-length rectocele and perineal body defect become evident.

If one is seeing the patient for the first time at this stage of her disease, it may be difficult to establish the site of primary damage. Sending for and reviewing the surgical dictation of the patient's past records may be, but is not invariably, helpful. However, determining the location of the major initial defect with reasonable certainty is important so that Bonney's precept of overrepair of the primary site can be

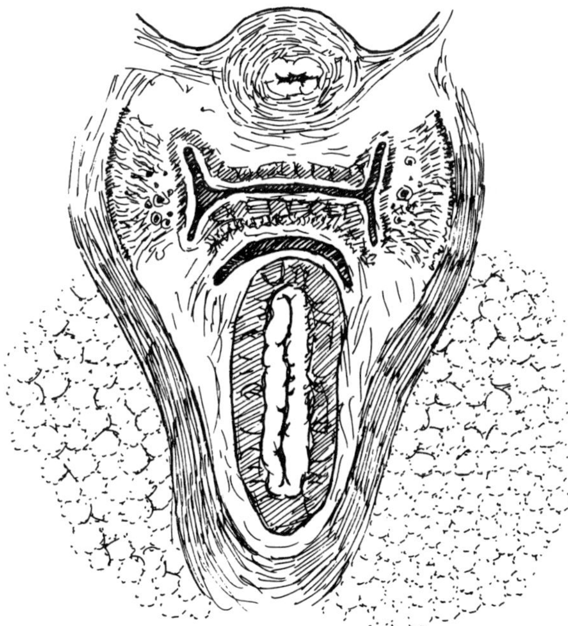

FIG 5–3.
A cross-section through the lower midportion of the pelvis is shown. Notice the fibers of Luschka that attach the lateral walls of the vagina to the fascia of the pelvic diaphragm. The pubococcygeus has a convex shape due to the pressure of the surrounding ischiorectal fat tissue, which helps to press it against the rectum. (Redrawn from Nichols DH, Milley P: Clinical anatomy of the vulva, vagina, lower pelvis, and perineum, in Sciarra J [ed]: *Gynecology and Obstetrics.* New York, Harper & Row, Publishers, 1977.)

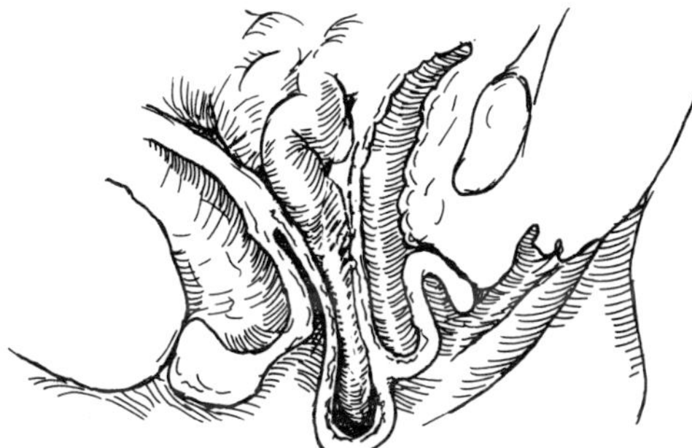

FIG 5–4.
Posthysterectomy eversion of the vagina is shown. There is rectocele, enterocele, and cystocele. The vaginal prolapse has stretched the attachments of the anterior fornix to the arcus tendineus, as well as elongated the attachments of the anterior vaginal wall to the urogenital diaphragm, producing a combined lateral and midline defect in support. (Redrawn from Nichols DH: *Obstet Gynecol* 1972; 40:257–263.)

accomplished to lessen the chance of recurrence. Examining the unanesthetized patient in a lithotomy position and gently replacing the prolapse within the pelvis, the examiner lets the tissue rest for 1 or 2 minutes, then asks the patient to strain and see what tissues appear first. If the cystocele and rectocele appear first, followed by the vaginal vault, the primary site of damage is probably in the supports of the lower portion of the vagina (i.e., the pelvic and urogenital diaphragms). If the vaginal vault appears first, followed by a cystocele and rectocele, the site of primary damage is probably in the upper suspensory system of the vagina and pelvis.

With an extreme degree of prolapse of the full length of the vagina, there is some stretching or avulsion of the paravaginal or lateral supporting tissues (Fig 5–4), including some of the fibers of Luschka which attach the anterior vaginal fornix to the arcus tendineus (Figs 5–5 to 5–7). This circumstance was first appreciated as a clinical problem by White in 1909.[1] The presence of this lateral detachment can be demonstrated by replacing the vaginal vault into the hollow of the sacrum, holding it there, and asking the patient to strain. This maneuver may demonstrate disappearance or descent of the lateral vaginal fornix. The lateral forniceal displacement is then reduced by mechanical or digital support, and the patient is asked to strain again while the examiner notes whether or not the cystocele returns. If it does not return, one has identified a probable defect in the lateral or paravaginal supporting tissues. If the cystocele persists with straining, even though the anterior fornix is supported on both sides, the defect is present in the midline supporting tissues of the vagina. The presence of significant lateral defect can be further evidenced with modification of this maneuver of Baden. Asking the patient to stand, the gynecologist holds the vault in its proper place in the hollow of the sacrum. With the free hand, the examiner lightly palpates the anterior fornix when the patient strains and once more when she voluntarily contracts her pubococcygei. Note is made of whether or not the vaginal fornix rises in concert with the contraction. If it does rise, some residual anatomic connection of the bridge between the

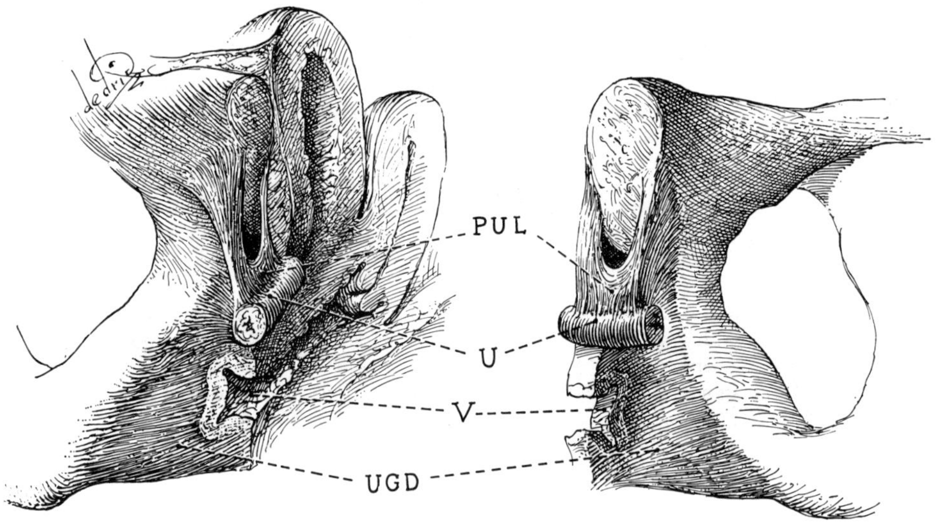

FIG 5–5.
The relationship between the pubourethral ligament *(PUL)* and the urogenital diaphragm *(UGD)* is shown in the sagittal drawing. Note further the relationship between the urethra *(U)* and vagina *(V)* to the urogenital diaphragm and to the bladder, which has been sketched into the drawing at the left. (From Milley PS, Nichols DH: *Anat Rec* 1971; 170:281–284. Used by permission.)

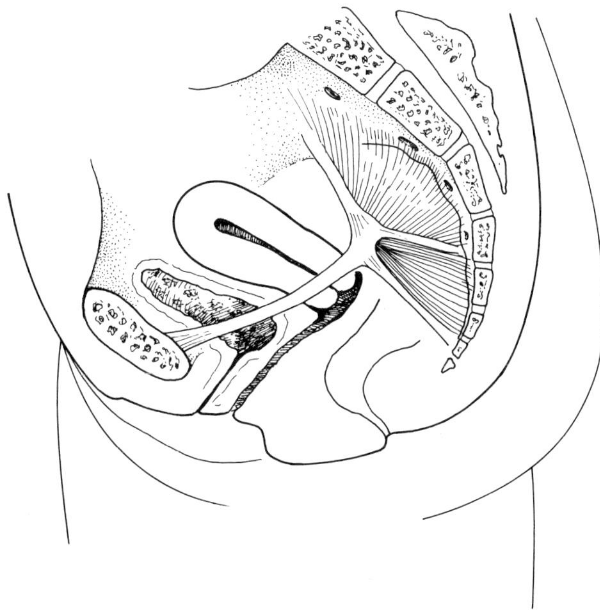

FIG 5–6.
The relationship between the arcus tendineus (one on each side of the pelvis) and the normal vaginal axis is shown in this schematic drawing. The anterior fornix is attached to the arcus tendineus by an intermediate bridge of connective tissue that varies in length between the proximal and distal portions of the vagina. (Redrawn from Nichols DH, Randall CL: *Vaginal Surgery,* ed 3. Baltimore, Williams & Wilkins Co, 1989, p 18.)

anterior fornix and the arcus tendineus is implied, but if it does not rise, it may be assumed that there is great likelihood of avulsion of the vaginal fornix from the arcus tendineus as such a site.

Pertinent specialized laboratory studies are related to an identification of possible disturbance in neuromuscular physiology. These may include a urethrocys-

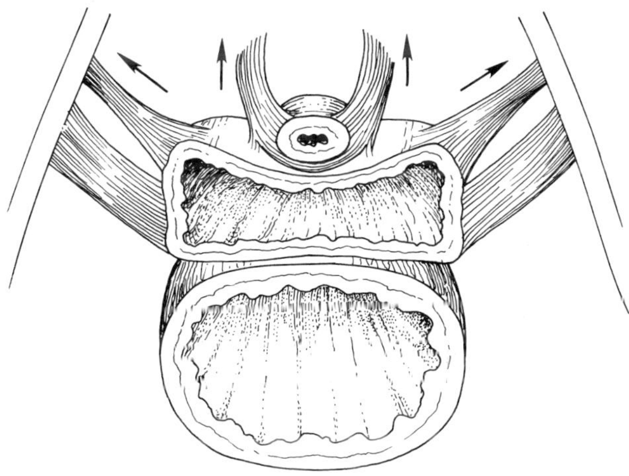

FIG 5–7.
The urethra is both suspended (by the urogenital diaphragm as shown by the *central placed arrows*) and supported by the anterior vaginal wall, which is itself attached to the arcus tendineus on each side by a connective tissue bridge, as indicated by the *lateral arrows.* (Redrawn from Nichols DH, Randall CL: *Vaginal Surgery,* ed 3. Baltimore, Williams & Wilkins Co, 1989, p 21.)

tometrogram if urinary continence is a question and an electromyography of the striated muscles of the pelvic floor and x-ray defecogram if rectal incontinence is present.

Disturbances in function of the voluntary muscles strongly suggest that contributory pudendal neuropathy is likely. If there is complete paralysis of the pelvic diaphragm and the external anal sphincter, rectal continence may be maintained solely through action of the involuntary internal anal sphincter, a sometimes fragile remaining source of continence, the integrity of which must be retained at all costs.

CHOICE OF OPERATION

Surgical reconstruction should involve a primary transabdominal approach, or a transvaginal one, or a combination of the two, depending on the experience of the operator and the availability of skilled surgical assistance. For the experienced reconstructive surgeon, the transvaginal approach holds many attractions. It permits appropriate enterocele excision, anterior and posterior colporrhaphy, including restoration of midline and paravaginal defects, and perineorrhaphy, all through the same operative exposure. If a perineal descent syndrome has been noted (see Chapter 15), a retrorectal levatorplasty may be performed as well.

Vaginal hysterectomy and repair may be the treatment of choice in the patient in whom the uterus is still present. Strong but surgically useful uterosacral ligaments may be shortened and employed to suspend the vault. A McCall-type cul-de-plasty will restore length and proper axis to the upper portion of the vagina (see Chapter 8). For the patient with previous hysterectomy, the uterosacral ligaments of a prolapsed vagina will generally have undergone atrophy and will be neither surgically useful nor dependable.

In some instances a primary abdominal approach for the support of the prolapsed vaginal vault is preferred. Indications for the abdominal route include the presence of an adenexal mass that must be investigated and the rare vaginal vault eversion in a patient with a short vagina that will not reach the sacrospinous ligament. The latter is usually the consequence of a significant iatrogenic change in the vaginal axis, such as the extreme anterior displacement of the vagina that may follow ventral suspension or less commonly the Burch procedure, in which a wide and unprotected cul-de-sac of Douglas was not separately obliterated.

Ventral fixation with obliteration of the cul-de-sac is an effective treatment for the parous prolapse patient born with bladder exstrophy, provided that the patient has been sterilized by either hysterectomy or tubal ligation.

TECHNIQUES OF RECONSTRUCTION

Vaginal Hysterectomy and Repair

The prolapse is carefully examined under anesthesia and a tenaculum placed on the posterior lip of the cervix to which traction is applied. Digital palpation carefully determines the site and width of the base of the cul-de-sac of Douglas and the length and strength of the uterosacral ligaments (Figs 5–8 and 5–13). In most instances, the latter will be strong, though elongated. If surgically shortened during the procedure, the uterosacral ligaments will be useful in supporting the vaginal

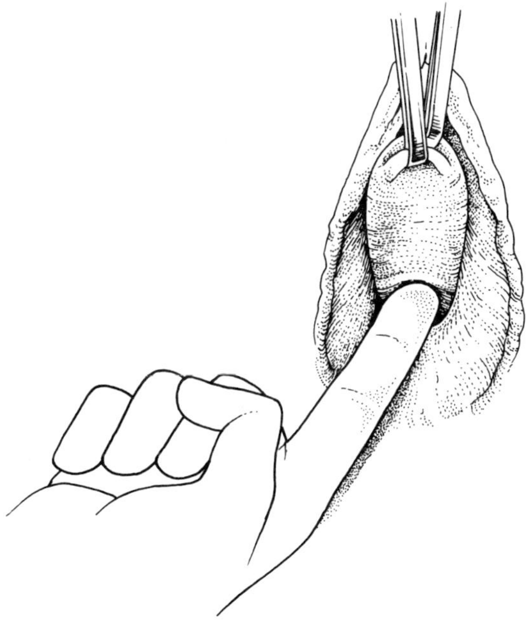

FIG 5–8.
When traction is made to a tenaculum applied to the posterior lip of the cervix, one can palpate both the length and strength of the uterosacral ligaments, as well as the base of the cul-de-sac of Douglas. (Redrawn from Nichols DH, Randall CL: *Vaginal Surgery,* ed 3. Baltimore, Williams & Wilkins Co, 1989, p 188.)

vault postoperatively. The surgeon then proceeds with a Heaney-type vaginal hysterectomy. If there has been a previous ventral suspension of the uterus, the fundus must be surgically detached from the underside of the anterior abdominal wall. The ovaries are carefully examined. They may be removed if there is any pathology present or, with her permission if the patient is postmenopausal, in the absence of pathology (Fig 5–9).

Any enterocele sac is carefully identified and dissected from the surrounding tissue up to the point where the yellow prerectal fat is attached to its underside (Fig 5–10). The excess peritoneum is excised. One or more McCall-type sutures are placed taking a bite through one side of the posterior vaginal vault, the cut edge of the peritoneum, and the peritoneal surface of the homolateral uterosacral ligament (see Fig 8–5). The suture is anchored to the prerectal peritoneum in the midline, then made to penetrate the same structures on the opposite side in reverse order. A second or third McCall stitch may be placed successively higher on the uterosacral ligaments as necessary.

If the posterior vaginal vault is unusually wide, it should be narrowed by excision of a V-shaped wedge (see Fig 8–6), the sides of which are approximated with full-thickness sutures (see Fig 8–7). The peritoneal cavity may be closed by one or more pursestring sutures (Fig 5–11). The McCall stitches are tied, bringing the posterior vault of the vagina into firm contact with the underside of the uterosacral ligaments grasped by the McCall stitches. The vagina is thus elongated and restored to its natural position in the hollow of the sacrum. Next, appropriate full-length anterior colporrhaphy is usually accomplished with special efforts expended to preserve and accentuate the cystourethral angle, so that it is restored to a posi-

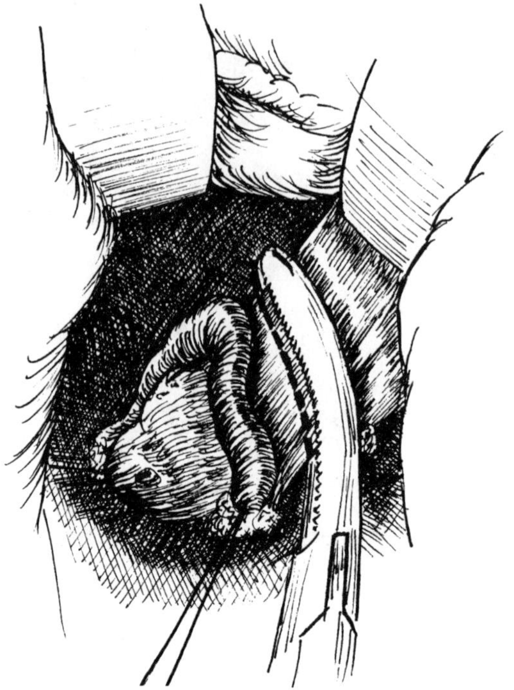

FIG 5–9.
A clamp is placed across the left infundibulopelvic ligament, when the latter is of sufficient length, and an incision is made as indicated by the *dashed line,* permitting removal of the ovary and tube. When the infundibulopelvic ligament is short, and visibility for surgical maneuvering is thereby restricted, the clamp may be placed alternately across the mesovarium and the ovary removed, sparing the tube. The clamp is replaced by a transfixion ligature.

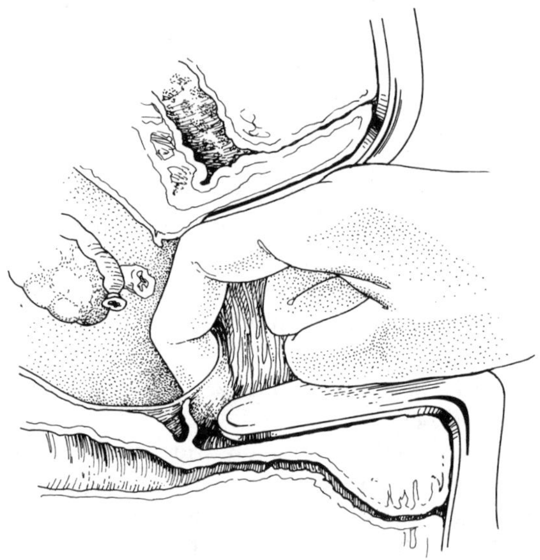

FIG 5–10.
Redundant peritoneum of the cul-de-sac that should be excised can be demonstrated by hooking a finger into this pocket of peritoneum. It should be mobilized and excised back to its junction with the peritoneum overlying the anterior surface of the rectum, indicated by the yellow prerectal fat attached to the underside of the peritoneum. (Redrawn from Nichols DH, Randall CL: *Vaginal Surgery,* ed 3. Baltimore, Williams & Wilkins Co, 1989, p 217.)

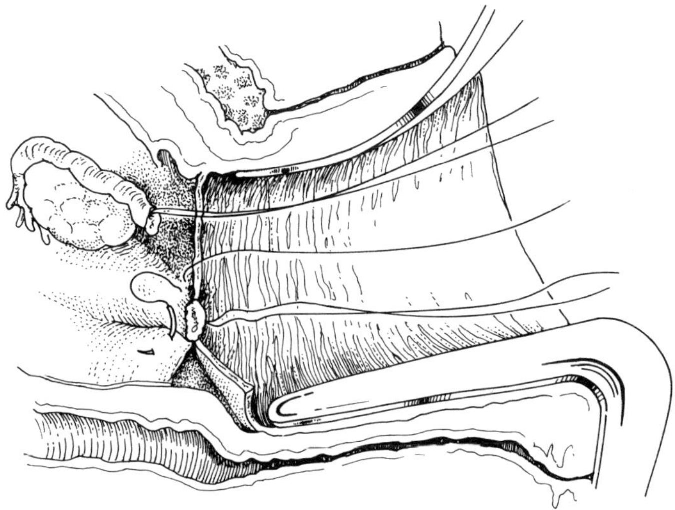

FIG 5–11.
High peritonealization is begun by a suture through the peritoneal side of the left uterosacral ligament, which proceeds in a clockwise fashion through the peritoneum overlying the rectum, the right uterosacral ligament, peritoneal side of the right round ligament, anterior peritoneum, and left round ligament. The suture avoids damaging the blood vessels within the cardinal ligament and brings together both the peritoneum and the subperitoneal retinaculum. (Redrawn from Nichols DH, Randall CL: *Vaginal Surgery*, ed 3. Baltimore, Williams & Wilkins Co, 1989, p 218.)

tion within the pelvis approximating the junction of the lower third and upper two thirds of the back of the pubis. Finally, any rectocele and perineal defect are repaired. At the conclusion of the operation, the patient should have an effective restoration of a normal vaginal depth and axis. Because of the increased proximity of the ureters to the operative field in genital prolapse, it is reassuring to verify ureteral patency at the end of the procedure. The patient is given one ampule (5 mL) of intravenous (IV) indigo carmine, the bladder emptied of urine, and 250 mL of sterile saline instilled. Observation cystoscopy is performed while the patient is still under anesthesia. Usually in less than 5 minutes from the time of IV indigo carmine injection, the operator will note violet-stained urine spurting from each ureteral orifice. Should patency not be thus demonstrated after a wait of 10 or 15 minutes, it is appropriate to investigate the reasons for apparent absence of ureteral patency. An infusion pyelogram may be performed while the patient is still on the operating table, and any obstruction can be confirmed by resistance to the passage of a ureteral catheter. If a ureter has been ligated, delegation without delay with probable catheterization of the ureter by a ureteral stent should be an effective remedy.

Transvaginal Sacrospinous Colpopexy

For patients in whom the uterosacral-cardinal ligament complex is too attenuated to be of use in supporting the vagina, transvaginal sacrospinous colpopexy is useful using the newer synthetic but nonabsorbable sutures (Fig 5–12). Coincident excision of any enterocele is easily done, and any necessary colporrhaphy may be performed through the same operative exposure.

Transvaginal sacrospinous colpopexy immediately following vaginal hysterec-

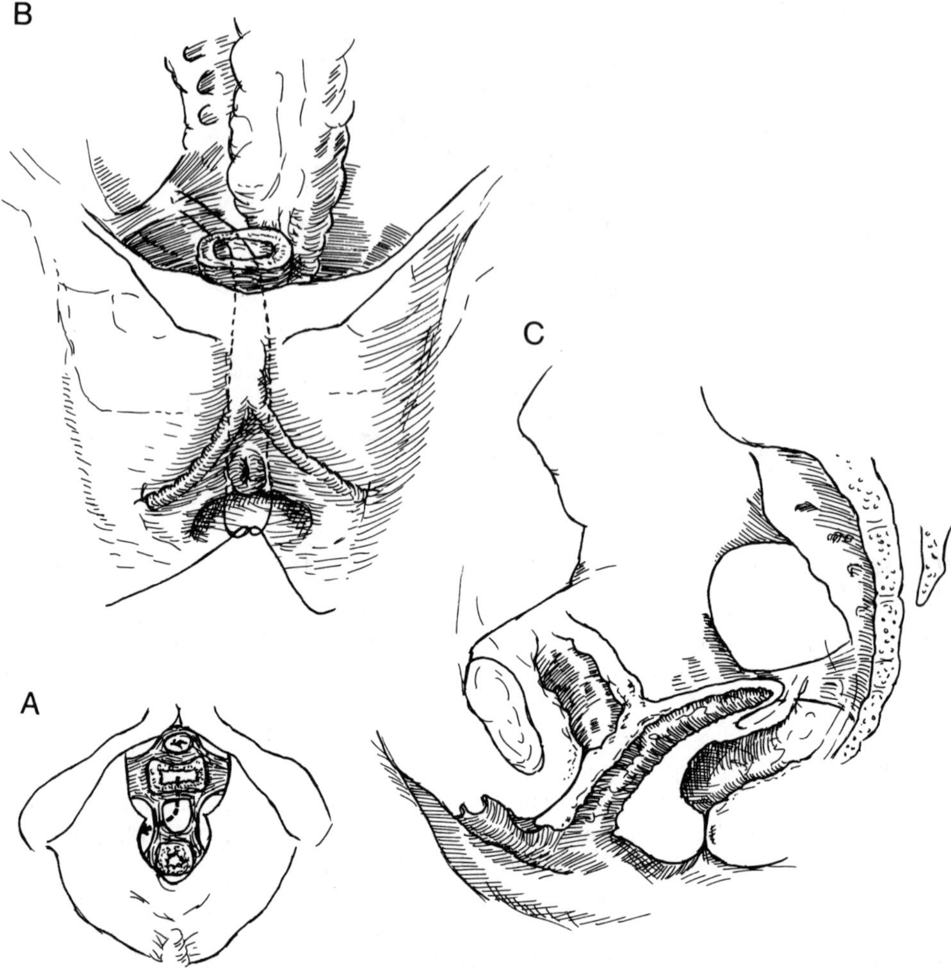

FIG 5–12.
Technique of right sacrospinous colpopexy. A path of dissection through the posterior vaginal wall into the rectovaginal space and then through a window in the descending rectal septum into the right pararectal space **(A).** The dissection always procedes toward the ischial spine in the lateral wall of the pararectal space. The vagina is sewn to the right sacrospinous ligament–coccygeus muscle complex at a point one and one half fingerwidths medial to the right ischial spine as shown in **B.** After the fixation stitches have been tied, the attachment of the vagina to the right sacrospinous ligament is shown in **C,** indicating after appropriate colporrhaphy, a fairly normal vaginal depth and axis.

tomy in patients with uterine prolapse without strong uterosacral-cardinal ligament support (Figs 5–13 and 5–14) is surprisingly easy. The operation can be accomplished within an additional 15 minutes of operating time. The sequence of events in this instance is as follows:

1. Vaginal hysterectomy.
2. Excision of any enterocele with high ligation of the sac and closure of the peritoneal cavity.
3. Anterior colporrhaphy.

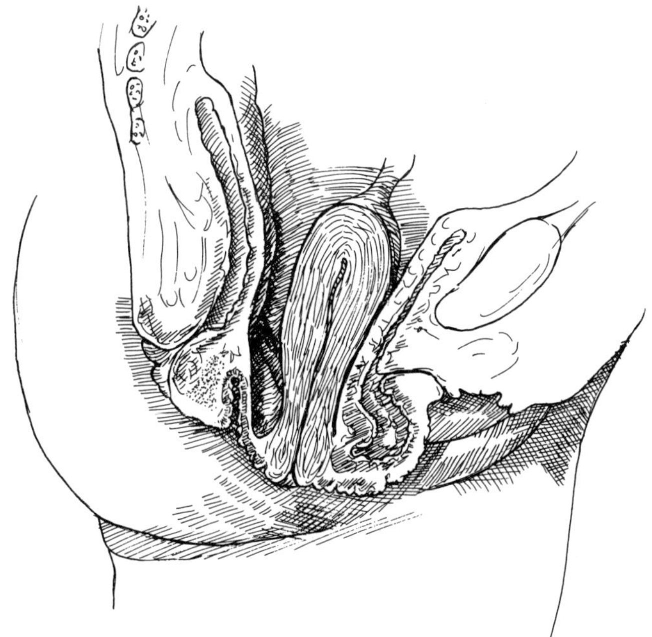

FIG 5–13.
The more common uterovaginal or sliding prolapse is shown. There is enterocele but no significant rectocele, because there is no direct involvement of the anterior rectal wall in this prolapse. The uterosacral ligaments are long and strong, and the cervix is elongated (Redrawn from Halban J, Tandler J: Änatomie und Atiologie der genitalprolapse beim Weibe. Vienna, Austria, Braumuller, 1907.)

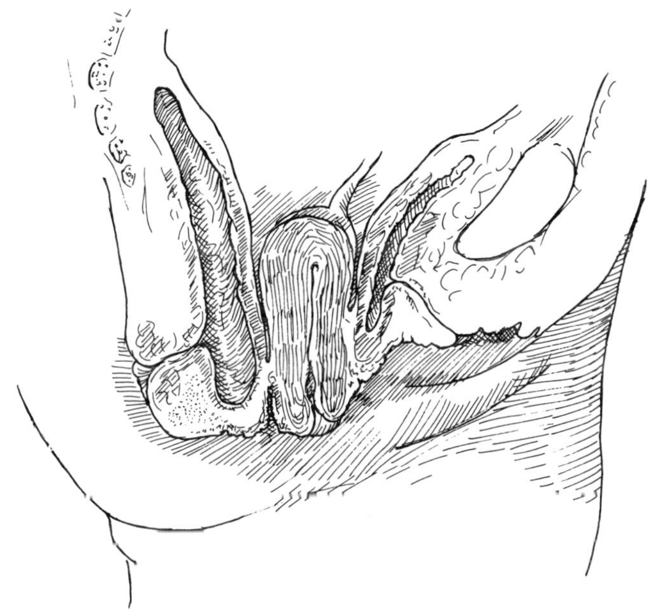

FIG 5–14.
The less common general postmenopausal prolapse is shown in sagittal section. All endopelvic supporting tissues are atrophied and weakened. A rectocele and a descent of the cul-de-sac are shown but no enterocele. There is an obvious defect in the supports of the anterior rectal wall. The uterosacral ligaments are weak and hard to define by palpation. The cervix is not elongated. (Redrawn from Halban J, Tandler J: Änatomie und Atiologie der genitalprolapse beim Weibe. Vienna, Austria, Braumuller, 1907.)

4. Posterior colporrhaphy through an incision in the perineum and opening of the rectovaginal space.
5. Penetration of the right rectal pillar overlying the right ischial spine to open the right pararectal space. (The ischial spine and the sacrospinous ligament–coccygeus muscle complex form a portion of the lateral wall of the pararectal space.)

In the likely event that the uterus has been removed before this procedure and there is massive posthysterectomy eversion of the vaginal vault, the sequence and techniques are as follows:

1. Initial surgical incision is through the perineum and posterior vaginal wall with entry into the rectovaginal space.

2. Any enterocele is identified and opened (Fig 5–15), and the neck of the enterocele sac is carefully palpated for any usable uterosacral ligament strength. Usually this is found lacking. The neck of the sac is closed by a pursestring suture, the sac is excised, and the operator may proceed with sacrospinous colpopexy.

3. When the rectum has been carefully displaced by an appropriate rectractor to the opposite side of the pelvis, the ischial spine is carefully palpated. To approach the sacrospinous ligament, the surgeon must make a window through the descending rectal septum over the ischial spine. This window can be established by blunt penetration with the operator's finger or by the closed tips of curved Mayo scissors or a sharp pointed hemostat (Fig 5–16).

4. Once established, the window is gently enlarged with the fingers in the axis of the vagina. This stretching of window provides a clear view and easy palpation of the upper surface of the pelvic diaphragm, the ischial spine, and coccygeus muscle. One retractor is placed in the 12 o'clock position holding the cardinal ligament containing the ureter out of harm's way. Another retractor holds the patient's rectum

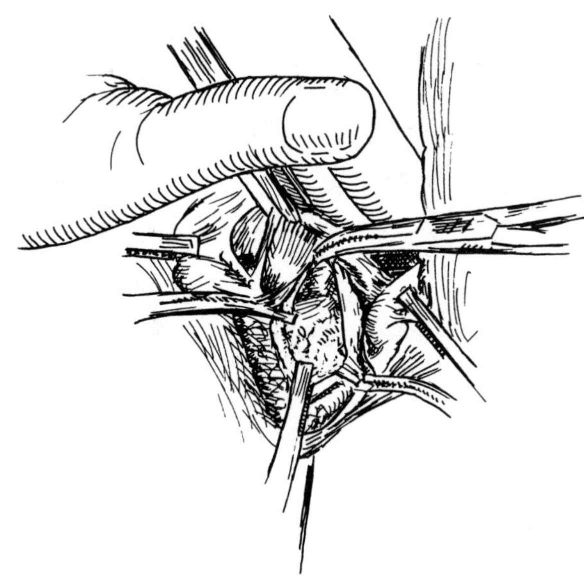

FIG 5–15.
An enterocele has been identified, opened, and mobilized before resection.

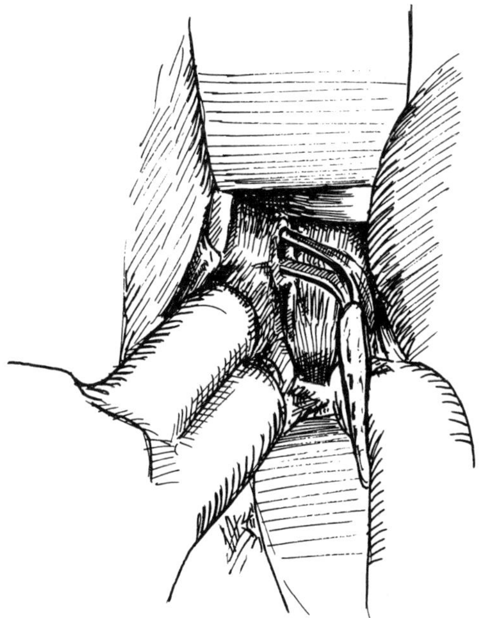

FIG 5–16.
While the upper retractor displaces the cardinal ligament and ureter and the lower retractor holds the rectum to the patient's left, the right rectal pillar has been penetrated by the tips of a long pointed forcep, providing entry to the right pararectal space at a point overlying the right ischial spine.

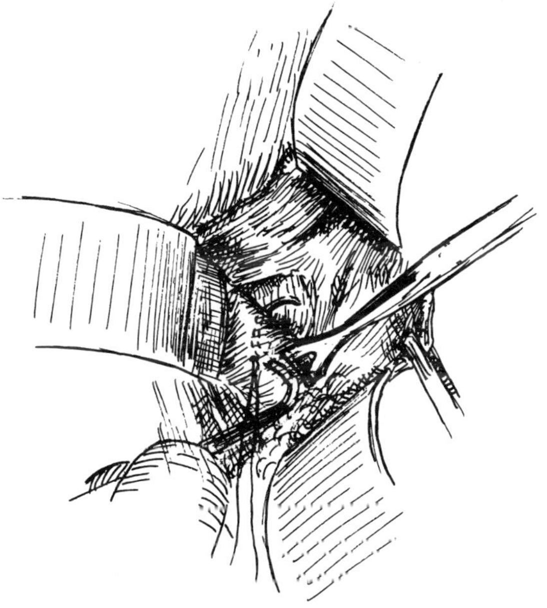

FIG 5–17.
The opening through the right rectal pillar has been enlarged and the sacrospinous ligament–coccygeus muscle complex grasped with a long Babcock clamp. At a point about one and one half fingerwidths medial to the right ischial spine, the sacrospinous ligament and coccygeus muscle have been penetrated by the suture-bearing tip of a long Deschamps ligature carrier

to the side opposite the dissection, and a shorter retractor may compress the distal portion of the pelvic diaphragm along the lateral wall of the pelvis. Because the surgeon is working in a confined area, essentially in the hollow of the sacrum, a fiberoptic headlight is useful.

5. At a point one and one half to two fingerbreadths medial to the ischial spine, the coccygeus muscle–sacrospinous ligament complex is penetrated by the blunt tip of a long-handled Deschamps ligature carrier (Figs 5–17 and 5–18) holding full lengths of a synthetic nonabsorbable suture, such as size 0 polypropylene (Prolene, Surgilene) or polytef (Gore-Tex), and a heavy polyglycolic acid suture, such as size 2 Dexon or Vienyl.

If visual exposure is difficult, penetration can be done safely by palpation using the following maneuver: If the penetration is made through the right sacrospinous ligament–coccygeus muscle complex, the index and middle fingers of the surgeon's left hand are inserted through the window in the rectal pillar into the pararectal space. The tip of the middle index finger is made to touch the medial surface of the right ischial spine.

The long-handled Deschamps ligature carrier, holding a proper suture, is grasped in the right hand, and the curved tip of the carrier is gently slid down the undersurface of the left index finger to the posteroinferior border of the sacrospinous ligament-coccygeal muscle complex at a spot one and one half to two fingerbreadths medial to the ischial spine, which is still being palpated by the middle finger of the left hand (Fig 5–19). Pressure is made pushing the tip of the ligature carrier beneath the under edge of the muscle complex, and the tip is rotated in a clockwise direction, a significant resistance should be encountered, indicating that the carrier has been placed *through* the ligament, and neither superficial nor deep to it. At the same time, the handle of the ligature carrier is moved in an indepen-

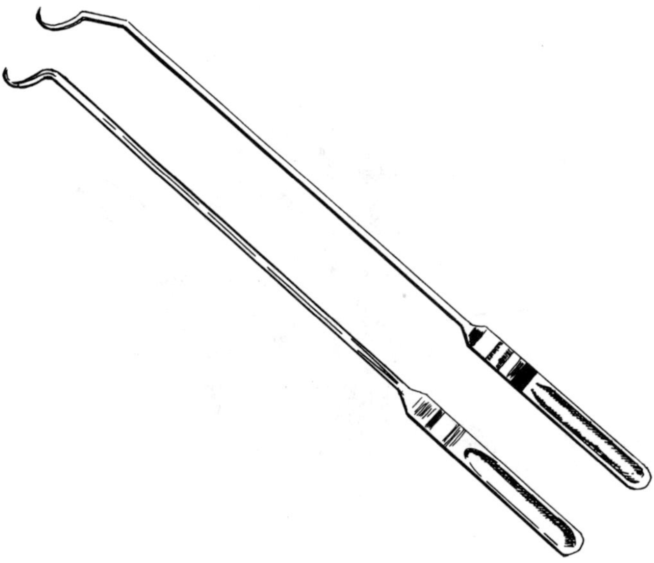

FIG 5–18.
Long Deschamps ligature carriers for the right hand are shown. The angled modification (suggested by Rosenshein) at the top is useful when the sacrospinous ligament is unusually deep. The handle must be swung through a wide arc. These instruments are available on special order from Codman and Shurtleff, Custom Device Department, New Bedford, MA 02745, or from William Merz, American V. Mueller Company, Chicago, IL 60648.

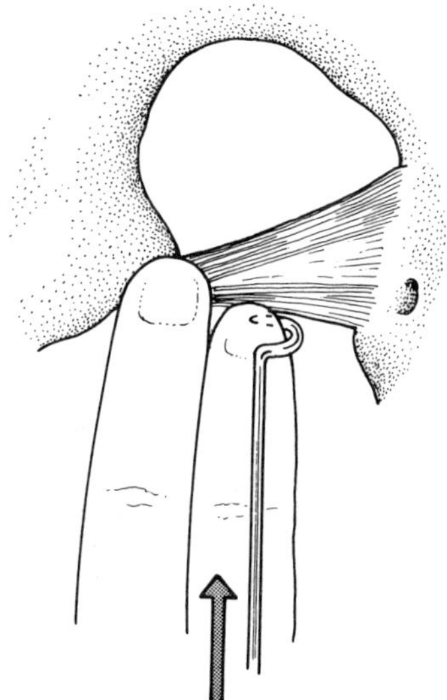

FIG 5–19.
Through a window between the rectovaginal space and the right pararectal space, the middle finger of the operator's left hand has been placed against the medial edge of the left ischial spine, and the tip of the Deschamps ligature carrier slid beneath the left index finger, as shown, until it is in contact with the lower border of the sacrospinous ligament–coccygeus muscle complex. It is pushed in the direction of the *arrow* beneath this complex at this point. (Redrawn from Nichols DH, Randall CL: *Vaginal Surgery,* ed 3. Baltimore, Williams & Wilkins Co, 1989, p 340.)

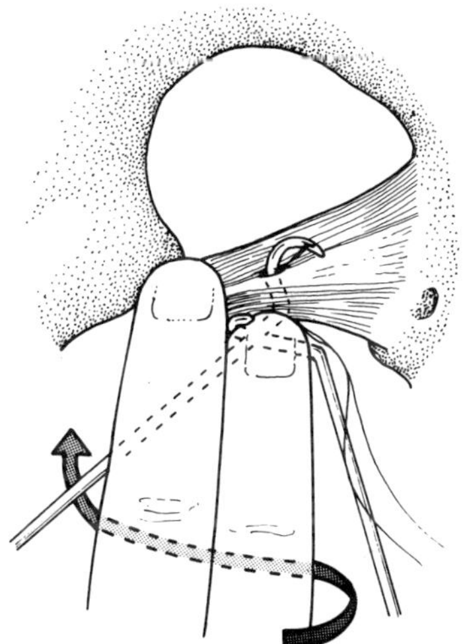

FIG 5–20.
The tip of the ligature carrier is rotated so as to penetrate this complex from below upward *(arrows)* at the same time as the handle of the ligature carrier is rotated in a clockwise direction *beneath* the palm of the left hand. (Redrawn from Nichols DH, Randall CL: *Vaginal Surgery,* ed 3. Baltimore, Williams & Wilkins Co, 1989, p 340.)

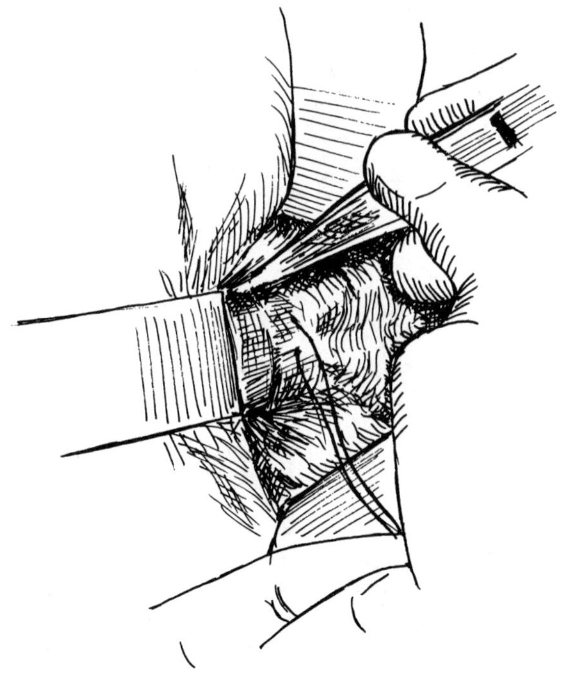

FIG 5–21.
The ligature carrier and Babcock clamp have been removed. The drawing shows the placement of the suture through the ligament-muscle complex. Traction to the suture will move the patient a slight amount on the table, indicating that the suture has been properly placed. The right ischial spine is at the tip of the forceps, indicating the position of the suture placement 2 to 3 cm medial to the ischial spine, and safely removed from the location of the pudendal nerve and artery.

dent clockwise direction permitting vertical penetration of the ligament (Fig 5–20). A gentle tug to the ligature carrier or to the suture (Fig 5–21), which has been grasped by a hook, should actually move the patient a small degree on the table. Proper placement of the suture through the substance of the sacrospinous ligament is thus indicated. Direct palpation of the suture and of the ischial spine confirms

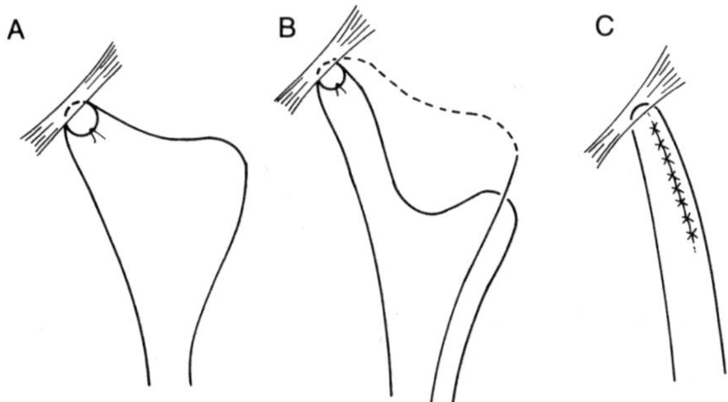

FIG 5–22.
A shows a wide vaginal vault illustrated at the left following sacrospinous colpopexy. The result of failure to narrow this wide vault is shown in **B** in which there may be prolapse of the left side. The result of narrowing this wide vault by excision of a proper width tissue from the anterior and posterior vaginal wall is shown in **C,** which has converted the shape of the vagina to that of a cylinder of more or less uniform diameter. It is now an instrument of coitus and not parturition. (Redrawn from Nichols DH, Randall CL: *Vaginal Surgery,* ed 3. Baltimore, Williams & Wilkins Co, 1989, p 338.)

the required distance between the two. If the suture seems too close to the ischial spine, traction is made on it, and a new suture is placed medial to the offending suture, which is then removed. An additional suture or two of a synthetic absorbable polyglycolic acid-type (no. 1 or 2 Dexon or Vicryl) can be inserted through the muscle-ligament complex medial to the first suture, if extra support is desired.

6. Although sacrospinous colpopexy may be performed on both sides if the vaginal vault is very wide, such a bilateral procedure is rarely done, because equally satisfactory results are obtained with a unilateral colpopexy, *provided that a wide vault is surgically narrowed* (Fig 5–22). The vagina, which is now an instrument of coitus and not for parturition, is thus converted to a cylinder of uniform diameter.

7. By a free needle, each suture is sewn to the undersurface of the midportion of the vaginal vault (Figs 5–23 to 5–25), but the colpopexy stitches are not tied until later in the operation.

8. Any necessary anterior colporrhaphy is accomplished. Full-length anterior colporrhaphy with special attention to the supports of the cystourethral junction is performed almost without exception. Such support usually includes plication of the pubourethral "ligament" portion of the urogenital diaphragm beneath the urethra (see Figs 6–7 to 6–9) using a long-acting absorbable suture such as polydiaxanone-type (PDS or Maxon). Colporrhaphy by this method will effectively treat or prevent postoperative urinary stress incontinence or prevent postoperative incontinence that could result from the change in the vaginal axis that occurs with the sacral colpopexy. A coincident uncommon low-pressure or low-compliant urethra may require a vesicourethral sling procedure to effectively elevate intraurethral pressure to a continent level.

9. The upper portion of the posterior colporrhaphy is begun at the vault of the vagina by a side-to-side, running spiral, subcuticular suture that incorporates the

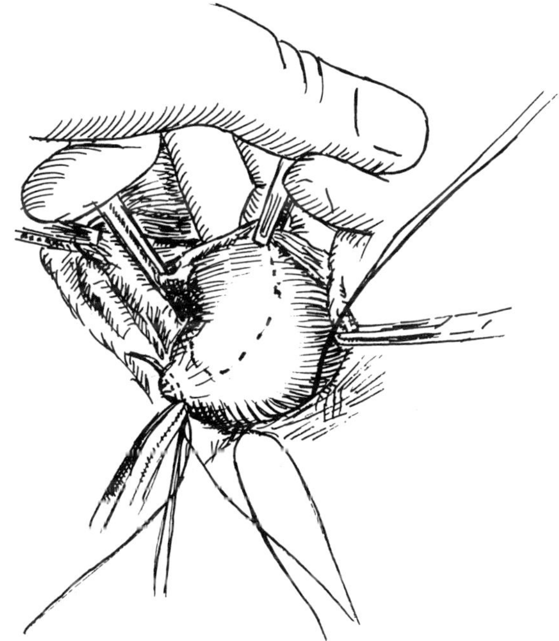

FIG 5–23.
The free end of the colpopexy suture is sewn through the undersurface of the fibromuscular wall of the vagina at the site of the new vaginal apex.

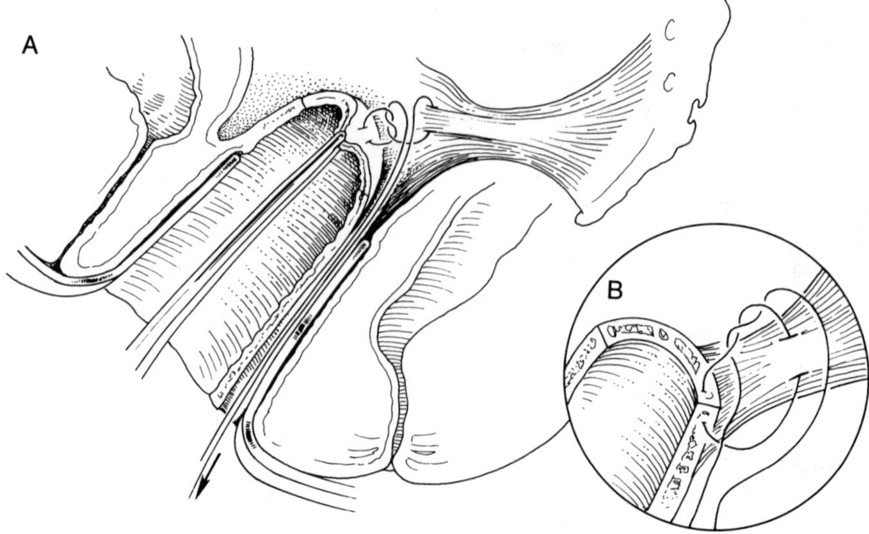

FIG 5–24.
The "pulley" stitch is shown. One end of the suture through the sacrospinous ligament has been sewn to the undersurface of the cut edge of the vaginal vault and the stitch tied **(A).** Traction to the other end of the suture draws the vagina up and laterally to the surface of the ligament. When the ends have been tied together, the vagina is fixed to the surface of the sacrospinous ligament–coccygeus muscle complex at this point **(B)**. A second or "safety" stitch for reinforcement of this attachment may be placed through the ligament. (Redrawn from Nichols DH, Randall CL: *Vaginal Surgery,* ed 3. Baltimore, Williams & Wilkins Co, 1989, p 345.)

full thickness of the posterior vaginal wall yet carefully avoids the anterior wall of the rectum to prevent obliteration of the rectovaginal space (see Fig 7–13). This stitch continues to the midportion of the posterior vaginal wall.

10. At this point, the sacrospinous colpopexy stitches are tied, firmly attaching the vagina to the surface of the coccygeus muscle–sacrospinous ligament complex with no intervening bridge of suture material (Fig 5–26).

11. The posterior colporrhaphy is completed.

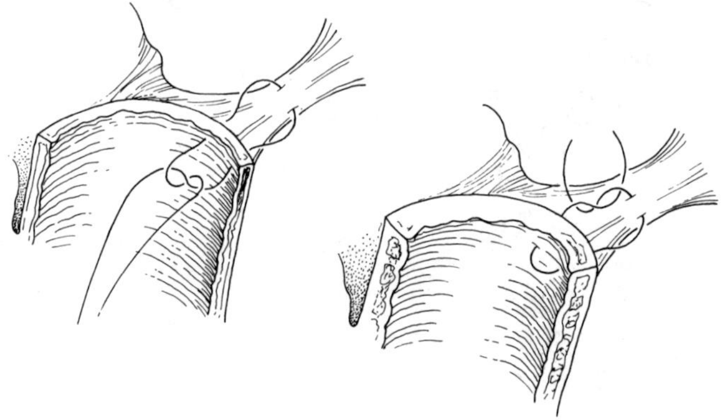

FIG 5–25.
The full thickness of a thin vaginal wall may be sewn to the surface of the complex, leaving the knot of an absorbable suture within the lumen of the vagina. If a monofilament suture has been used, the knot is buried beneath the vagina *(inset).* (Redrawn from Nichols DH, Randall CL: *Vaginal Surgery,* ed 3. Baltimore, Williams & Wilkins Co, 1989, p 345.)

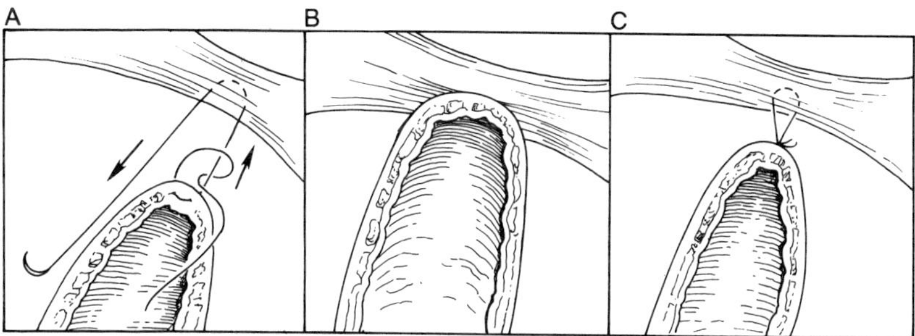

FIG 5–26.
The pulley stitch. After the suture has been placed through the ligament-muscle complex **(A)**, one end is fixed to the underside of the vagina by a stitch tied with a single half-hitch. Traction to the free end of the stitch will bring it to the surface of the complex **(B)**. Failure to tie this snugly will result in a suture bridge **(C)**, which should be avoided, if possible, because the weak scar that results threatens the security of the attachment. (Redrawn from Nichols DH, Randall CL: *Vaginal Surgery*, ed 3. Baltimore, Williams & Wilkins Co, 1989, p 354.)

12. Any necessary perineorrhaphy is accomplished.
13. Rectal examination confirms the integrity of the rectum, and a vaginal packing may be inserted overnight, if desired.

When the patient has a history of previous surgery in this area, the anatomic relationships are often distorted by fibrosis and adhesions. This distortion complicates the ease with which the surgeon can find the lateral wall of the pararectal space. Nevertheless, when one follows the previous steps, identification and entry into the pararectal space is anatomically and surgically precise. Alternatively, the space and structure of the patient's left side may be used.

Transabdominal Repair

If the operator is more comfortable with transabdominal surgery, and especially if there is some pressing reason for a transabdominal approach such as the presence of a suspicious lesion of the adnexa, hysterectomy and colpopexy can be performed by the abdominal route. When there is a minor degree of vault prolapse, the McCall-type cul-de-plasty can be used transabdominally as well with great effectiveness, provided that the uterosacral ligaments are strong. Any pathologic widening of the vaginal vault should be corrected by excision of an appropriate wedge from either posterior or anterior vaginal wall, with reapproximation of the cut edges of each by a running suture. A deep cul-de-sac should be obliterated by either the sagittally placed sutures of Halban (see Fig 8–4) or the circumferential sutures of Moschowitz, either of which will lessen the tendency toward future enterocele. Any remaining cystocele or rectocele should be repaired by appropriate colporrhaphy, whether the hysterectomy was transvaginal or transabdominal. With transabdominal hysterectomy and the McCall or New Orleans–type cul-de-plasty, the surgeon must be particularly mindful of the possibility of interference with the path of the ureter, because it is more vulnerable in the transabdominal approach. The position of the ureter should be verified before the passage and tying of each stitch. At the conclusion of the procedure, it is helpful to give the patient 5 mL of IV indigo carmine and perform an observation cystoscopy 5 or 6 minutes later to observe the efflux of dye from each of the ureteral orifices (see Chapter 13). Such verification of ureteral patency is easily accomplished if the abdominal procedure has been performed with the patient in Allen stirrups.

If the patient's prolapse is due primarily to an enlarged cervix and the patient is desirous of preserving her reproductive potential, the situation may be remedied by a Manchester (Fothergill) type of operation. This procedure includes cervical amputation, crossing of the cardinal-uterosacral ligaments in front of the remaining cervical stump, and an appropriate anterior and posterior colporrhaphy. The uterus is preserved; however, future reproduction may be handicapped by unexpected premature labor or dystocia from compromise of vaginal width by the attendant colporrhaphy. Consequently, few gynecologists in the United States employ this procedure for patients whom future childbirth is likely.

An alternate procedure that also preserves the uterus is the transabdominal construction of a sacrocervical ligament. In this instance, a ligament of transplanted fascia lata is attached securely to the posterior surface of the cervix, run through a retroperitoneal presacral tunnel, and attached to the midportion of the presacral ligament to bring the uterus back into the hollow of the sacrum.

In a patient with massive posthysterectomy eversion of the vagina in whom a transabdominal approach is desired, it is similarly possible to support the vault of the vagina by a ligament attaching it to the periosteum in the hollow of the sacrum

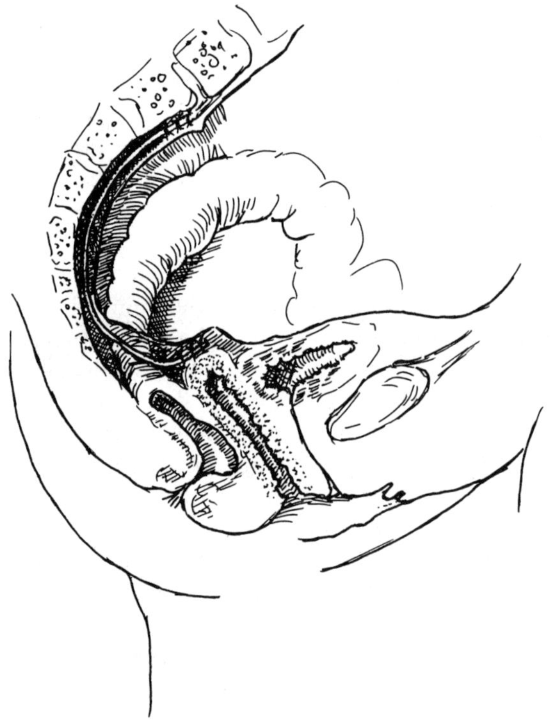

FIG 5–27.
Transabdominal sacrocolpopexy is shown in sagittal section. By use of an intermediate bridge of Mersilene mesh or fascia lata, the vault of the vagina has been fixed by a retroperitoneal tunnel to the sacral periosteum. Any necessary coincident colporrhaphy should be performed as a separate transvaginal procedure. (Redrawn from Nichols DH: Repair of enterocele and prolapse of the vaginal vault, in Barber H [ed]: *Goldsmith's Practice of Surgery.* Philadelphia, JB Lippincott Co, 1981.)

through a retroperitoneal tunnel. In this transabdominal sacral colpopexy, the surgeon may once again use fascia lata, but many will prefer to save the patient the attendant painful leg and use a synthetic plastic such as a Mersilene mesh. The mesh should be attached by multiple nonabsorbable sutures both to the vaginal vault and to the presacral ligament (Fig 5–27). Simultaneous appropriate colporrhaphy may correct any significant cystocele and rectocele, and coincident enterocele can be excised along with the primary procedure.

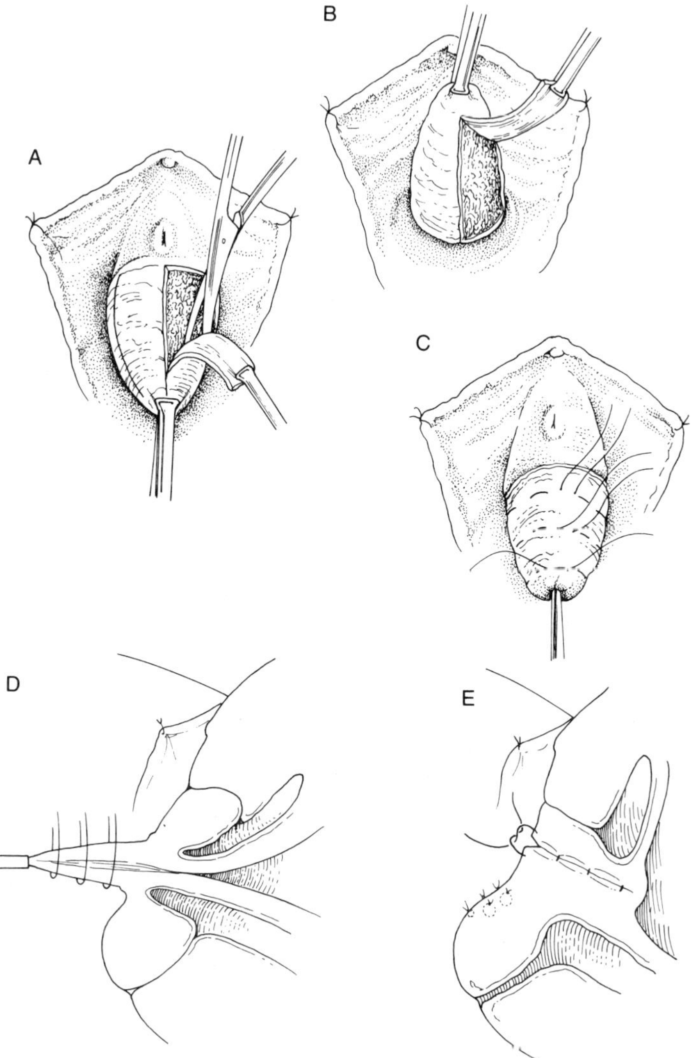

FIG 5–28.
The technique of total colpectomy. After subcutaneous infiltration by 0.5% lidocaine in 1:200,000 epinephrine solution, the vagina is circumscribed by an incision at the hymen and marked into quadrants, each of which is separately removed by sharp dissection (**A** and **B**). A series of purse-string, synthetic absorbable sutures are placed **(C)** and tied, with progressive inversion of the soft tissue before tieing each suture **(D)** so that the final result is as shown in **E.** An appropriate perineorrhaphy may complete the operation. (Redrawn from Nichols DH, Randall CL: *Vaginal Surgery,* ed 3. Baltimore, Williams & Wilkins Co, 1989, p 334.)

Other Techniques

For the occasional patient, often one who is bedridden, is infirm, and can no longer wear an intravaginal pessary, conservation of vaginal function may no longer be a prerequisite. In such cases, there is a place for the LaFort colpocleisis if the uterus is present, or colpectomy (Fig 5–28) if the uterus has been removed. Rarely, the surgeon may elect vaginal hysterectomy with colpectomy as a means of providing permanent obliteration of the vaginal canal.

With LaFort colpocleisis (or partial colpectomy), a rectangle of tissue is removed from the upper anterior vaginal wall and the upper posterior vaginal wall. The posterior surface of the bladder is then sewn directly to the anterior surface of the rectum, leaving a permanent lateral drainage canal across the vault and along both sides of the centrally obliterated vagina.

The operation is relatively simple, but has three principal disadvantages:

1. The coital use of the vagina and the patient's concept of her vagina as a part of her intrinsic femininity may be destroyed.
2. If there is an enterocele present, it will still be present postoperatively, because the operation is essentially extraperitoneal. The persistent enterocele may progress and ultimately continue downward to distend the perineum, with as many symptoms as were present with the original prolapse.
3. Occasionally a patient will develop postoperative urinary stress incontinence following a LaFort colpocleisis. This can be most difficult to treat, because the base of the bladder will be fused to the anterior surface of the rectum, straightening out the cystourethral angle.

A disadvantage of colpectomy, on the other hand, is the sometimes generous blood loss associated with transection of the vaginal blood supply at its lateral margins. To combat this problem, the surgeon may, following excision of the vagina, bring together the covering fascia of the levatores ani in the midline and thoroughly pack the remaining pelvic cavity with iodoform gauze. Starting on the fifth postoperative day, the gauze packing is gradually removed a little bit at a time over a period of several days. The residual cavity will quickly shrink, become covered with healthy granulation tissue, and finally obliterates over a period of several weeks. The process is less complicated than seeking to obliterate the vaginal cavity by sewing it tightly shut in its entirety. This latter feat is rather difficult to achieve without leaving little pockets of dead space into which troublesome postoperative hematoma or seroma may form.

BIBLIOGRAPHY

Baden WF, Walker TA: Physical diagnosis in the evaluation of vaginal relaxation. *Clin Obstet Gynecol* 1972; 15:1060.

Burch JC: Urethrovaginal fixation to Cooper's ligament for stress incontinence. *Am J Obstet Gynecol* 1961; 81:2.

Nichols DH: Sacrospinous fixation for massive eversion of the vagina. *Am J Obstet Gynecol* 1982; 142:901.

Nichols DH, Milley PS, Randall CL: Significance of restoration of normal vaginal depth and axis. *Obstet Gynecol* 1970; 36:241–246.

Nichols DH, Randall CL: *Vaginal Surgery*, ed 3. Baltimore, Williams & Wilkins Co, 1989.

Parsons L, Ulfelder H: *An Atlas of Pelvic Operations*, ed 2. Philadelphia, WB Saunders Co, 1968, pp 280–283.

Richter K, Albrich W: Long-term results following fixation of the vagina on the sacrospinal ligament by the vaginal route (vaginaefixatio sacrospinalis vaginalis). *Am J Obstet Gynecol* 1981; 141:811.

Symmonds R, Williams TJ, Lee RA, et al: Posthysterectomy enterocele and vaginal vault prolapse. *Am J Obstet Gynecol* 1981; 140:852.

White GR: An anatomical operation for the cure of cystocele. *JAMA* 1909; 53:1707–1710.

Chapter 6

Recurrent Cystocele

David H. Nichols, M.D.

Recurrent cystocele is an entity that is not as simplistic as the name implies. In most instances, it is asymptomatic; however, the patient may have noticed and reported a recurrent bulging in the vagina with an ill-defined feeling of fullness and weakness. The fullness and weakness become worse with bearing down or at the end of the day and are relieved by lying down. When the condition is demonstrated, it must be followed by periodic reexamination and certain questions answered.

The time when the cystocele was first noted becomes significant in determining whether it is truly a recurrent cystocele or whether it is, in fact, a persistent one. If the cystocele is noted at the first postoperative examination, it is probably the consequence of an initially inadequate anterior colporrhaphy. In evaluating the problem, one should consider whether the recurrence is due to an incorrectly chosen initial procedure, whether the surgery was inexpertly performed, or whether, for example, the choice of a short-acting catgut suture rather than a long-lasting synthetic or even permanent suture material could account for the failure.

On the other hand, if the cystocele is seen for the first time 2 or more years after the original surgery, it is more likely to be recurrent. One should ask if it developed over a period of time postoperatively and whether it is continuing to progress. Is it accompanied by any other signs of endopelvic herniation or weakness? Is it a consequence of the continuation of the normal aging process or of a lifestyle persistently characterized by increased intra-abdominal pressure (e.g., heavy lifting, chronic respiratory disease, or smoking)? Do the findings represent extension of a herniation process beyond that which was present at the time of the initial surgery? To make such determination, one should obtain a copy of the surgical report from each previous operative experience so that they may be correlated with the present findings on examination.

One should determine with precision any symptoms related to the bladder. Is there inability to empty the bladder completely? Is there urinary stress incontinence present? If so, is it a new symptom, recurrence of an old symptom, or persistence of an old symptom? Is the patient bothered by urinary urgency, frequency, or both? Are there episodes of recurrent cystitis? If so, what seems to trigger them?

Is there nocturia? Is there constipation? Does the patient spend much of her time bearing down excessively to achieve a bowel movement? Is the patient sexually active? Is she bothered by dyspareunia or vaginal dryness? If she is postmenopausal, is she receiving estrogen supplementation? If so, is the dose appropriate for her needs? Might the recurrent cystocele represent the consequence of a failure to repair coexistent accessory damages such as a large rectocele or perineal defect that were present at the time of the initial operation?

TYPES OF RECURRENT CYSTOCELE

There may be a somewhat diverse origin or combination of factors determining cystocele. It is fundamentally a hernial weakness of the vagina and its supporting tissues. The bladder only follows the altered vaginal contour. Thus, primary care must be directed to the vagina and its supports.

The cystocele that is seen may represent one or a combination of varying types of defects in the anterior vaginal wall. Anterior cystocele,[1] occurring anterior to Mercier's bar or the interureteric ridge, is fundamentally a rotational descent of the bladder neck and represents a significant alteration in the supports of the vesicourethral junction (Fig 6–1). It may occur with or without urethral funneling (Fig 6–2). When the latter is present, the incidence of coincident urinary stress incontinence is increased.

Posterior cystocele,[1] on the other hand, represents herniation of the bladder into the vagina behind the interureteric ridge (Fig 6–3). It may be the consequence of overdistention at childbirth with compromise of the normal elasticity of the vagina. Diminution in rugal folds of the vagina and thinness of the central portion of the vaginal wall are often a feature. The defect is literally a hernial weak spot, or "blowout," in the vaginal wall itself. Posterior cystocele and urethral detachment may coexist (Fig 6–4).

Compromise of the connective tissue bridge between the vagina and the arcus tendineus (Fig 6–5), either by stretching or avulsion, is not rare and can be deter-

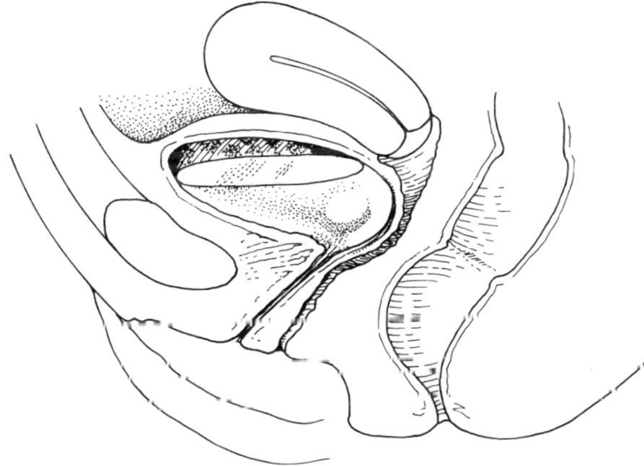

FIG 6–1.
Rotational descent of the vesicourethral junction. Notice the loss and straightening of the posterior urethrovesical angle. (Redrawn from Nichols DH, Randall CL: *Vaginal Surgery,* ed 3. Baltimore, Williams & Wilkins Co, 1989, p 240.)

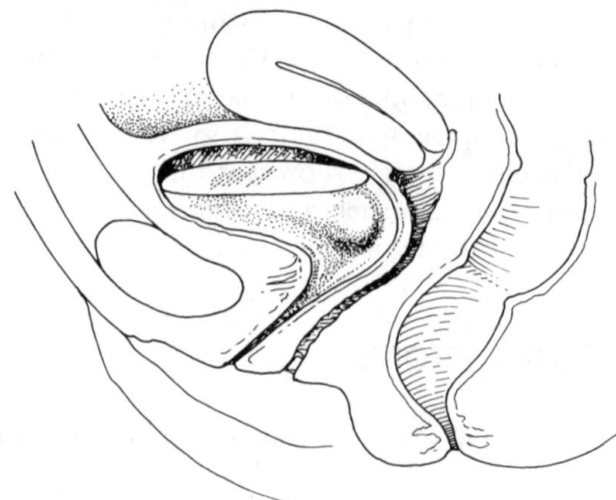

FIG 6–2.
Funneling of the urethra and rotational descent of the vesicourethral junction. (Redrawn from Nichols DH, Randall CL: *Vaginal Surgery,* ed 3. Baltimore, Williams & Wilkins Co, 1989, p 241.)

mined by noting the disappearance of the anterior fornix of the vagina on one or both sides and by the inability of the tissue in this area to elevate when the patient voluntarily contracts her pubococcygeus muscles. The paravaginal defect may occur at any level in the vagina or at all levels (Fig 6–6).

Its presence can be demonstrated by elevating the anterior vaginal wall with the tips of a modified sponge or dressing forceps held adjacent to the arcus tendineus. The patient is asked to strain, and one observes whether or not the cystocele persists. If the cystocele is eliminated by this maneuver, the defect is primarily in the paravaginal tissues.[2] If it persists, the defect must be in the central portion of the vaginal wall.

Eversion of the vault of the vagina gives rise to a displacement cystocele. The eversion may be unsuspected, but even so, it is by no means an uncommon finding. Best seen when the patient is examined while she is standing, it is usually a partial eversion of the vaginal vault that brings with it the underlying bladder anteriorly.

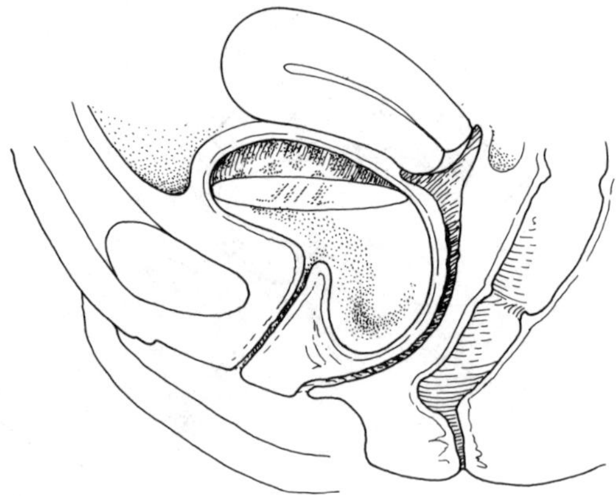

FIG 6–3.
Posterior distention-type cystocele. (Redrawn from Nichols DH, Randall CL: *Vaginal Surgery,* ed 3. Baltimore, Williams & Wilkins Co, 1989, p 242.)

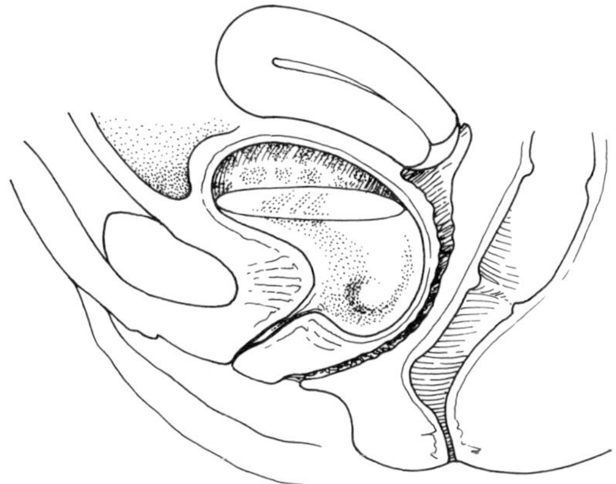

FIG 6–4.
Urethral detachment may coexist with cystocele. (Redrawn from Nichols DH, Randall CL: *Vaginal Surgery*, ed 3. Baltimore, Williams & Wilkins Co, 1989, p 243.)

Its occurrence is so frequent, particularly in the patient who has had hysterectomy, that it should be looked for again in the operating room by traction on the vault of the vagina with one or more Allis clamps applied to the site to which the uterus had been attached. When traction pulls the vault down into the midportion of the vagina, a partial eversion of the vault is assuredly present, and the cystocele is thus recognized to be due to displacement.

Recurrent cystocele is frequently the consequence of a number of these weaknesses, which may appear in an almost limitless variety of combinations. The most successful surgeon will have recognized each of the contributing factors and anatomic weaknesses

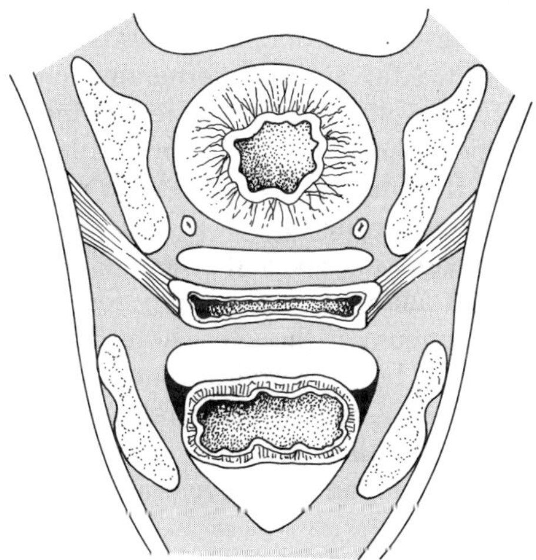

FIG 6–5.
Connective tissue septa and spaces of the pelvis. Notice particularly the vesicovaginal space, between bladder and vagina, and the rectovaginal space between the vagina and the rectum. There is an attachment of the vaginal sulci to the arcus tendineus and levator ani at the sidewall of the pelvis. (Redrawn from Nichols DH, Randall CL: *Vaginal Surgery*, ed 3. Baltimore, Williams & Wilkins Co, 1989, p 33.)

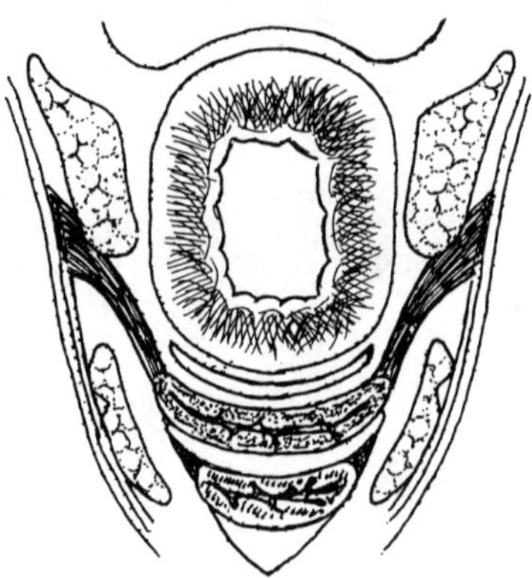

FIG 6–6.
Notice the marked elongation of the attachment of the vaginal sulci to the arcus tendineus and levator ani, constituting a paravaginal support defect.

Care should be taken to ensure that a cystocele is not incorrectly diagnosed when, in fact, none exists. "Apparent cystocele" is an entity in which a pathologic exposure of the anterior vaginal wall because of an unrepaired but marked perineal defect suggests cystocele, but examination reveals that the tissues do not extend caudal to the inferior margin of the pubis. Thus, apparent cystocele is a visual misconception of the consequence of overexposure of the anterior vaginal wall.

Anterior enterocele (see Fig 8–9) is another defect occasionally seen masquerading as a cystocele.[3] It may be accompanied by the same feeling of pelvic pressure and fullness when the patient is on her feet and straining. It is often the consequence of incomplete repair of an enterocele found at the initial surgery or of a failure to have resected excess anterior perineum on removing the uterus at the time of hysterectomy. In the latter circumstance, the surgeon may have encountered some difficulty in identifying the anterior vesicouterine peritoneal fold at the time of hysterectomy and dissected the anterior perineum from the lower uterine segment and body of the uterus well above the vesicouterine perineal fold before entering the peritoneal cavity. There is nothing wrong with this approach to the anterior colpotomy, as long as the surgeon recognizes the presence of this excess peritoneum and excises it carefully at the time of peritonealization.

Anterior enterocele is often unsuspected preoperatively but may be recognized at the time of the planned anterior colporrhaphy for "recurrent cystocele." The surgeon finds a sac of peritoneum at the site where the bladder was presumed to be. When its exact nature has been proved beyond a shadow of a doubt, often by delineating the bladder margin with a transurethral uterine sound, the sac is opened and the true nature of the herniation determined. The treatment is by mobilization of the sac, high ligation of its neck, and resection of the excess peritoneum.

The presence of an unrecognized defect in the lateral or paravaginal supports at the time of the original anterior colporrhaphy is another nemesis leading to recurrent cystocele. The patient's surgeon will usually have performed a midline colporrhaphy without realizing that the attachments of the anterior vaginal fornix to the connective tissues bridging them to the arcus tendineus have been torn or stretched. Paravaginal reattachment during the original repair would probably have aborted a recurrence.

SURGICAL ANATOMY

The vagina is a fibromuscular tube lined by stratified squamous epithelium with rugal folds, permitting some accordion-like distensibility without laceration. A thin but dense layer of elastic fibers is found immediately beneath the epithelium. The fibromuscular layer is a meshwork of smooth muscle fibers oriented predominantly in a longitudinal direction in the innermost layer but arranged circularly toward the periphery. The fibrous connective tissue capsule external to this muscular coat is rich in elastic fibers and large venous plexuses. The vagina is attached to the lateral pelvic wall by condensations of connective tissue and smooth muscle intimately adherent to the adventitia of the vaginal blood vessels. The rectovaginal septum is fused with the undersurface of the posterior vaginal wall as the anterior lining of the rectovaginal space.[3]

Since the cervix is incorporated in the anterior vaginal wall, the length of the anterior wall plus cervix approximates the length of the posterior wall. The connective tissue adventitia of the vagina is continuous with that of the cervix. The connective tissue lateral to the lower third of the vagina is attached to the pubococcygeal muscle by the fibers of Luschka. At the vesicourethral junction, it is fused with the fibers of the urogenital diaphragm.

The blood vessels enter the vagina from each side. Their surrounding connective tissue condensations and perivascular sheaths are arranged laterally in tissue that also includes some smooth muscle. The anterior portion of this connective tissue bridge is attached to the arcus tendoneus, which is the site of origin of the lateral portions of the levator ani from the surface of the obturator internus.

There is an avascular plane or potential space between the connective tissue capsule of the anterior vagina and the adventitia of the bladder. This vesicovaginal space has strong functional significance in that it permits the bladder and vagina to distend and function independently of each other. The space ends caudally at the vesicourethral junction, since the urethra acts mainly as a conduit of urine, and requires limited distensibility.

The upper limit of the vesicovaginal space is the fusion between the connective tissue capsule of the vagina and that of the bladder near the cervix. This area of fusion is called the *supravaginal septum.*[4]

The urethra is secured laterally by fibers of the urogenital diaphragm. A condensation of fibers in the urogenital diaphragm forms the so-called pubourethral ligaments. These attach primarily to the lateral sides of the urethra, but the condensations run to the back portion of the pubis (see Fig 5–5) as well and have two components: (1) an anterior ligament, the homologue of the suspensory ligament of the penis; and (2) a posterior ligament that runs to the vesicourethral junction. The posterior pubourethral ligaments aid significantly in the midline support of the proximal urethra.[5, 6] Because they contain smooth muscle fibers, the ligaments are capable of relaxation during the normal voiding process and thus permit a physiologic descent of the vesicourethral junction.[7] They are susceptible to damage from obstetric trauma and, when pathologically elongated, permit a rotational descent of the bladder neck even in the resting phase. This anatomic situation is conducive to a decreased urethral tone and in some patients is etiologically significant in the production of urinary stress incontinence, because the urethrovesical junction has been removed from its retropubic position where it can be responsive to increases in intra-abdominal pressure coincident with laughing, sneezing, coughing, or changing position.

In addition, the urethra receives considerable support from the underlying anterior vaginal wall. The anterior fornix of each side of the anterior vaginal wall is normally attached to the arcus tendineus on each side by an intermediate bridge of connective tissue, which can similarly be damaged by a number of factors. Obstetric trauma is the principal culprit, but chronic increases in intra-abdominal pressure may also play a role. Thus, the urethra is both suspended and supported: suspended by the pubourethral portion of the urogenital diaphragm and supported by the anterior vaginal wall.[3]

The pubococcygeus muscle plays a considerable role in the normal voiding mechanism, as was described by Muellner, who emphasized the importance of voluntary skeletal muscle in the mechanism of continence[8]:

> Before urination begins, the diaphragm and the muscles of the abdominal wall contract. The intra-abdominal pressure rises, and the pubococcygei relax. As the pubococcygei relax, the neck of the bladder moves downward. This downward movement activates or initiates the contraction of the detrusor. At the same time, the contraction of the longitudinal fibers of the urethra, which are continuous with those of the detrusor, shortens the urethra and thereby widens and opens the internal urethral orifice. Urine is then expelled from the bladder.
>
> At the conclusion of voiding, a contraction of the pubococcygei raises the neck of the bladder, the detrusor and urethral musculature relax, the urethra lengthens, the internal urethral orifice narrows and closes, and urination stops.

More recently, Gosling has described the relationship between the levator ani muscles and the urethral wall and urethral junction[7]:

> The medial parts of the levator ani muscles (spincter vaginae) are related to (but structurally separate from) the urethral wall. These periurethral fibers consist of an abundance of large-diameter fast-and slow-twitch fibers, together with muscle spindles. Therefore, unlike the rhabdosphincter, periurethral muscle possesses morphologic features that are similar to other "typical" voluntary muscles.
>
> The levator ani plays an important part in urinary continence by providing an additional occlusive force on the urethral wall, particularly during events that are associated with an increase in intra-abdominal pressure, such as coughing and sneezing. This urethral occlusive force in the female is maximal at the level immediately distal to the maximum urethral pressure generated by the external urethral spincter. Thus, in addition to providing support for the pelvic viscera, the periurethral parts of the levator ani also play an important active role in the urethral mechanisms that maintain continence of urine.
>
> For micturition to occur, the pressure differential between the bladder and urethra muscle overcome the elastic resistance of the bladder neck. Immediately before the onset of micturition, the tonus of the rhabdosphincter is reduced by central inhibition of its motor neurons located in the second, third, and fourth sacrospinal segments. Such inhibition is mediated by descending spinal pathways originating in higher centers of the central nervous system. Concomitantly, other descending pathways activate (either directly or via sacral interneurons) the preganglionic parasympathetic motor outflow to the urinary bladder. This central intergration of the nervous control of the bladder and urethra is essential for normal micturition. . . . Periurethral fibers are innervated by the pudendal nerve and consist of an admixture of large-diameter fast-and slow-twitch fibers.

CONSERVATIVE MANAGEMENT

Prevention of recurrent cystocele should be achieved when at all possible. The avoidance of unnecessary heavy lifting is important, as is the use of timely and adequate episiotomy, properly repaired, in the obstetric patient with reduced tissue elasticity (e.g., the primigravida more than age 25, years). When a postmenopausal patient demonstrates atrophy of the vaginal skin, one may presume that the subepithelial tissues also are hypoestrogenic with a reduction in subepithelial elastic tissue as well as in blood supply. These atrophic changes can be slowed, arrested, and at times reversed by long-term adequate estrogen supplementation or replacement. Attention to posture is important. Keeping the back and shoulders straight permits the pelvis to rotate to a more effective axis. Lifting should be accomplished by the patient bending her knees while keeping her back straight rather than by bending at the waist. For a patient with poorly developed or hypofunctional pubococcygei, Kegel perineal resistive exercises are useful and should be employed as a long-term habit. An appropriate regimen consists of 15 strong, 3-second isometric pubococcygeal squeezes in a row, performed 6 times daily. After 2 or 3 months, there will be a considerable improvement in pubococcygeal strength, which will many times help in the support of the vagina and indirectly in the support of the bladder and urethra. For the symptomatic patient who refuses surgery, an intravaginal pessary, such as the Gellhorn or rubber doughnut, can be used. The pessary must, however, be taken out, the vagina inspected for irritation or ulceration, and the pessary replaced at intervals for the balance of the patient's life. Compared with surgery, it is a poor second choice.

Finally, it should be remembered that pregnancy, labor, and delivery all traumatize the supports of the anterior vaginal wall. Therefore, colporrhaphy should generally be reserved for the patient who has finished her childbearing. Repeated surgery after subsequent obstetric damage to these tissues is never as effective as a properly executed primary procedure. Reoperation in the former case necessitates dealing with alterations caused by postsurgical scar tissue. In the latter case, scarring is nonexistent or at least not as extensive.

SURGICAL MANAGEMENT

An important goal of surgery is the reestablishment of normal anatomic relationships between the vagina, bladder, urethra, and their supporting structures, including the urogenital diaphragm and pelvic diaphragm, cardinal ligaments, other genital organs, and the bony pelvis. Careful and thorough preoperative physical evaluation should be performed and the findings correlated with the patient's symptoms. The surgeon should identify all sites of weakness, including urethral detachment, vaginal detachment, uterine prolapse, prolapse of the vaginal vault, enterocele, rectocele, and perineal defect. The axis and depth of the vagina should be determined with the patient at rest, then straining in a Valsalva maneuver. Using a single examining finger, the surgeon should note the strength, symmetry, and effectiveness of the pubococcygei, first with the patient at rest, then with the patient voluntarily making a vigorous and sustained contraction of the muscles, and finally with the patient straining in a Valsalva maneuver. Palpation of the pelvic diaphragm via the vaginal hiatus while the patient is contracting or "holding" will frequently identify a defect in the integrity of the pelvic diaphragm, often the result of avulsion during childbirth many years ago. During a repetition of these maneuvers (i.e., with the patient relaxing, then squeezing, then holding), the surgeon palpates the anterior vaginal fornices[2] to identify any lateral detachment of the vaginal and periurethral tissues from the bridge of connective tissue that attaches the vagina to the arcus tendineus. Note should be made of whether there is damage on one or both sides. This assessment may be aided by using an open ovum forceps or specially designed paravaginal elevator (Fig 6–7) to hold the vaginal fornices bilaterally against the arcus tendinei to access the degree to which the cystocele is corrected by this manuever. The recurrent cystocele is thus seen to be due to a midline defect, paravaginal defect, or a combination of the two, with or without vault prolapse.

Pelvic examination is then repeated with the patient in a standing position. All of these observations are confirmed or modified. The standing position is, of course, the one in which the effects of gravity are added to the patient's demonstrated weaknesses. The most important single consideration is whether or not the vault of the vagina descends either to mimic a cystocele or by bringing with it portions of the anterior vaginal wall to cause a displacement-type cystocele. The only treatment for a vault prolapse is effective colpopexy,[3] usually by the transvaginal route, but occasionally by the transabdominal approach (see Chapter 5).

The surgeon should note the extent to which the bladder sags beneath the inferior margin of the pubis when the patient strains. If the descent is less than 4 cm, much can be expected from a course of Kegel's perineal resistive exercises. If the bladder descends more than 4 cm beneath the inferior margin of the pubis, Kegel has suggested that surgery becomes the treatment of choice for the symptomatic patient. With the patient in the standing position, the rectum is examined for weakness of the posterior vaginal wall and coincident rectal prolapse. If the surgeon places one finger in the patient's rectum and the thumb in the vagina and has the patient strain (see Fig 7–6), not only can the presence of a previously unsuspected

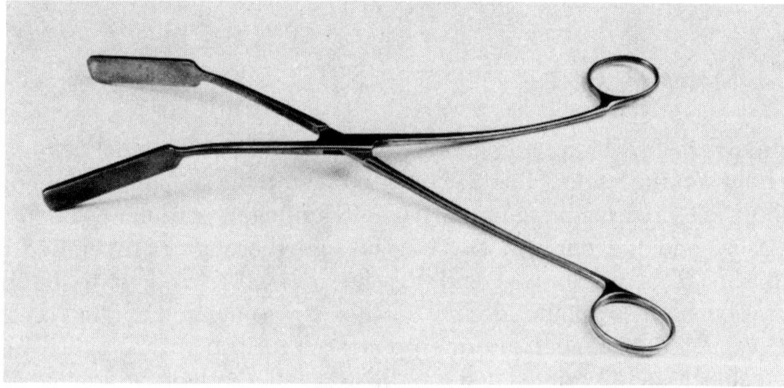

FIG 6–7.
Baden vaginal elevating forceps. When they are inserted into the vagina and opened, they press each anterior vaginal fornix against the arcus tendineus. The observer should note what happens to the cystocele in this circumstance. If it disappears, there is probably a defect in the paravaginal supporting tissue. If it does not, there is a midline defect. Occasionally both are present. The instrument is available from the Special Order Department, Codman-Shurtleff Inc., New Bedford, MA 02745.

and undetected vault prolapse be determined, but enterocele can be palpated between the operator's thumb and index finger.

The choice of the procedure or combination of procedures to be performed for an individual patient depends on the types and extent of the various defects that are present. There is no such thing as a standard patient or a standard procedure. Each case must be individualized. Some general guidelines are in order, however.

For the patient with a uterus who has a partial or complete prolapse of the vaginal vault accompany her recurrent cystocele, effective treatment must reestablish the support of the vault. If the cardinal-uterosacral ligament complex is strong, the simplest way to correct the prolapse is via vaginal hysterectomy with shortening of the cardinal-uterosacral ligament complexes, which are then reattached to the vaginal vault. A McCall or New Orleans type of cul-de-plasty will reinforce the reconstruction and act to prevent subsequent enterocele formation.[3] Appropriate colporrhaphy is then carried out.

For the patient in whom retention of the uterine corpus is requested or desired for future reproduction, a Manchester-Fothergill procedure may be indicated, if the prolapsed vault is of the uterovaginal type with demonstrable cervical elongation.[3] The uterosacral and cardinal ligaments are mobilized, the cervix is amputated, and the shortened ligaments are crossed in front of the remaining cervical stump to aid in its support. Appropriate anterior and posterior colporrhaphy follows. This procedure is not as popular in America as it once was. If the premenopausal patient understands the hazards of cervical amputation with its increased risk of premature labor, infertility, dysmenorrhea, and possible difficulty of assessing future uterine bleeding because of cervical stenosis, the procedure may be considered for her.

When it is evident that the cardinal-uterosacral complex is weak and cannot be relied on with confidence to support the vaginal vault, an alternative method of colpopexy should be considered. For the experienced vaginal surgeon, the procedure of choice is usually a transvaginal sacrospinous colpopexy, in which the vaginal vault is attached to sacrospinous ligament at a point one or more fingerbreadths medial to the ischial spine. If the vaginal vault is widened, the procedure may be accomplished bilaterally. An equally good result is achieved, however, when it is performed unilaterally and the vaginal cylinder narrowed to an appropriate width during the coincident colporrhaphy (see Chapter 5).

In cases of pure displacement cystocele, reconstructive surgery to support the vaginal vault may be all that is required to reduce the cystocele. If one chooses not to perform a coincident colporrhaphy, however, one must be confident that straightening of the anterior vaginal wall from the colpopexy will not result in urinary stress incontinence.[9]

In spite of the preoperative assessment in the examining room, the extent of colporrhaphy required to correct the recurrent cystocele must be reconfirmed during the examination under anesthesia as well. The effect of vaginal vault suspension on the anterior vaginal wall becomes apparent when a tenaculum, such as a long Allis clamp, is attached to the vaginal vault at the site that will become the new apex, and the vault is replaced into the hollow of the sacrum adjacent to the ischial spine. If the patient is awake under spinal anesthesia, she can be asked to strain or cough. The extent to which residual cystocele is apparent after replacement of the vault is the extent to which the displacement cystocele will require coincident colporrhaphy to effect an adequate repair. When performed along with a sacrospinous colpopexy, the anterior colporrhaphy is usually carried out first, hence the need for skillful judgment so that the vagina will not end up too large or too small. The former case would encourage recurrent prolapse, the latter, dyspareunia.

If the surgeon is uncomfortable with the transvaginal colpopexy, the transabdominal route may be chosen in transabdominal sacral colpopexy. The apex of the vagina is attached to the periosteum of the sacrum just caudal to the sacral promontory via an intervening bridge of fasica lata, synthetic mesh such as uncoated polyester (Mersilene), or lyophylised dura mater.[3] Although sacral colpopexy will to some degree eliminate a displacement cystocele and rectocele, it will not effectively treat the more common coincident distention type of cystocele and rectocele. These must be treated separately by colporrhaphy. Even though it will necessitate a two-stage procedure, most operators will prefer to perform the colporrhaphy vaginally since only the transvaginal route will allow the concomitant repair of a low rectocele and perineal defect.

Alternatively, a high cystocele and rectocele can be repaired from above (transabdominally) by excising a wedge of tissue from the anterior and posterior walls of the vagina, respectively. Since the sacral colpopexy has a tendency to straighten the urethrovesical junction, a prophylactic urethropexy, such as the Marshall-Marchetti-Krantz or the Burch procedure, may be performed in such a case before the abdomen is closed. If a paravaginal defect has been demonstrated, a transabdominal paravaginal repair attaching the anterior vaginal fornices to the arcus tendineus can be carried out.[10]

Transvaginal Colporrhaphy

It is important for the surgeon to estimate the extent to which there is an excess of anterior vaginal wall so that excision of an appropriate amount can be effectively gauged before any vaginal wall has been excised. The surgeon should similarly establish whether the damage for which reoperative surgery is being performed involves primarily the midline suspensory tissues, a hernial weakness in the central part of the anterior vaginal wall, or a paravaginal defect. Although the latter is suspected from the initial pelvic examination, it can be confirmed in the operating room as well by placing each anterior vaginal fornix adjacent to the tissues of the arcus tendineus on each side and observing what happens to the anterior vaginal wall. In the event of demonstrated paravaginal or lateral vaginal contributory weakness, coincident paravaginal colpopexy can be incorporated in the operative procedure.

Midline Defects

For adequate mobilization of the affected tissues, the operator should proceed directly into the vesicovaginal space so that the full thickness of the anterior vaginal can be identified, mobilized, resected, and repaired (see Fig 7–2). Sometimes this space will have been compromised by scarring from the previous surgery, so the operator must proceed with great caution lest an unintentional cystotomy be produced. The bladder is emptied of urine. An indwelling no. 16 silicone Foley catheter is inserted for identification of the vesicourethral junction and urethra during the course of surgery. The midpoint of the anterior vaginal wall underlying the cystocele is grasped between two transversely placed Allis clamps about 1.5 cm apart. The anterior vaginal wall between the clamps is massaged to help break up any ad-

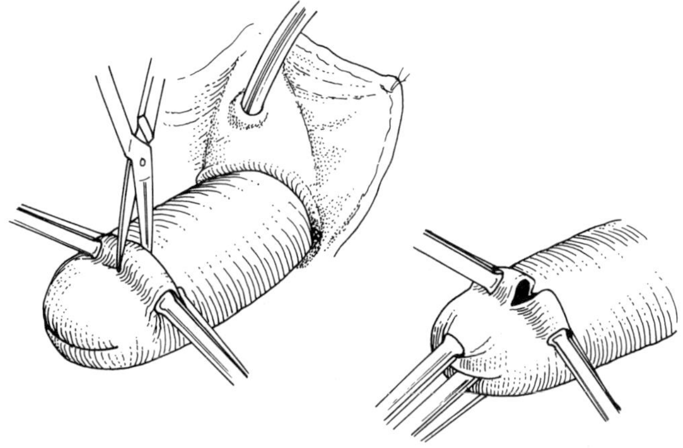

FIG 6–8.
The anterior vaginal wall is grasped between two Allis clamps that overlie the vesicovaginal space that separates the bladder from the thickened anterior vaginal wall **(A).** An incision is made between these clamps opening directly into the vesicovaginal space **(B).** (Redrawn from Nichols DH, Randall CL: *Vaginal Surgery,* ed 3. Baltimore, Williams & Wilkins Co, 1989, p 249.)

hesions between the vagina and bladder. A vertical incision through the anterior wall is made between the Allis clamps directly into the vesicovaginal space (Fig 6–8). The position of the Allis clamps is changed so that they now grasp the full thickness of the anterior vaginal wall, which is incised for the full length of the vesicovaginal space beneath the cystocele.[3] The surgeon next establishes a plane of cleavage between the anterior vaginal wall and urethra and separates the vaginal wall from the undersurface of the urethra for most of its length, to within 1 or 1.5 cm of the external urethral meatus. Appropriate Allis clamps are placed along the edges of the vaginal wall for traction and exposure. The vagina is freed from the undersurface of the urethra down to the site of the urogenital diaphragm, being careful to avoid skeletonizing the urethra lest one compromise its blood and nerve supply. Any urethral funneling that has been demonstrated (Fig 6–9) is corrected by one or more Kelly-type[11] urethral wall plication stitches (Fig 6–10) using a long-

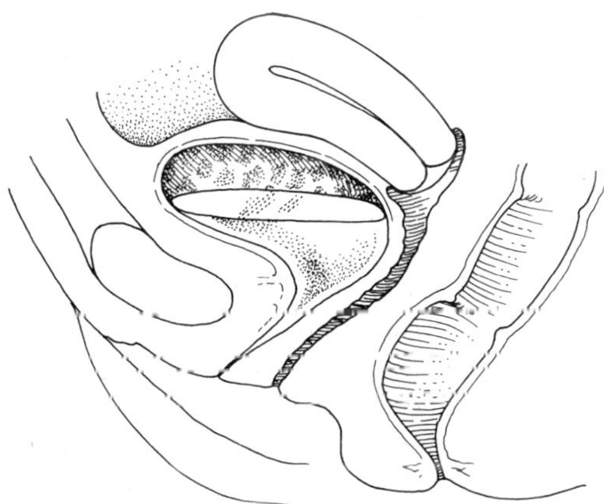

FIG 6–9.
Funneling or vesicalization of the urethra is shown in the sagittal view. (Redrawn from Nichols DH, Randall CL: *Vaginal Surgery,* ed 3. Baltimore, Williams & Wilkins Co, 1989, p 253.)

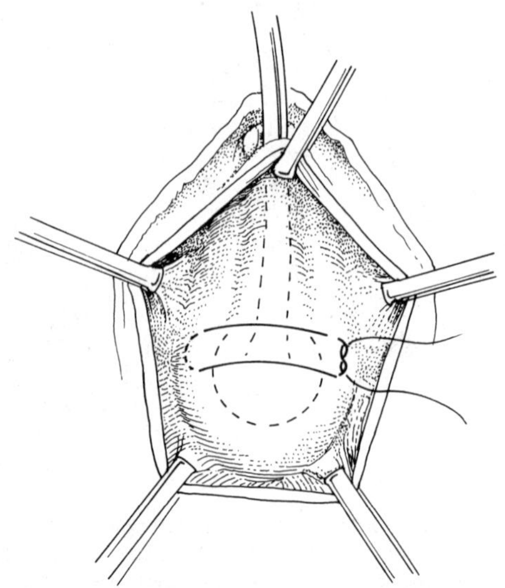

FIG 6–10.
The original Kelly stitch. It had been introduced to plicate a presumed internal urethral sphincter. One or more may be placed at the vesical neck. Note the inflated bulb on the Foley catheter *(dashed line)*. (Redrawn from Nichols DH, Randall CL: *Vaginal Surgery,* ed 3. Baltimore, Williams & Wilkins Co, 1989, p 254.)

acting synthetic suture material of the polyglycolic acid type. A gentle tug on the Foley catheter will identify the vesicourethral junction. If there is hypermobility of the urethra with coincident rotational descent of the bladder neck, this should be repaired by pubourethral ligament plication[5] (Fig 6–11) using a long-lasting or a nonabsorbable synthetic suture, which, when tied, should displace the vesicourethral junction cranially until it is once again retropubic at about the junction of the lower third with the upper two thirds of the back of the pubis. If one suture is insufficient to achieve this goal, a second should be placed lateral to the first. The suture is tied, but the ends are held for use again later in the operation.

The vesicovaginal space is dissected the full limits of its lateral extent to separate fully the unsplit anterior vaginal wall from the underlying bladder. The width and length of the connective tissue capsule of the bladder are reduced by one or more layers of running locked sutures of polyglycolic acid or catgut. Occasionally this bladder plication is accomplished using a "tobacco pouch" pursestring suture. The neck of such a pursestring suture must always be reinforced by an additional layer of mattress sutures in case strength is lost at the time of absorption of the suture material of the purse string.

It is important for the operator to correct most of the secondary damage to the wall of the bladder by this colporrhaphy but to guard carefully against overcorrection lest the posterior urethrovesical angle be straightened out pathologically and the patient given an anatomic predisposition for postoperative urinary stress incontinence (Fig 6–12).[9] If a sacrospinous colpopexy is to be performed, the extent of excess anterior vaginal wall can be very carefully estimated by holding the vaginal vault adjacent to the ischial spine, and the full thickness of the excess vagina can be excised. The vaginal walls are then reapproximated in the midline by a spiraling subcutaneous subcuticular suture of size 00 polyglycolic acid suture. The suture starts at the urethral end of the dissection and brings the sides of vagina together

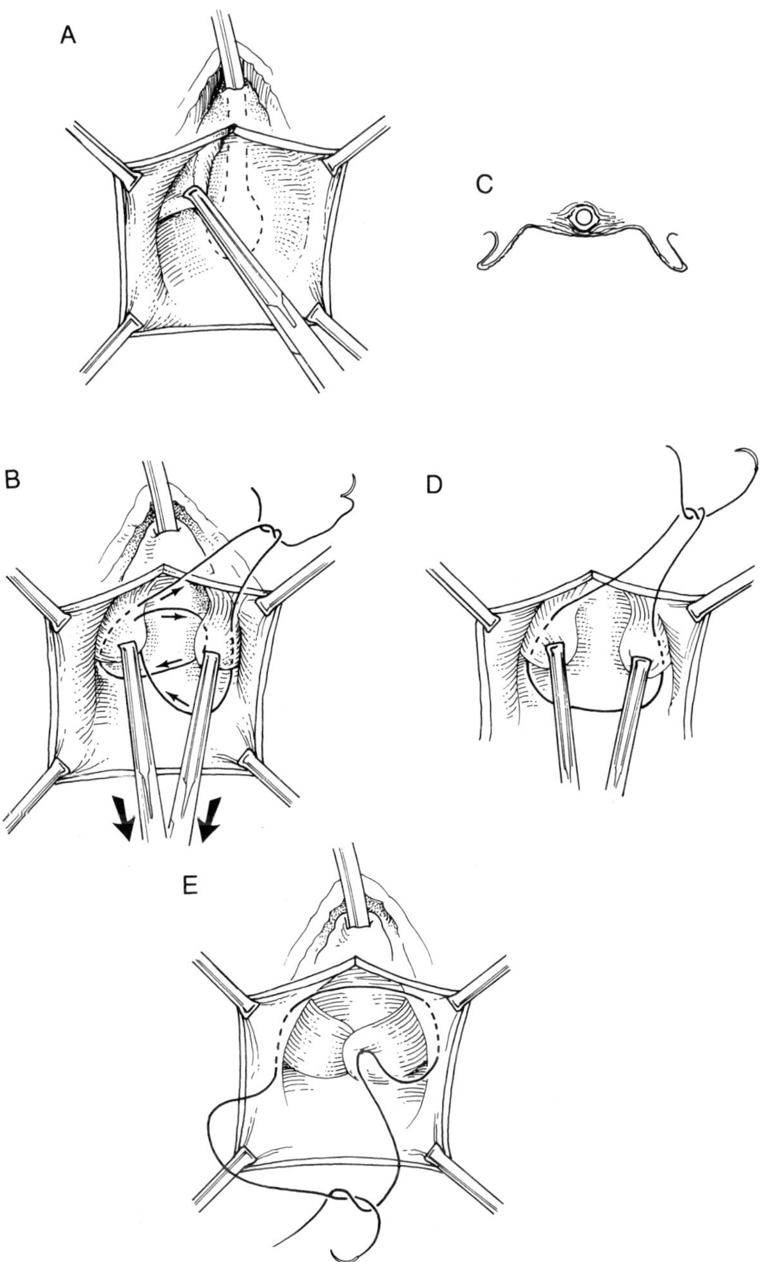

FIG 6–11.
Pubourethral "ligament" plication. The anterior vaginal wall has been incised in the midline into the vesicovaginal space and the dissection carried anteriorly beneath the urethra **(A** and **B)**. Notice that the proper depth of urethral dissection does not skeletonize the urethra **(C)** so as not to overly disturb its blood and nerve supply. In **A** the paraurethral tissue of the urogenital diaphragm has been grasped in a Kocher hemostat closed only one notch of its ratchet. Traction to the forceps in the line indicated by the *arrows* **(B)** will actually move the patient a small degree on the table. A polydioxanone suture is placed through each side of the "ligament" **(B)** in a far-near-near-far configuration. An alternate method **(D)** may be used when synthetic nonabsorbable sutures are applied. After the "ligaments" have been plicated, the same suture takes a bite of the vaginal wall **(E)**, reestablishing the fusion between vagina and urogenital diaphragm. (Redrawn from Nichols DH, Randall CL: *Vaginal Surgery,* ed 3. Baltimore, Williams & Wilkins Co, 1989, p 256.)

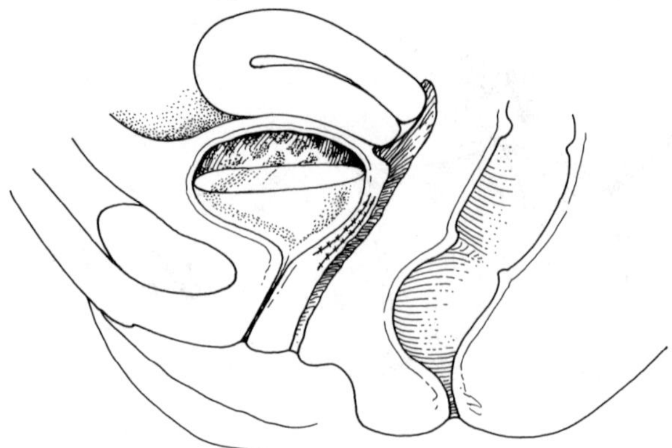

FIG 6–12.
Overcorrection of cystocele has thoughtlessly straightened the posterior vesicourethral angle. (Redrawn from Nichols DH, Randall CL: *Vaginal Surgery,* ed 3. Baltimore, Williams & Wilkins Co, 1989, p 250.)

for the full length of the incision. Each pass of the suture incorporates the full thickness of the vaginal wall with the exception of penetration of the outermost layer of the epithelium; that is, the suture material remains subcuticular and does not actually perforate the "mucosa." Since the vaginal wall has not been split, its blood supply has not been disturbed, and the integrity of the subepithelial coat of the vagina adds its full strength to the repair.

Paravaginal Defects

If the recurrent cystocele demonstrates a coincident paravaginal defect, before any vaginal wall is resected, the dissection of the anterior vaginal wall from the bladder is continued laterally beyond the lateral margins of the vesicovaginal space to expose the obturator internus and the arcus tendineus. Interrupted stitches (usually synthetic absorbable sutures) are placed in series in the tissues of the arcus tendineus. The sutures, which are held long, are then individually sewn to the

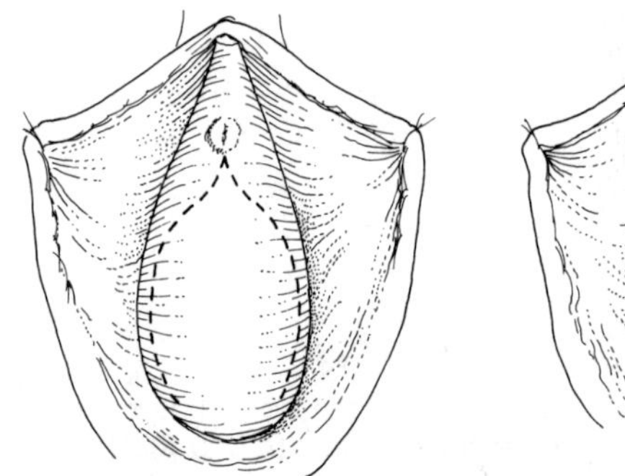

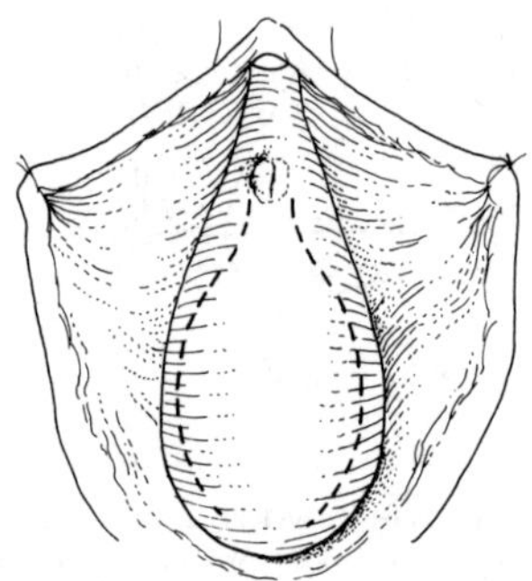

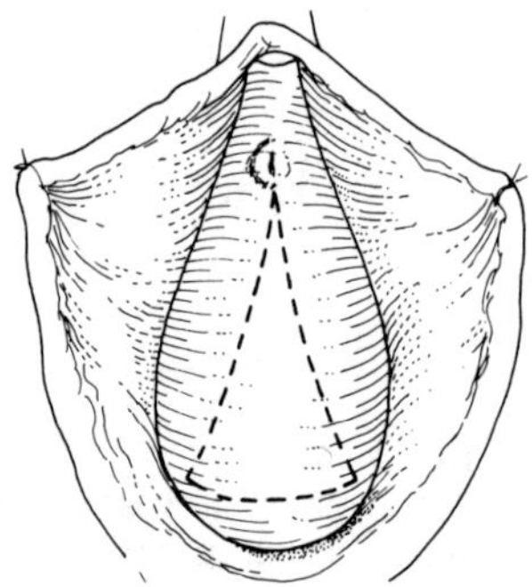

FIG 6–13.
An incision for correcting simultaneous midline and lateral defects of the anterior vaginal wall support is shown by the *dashed line* **(left).** White's original bilateral incisions from the site of the ischial spine to the urethra is used for correcting lateral support defects **(middle).** An incision for correcting midline defects is shown on the **right.** Excess vaginal wall will be excised as shown within the *dashed lines.* (Redrawn from Nichols DH, Randall CL: *Vaginal Surgery,* ed 3. Baltimore, Williams & Wilkins Co, 1989, p 264.)

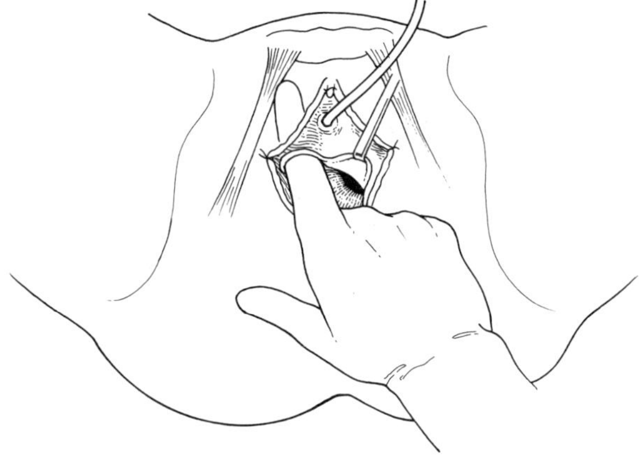

FIG 6–14.
An opening has been made through the anterior vaginal wall, and the operator's index finger, having swept the bladder and urethra medially, palpates and by blunt dissection exposes the arcus tendineus on the patient's right. A similar dissection will be performed on the patient's left. (Redrawn from Nichols DH, Randall CL: *Vaginal Surgery,* ed 3. Baltimore, Williams & Wilkins Co, 1989, p 265.)

subepithelial fibromuscular wall of the vagina. After the sutures, on one side, have been individually tied, a similar fixation is accomplished on the opposite side, as is usually necessary. Only after paravaginal repair is complete is any excess anterior vaginal wall trimmed for repair of any remaining midline defect. The surgeon then closes the midline incision with the spiraling subcutaneous suture.

For the patient without a demonstrable midline defect, the paravaginal repair is approached through parallel incisions in the anterior vaginal wall (Figs 6–13 and 6–14),[12] as originally suggested by White.[13] Preliminary infiltration of the area with a liquid tourniquet such as 1:200,000 epinephrine-lidocaine solution will diminish the blood loss during the dissection. The stitches in the arcus tendineus are placed,[14] then brought through the cut edges of the vagina (Fig 6–15). When all have been placed, they are tied one by one. This is completed first on one side and then on the other.

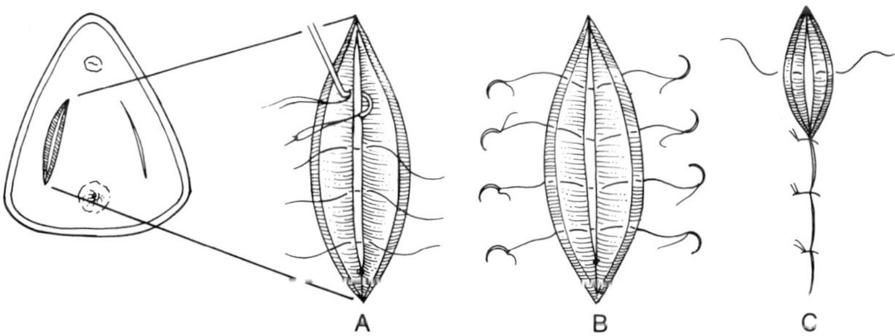

FIG 6–15.
White's method of transvaginal paravaginal fixation. The vagina is shown to the far left. Notice the urethra at the 12 o'clock position and the cervix at the 6 o'clock position. Bilateral incisions are made through the full thickness of the vaginal wall at a site overlying the arcus tendineus **(A).** A Deschamps ligature carrier is used to place a number of stitches in the arcus tendineus **(B).** Each free end is passed through the full thickness of the vaginal wall **(C).** When all have been placed, they are tied as shown to the far right. (Redrawn from Nichols DH, Randall CL: *Vaginal Surgery,* ed 3. Baltimore, Williams & Wilkins Co, 1989, p 265.)

Unusually Thin Vagina

One will occasionally encounter a patient who has undergone numerous procedures and who has marked atrophy and thinning of the anterior portion of the vagina that has not responded sufficiently enough to estrogen supplementation to have restored adequate thickness to the vaginal wall. The patient, who is usually postmenopausal, may be sexually active, making the surgeon most reluctant to resect any more vaginal tissue. Too much may already have been removed by previous colparrhaphy to permit bilateral paravaginal fixation. One alternative repair for such a large thin-walled cystocele is that of using a subepithelial prosthetic mesh such as Mersilene to create an additional tissue layer.[3] When cut to size, the Mersilene mesh is fixed in place by interrupted nonabsorbable sutures and insulated from the overlying vaginal wall by either a vaginal lapping operation (Fig 6–16) or by the use of a broad-based bulbocavernosus fat pad transplant.[3] The anterior vaginal wall should then be closed without tension, usually with interrupted sutures. If there is any question as to the presence of tension in this suture line, bilateral vaginal relaxing incision should be made at the 3 or 9 o'clock position as described in Chapter 22. These will effectively take the tension from the anterior suture line.

Another interesting alternative procedure in such a patient, should she still retain a well-supported uterus, would be the Acejo[15] modification of the Watkins-Wertheim bladder transposition operation. In this procedure, the fundus of the uterus, from which all endometrium has been excised, is interposed between the bladder and the anterior vaginal wall. The excision of the endometrium removes the site and source of future uterine bleeding and its attendant problems.

Posterior Colporrhaphy

The length of the urethra is approximately the same as the length of the perineal body. If, therefore, the patient who is undergoing anterior colporrhaphy for a recurrent cystocele has a coincident defect of the perineum or posterior vaginal wall, the coincident rectocele or perineal defect should be repaired, because such a repair will aid considerably in the postoperative long-term support of the anterior vaginal wall.

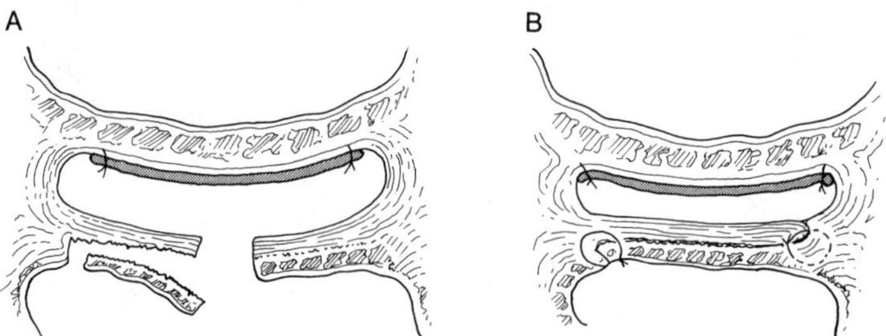

FIG 6–16.
The vaginal lapping technique has been applied to insulate a patch of Mersilene mesh that has been sewn in place to the undersurface of the bladder muscularis. The vaginal flap has been split and the superficial membrane and skin excised **(A).** The now denuded fibromuscular layer of vagina is sewn to the undersurface of the unsplit vaginal flap on the opposite side **(B).** The cut edge of the full thickness of the unsplit vaginal flap is sewn to the cut epithelial edge of the opposite side with a series of interrupted, absorbable sutures. (Redrawn from Nichols DH, Randall CL: *Vaginal Surgery,* ed 3. Baltimore, Williams & Wilkins Co, 1989, p 267.)

POSTOPERATIVE CARE

Wound healing seems to be improved by postoperative administration of 500 mg of ascorbic acid daily for 3 to 6 months, minimum time. A long-term course of voluntary perineal resistive exercises, as described earlier, should continue at least 3 months postoperatively. Suitable estrogen replacement (in every postmenopausal patient) either systemically or with intravaginal estrogen cream should be used unless contraindicated. The patient should be cautioned that convalescence is a slow process. Physical activities should be rather conservative for the first month after surgery. If the patient has been prone to unnecessary heavy lifting in her daily life, this should be amended. If her posture is faulty, it should be effectively corrected.

REFERENCES

1. Ball TL: Anterior and posterior cystocele. *Clin Obstet Gynecol* 1966; 9:1062–1069.
2. Baden WF, Walker TA: Evaluation of the stress incontinent patient, in Canton EG (ed): *Female Urinary Stress Incontinence.* Springfield, Ill, Charles C Thomas, Publisher, 1979, p 157–158.
3. Nichols DH, Randall CL: *Vaginal Surgery,* ed 3. Baltimore, Williams & Wilkins Co, 1989.
4. Von Peham H, Amreich J: *Operative Gynecology.* (Translated by Ferguson LK.) Philadelphia, JB Lippincott Co, 1934.
5. Nichols DH, Milley PS: Identification of pubourethral ligaments and their role in transvaginal surgical correction of stress incontinence. *Am J Obstet Gynecol* 1973; 115:123.
6. Zacharin RF: The suspensory mechanism of the female urethra. *J Anat* 1963; 97:423–427.
7. Gosling JA: The structure of the female lower urinary tract and the pelvic floor. *Urol Clin North Am* 1985; 12:207–214.
8. Muellner SR: The anatomies of the female urethra. *Obstet Gynecol* 1959; 14:429–434.
9. Symmonds RE, Jordan LT: Iatrogenic stress incontinence of urine. *Am J Obstet Gynecol* 1961; 82:1231–1237.
10. Richardson AC, Lyons JB, Williams NL: A new look at pelvic relaxation. *Am J Obstet Gynecol* 1976; 126:568.
11. Kelly HA: Incontinence of urine in women. *Urol Cutan Rev* 1913; 1:291–293.
12. Word BH Jr, Montgomery HA: Paravaginal fascial repair. Film and personal communications, 1986.
13. White GR: Cystocele—a radical cure by suturing lateral sulci of vagina to the white line of pelvic fascia. *JAMA* 1909; 53:1707–1709.
14. Figuranov KM: Surgical treatment of urinary incontinence in women. *Akush Ginekol (Mosk)* 1949; 6:7–13.
15. Gallo D: Ocojo modification of interposition operation, in *Urologica Ginecologica.* Guadalajara, Mexico, Gallo, 1969.

Chapter 7

Recurrent Rectocele

David H. Nichols, M.D.

Recurrent rectocele is a frustration for both the patient and her surgeon. Although it may be an extension of the naturally progressive aging process, it usually indicates either an initial misdiagnosis as to the extent of the patient's weakness, failure to have correlated the anatomic damages with the patient's symptoms, or performance of an inadequate repair. The surgeon must decide whether only the patient's symptoms are recurring or whether an actual rectocele and/or perineal defect has recurred.

Posterior vaginal repair is among the most poorly understood and poorly performed of the common gynecologic surgical procedures. Although rectocele is fairly common among multiparous women, there is considerable confusion and divergence of opinion concerning not only the related symptoms and indications for repair but also the anatomic goals sought by the repair and, therefore, the specific techniques used to achieve them. Perineal defect generally is identified by a gaping perineum and may occur with or without coincident rectocele (Fig 7–1). Rectocele may be found in the lower third, middle third, or upper third of the vagina or all three, and it may or may not coexist with enterocele. When it is symptomatic, all elements of weakness should be repaired as part of the initial operation, or those sections left unrepaired will generally progress, requiring future surgical attention. Rectocele is fundamentally a defect of the vagina, and the dilated rectum follows the vaginal defect rather passively, although the secondary damage to the wall of the rectum may become extreme over a long period of time. Since the vagina is the primary site of damage, it is to the vagina that primary attention should be given and reconstruction directed when the patient is symptomatic.

SYMPTOMS

Surprisingly, constipation is not necessarily a symptom of rectocele, though it may coexist. There are many women with constipation without rectocele, many more with rectocele who are not constipated, and some women with constipation who have rectocele. Posterior colporrhaphy, therefore, will not necessarily relieve constipation, which is essentially a functional disorder.

The primary symptoms of rectocele include an inability to completely empty the bowel with defecation, often requiring manual vaginal or perineal expression to

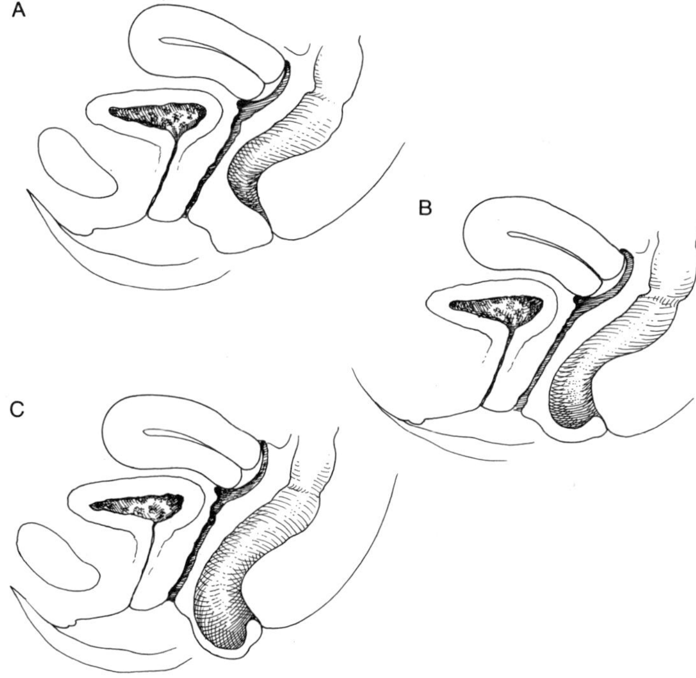

FIG 7–1.
A, a normal relationship between the vagina, perineum, and rectum. **B,** a major perineal defect. There is no rectocele but restoration of the perineal body is indicated. **C,** a major perineal defect with rectocele. In this circumstance, perineorrhaphy should be accompanied by an appropriate posterior colporrhaphy. (Redrawn from Nichols DH, Randall CL: *Vaginal Surgery,* ed 3. Baltimore, Williams & Wilkins Co, 1989.)

complete the process. Evacuation is often followed by postevacuation rectal discomfort probably related to venous engorgement consequent to straining. Such a tendency toward passive congestion may interfere with perineal circulation, and coincident hemorrhoids are frequent. Constipation per se is more likely the result of deranged bowel habits in which the patient has difficulty "unlocking" the anorectal valve and relaxing the internal anal sphincter.

It is important to review briefly the mechanism of rectal continence. The levator ani, or muscular portion of the pelvic diaphragm, is unique among human striated muscle in that it maintains sensory receptors that are stimulated by coincident rectal fullness. Stimulation of these sensors may reflexly influence the tone of the voluntary muscles of the pelvis but may also convey to the patient's sensorium a message of fullness. Although the levator ani is a voluntary muscle and can be contracted at will by the patient, it maintains a voluntary tone that is reflexly greater with increased rectal distention.

Both the levator ani and the external anal sphincter are innervated by the pudendal nerve and, most of the time, act in synergy. This reflex tone is involuntary and constant, and for this reason we do not soil ourselves during the night, even though peristalsis constantly propels our intestinal content toward its ultimate site of expulsion. As it continues downward, the muscular wall of the large bowel becomes the internal anal sphincter, composed of smooth involuntary muscle. The internal sphincter is the backup system of continence to that offered by the external anal sphincter.

At certain times, usually in the morning, and following initiation of the gastrocolic reflex, a sensation of rectal fullness is conveyed to the sensory nervous system, and the patient may experience a desire to evacuate. If this desire is heeded, the patient in the course of evacuation relaxes the external anal sphincter and levator ani, straightening out the anorectal angle, and permitting direct access of intestinal content to the distal portion of the intestinal system. With intra-abdominal pressure increased by a gentle voluntary Valsalva maneuver, this bolus is propelled, the internal anal sphincter relaxes, and defecation occurs.

If any step of this process is deliberately or accidentally circumvented, the normal reflex pattern is disturbed, the internal anal sphincter will not unlock, and the tone of the levator ani and external sphincter system increases to avoid incontinence. When the patient persists in habitual inhibition over a long period of time, the sensory mechanism is suppressed, and it may be difficult to reinitiate the reflexes leading toward evacuation. When these problems have been present for some time, the patient may develop a habit of overcoming them by excessive straining at stool. Voluntary massive increase in intra-abdominal pressure by contraction of the anterior abdominal muscles to force content out of the bowel can result in damage to the resisting pelvic diaphragm and levator ani.

Once the normal evacuation system has been suppressed by voluntary interference with this normal reflex activity, it is difficult to reestablish a useful bowel pattern but is worth the trouble if the patient is to be cured of an annoying constipation. In hope that it will act as an intestinal stimulant, additional bulk in the stool may be provided by increased dietary fiber or various preparations. Peristalsis may be stimulated by the use of a laxative or cathartic. It is important that the patient maintain an adequate dietary liquid intake. Because thirst decreases with age, the older woman usually will consume less liquid in her diet than she did in her earlier and thirstier years. This relative dehydration promotes fecal hardness as the colon seeks to extract every possible bit of water from its content.

Since a long history of evacuation straining is associated with increases in intracolonic pressure, patients with this problem may also suffer from diverticulosis, which increases in frequency with age as well. Inducing adequate bulk by an increase in dietary fiber, such as bran, may coincidentally improve intestinal dysfunction associated with diverticulosis.

Another symptom of rectocele may be the partial retention of stool. The problem is mechanical, related not to constipation but to the trapping of stool in a pocket, which functions as a rather massive diverticulum of the anterior rectal wall. The harder the patient strains, the more intensely stool is packed into this pocket, preventing easy expulsion but producing congestion and discomfort.

Perineal Descent Syndrome

In the evaluation of the patient, it is important to note any tendency toward dropping of the perineum, which is called the perineal descent syndrome, because this may have great importance to the patient's future comfort (see Chapter 15).[1,2]

Perineal Defect

Rectocele and perineal defect are anatomically separate, but they may coexist. For an appropriate reconstruction, symptoms referrable to each should be evaluated in concert with the specific anatomic pathology demonstrated. Perineal defect may produce a wide and gaping perineum, which may at times subtract from coital satisfaction. The latter can be restored by perineorrhaphy, but the surgeon must be careful not to overtighten the outlet, because it may induce an anatomic marital obstruction. Perineorrhaphy, however, will not correct any marital discontent that is the result of interpersonal dissatisfaction or conflict, despite a patient's preoperative insistence to the contrary.

NORMAL ANATOMY OF POSTERIOR VAGINAL WALL AND ITS SUPPORTS

The S-shaped curve of the vagina terminates just anterior to the hollow of the sacrum (Fig 7–2). The vagina is separated from the rectum by the avascular rectovaginal space, more a potential space than an actual cavity. Because it permits the rectum and vagina to function independently of one another, the rectovaginal space should be preserved following surgery. The thin membrane-like connective tissue, the fascia of Denonvilliers, is fused to the underside of the posterior vaginal wall.[3] It extends from the bottom of the cul-de-sac of Douglas to an attachment at the upper margin of the perineal body (Fig 7–3). When this attachment has been avulsed from the perineal body, the latter is destabilized anteriorly. Such a weakness is one cause of low rectocele and should be remedied by surgical reattachment during posterior repair.

The fascia of Denonvilliers has sufficient strength that it may be used effectively during posterior colporrhaphy to strengthen the posterior vaginal wall. It represents a peritoneal fusion layer of the obliterated extension of the cul-de-sac to the perineal body during fetal life. Failure of fusion of these two layers of perito-

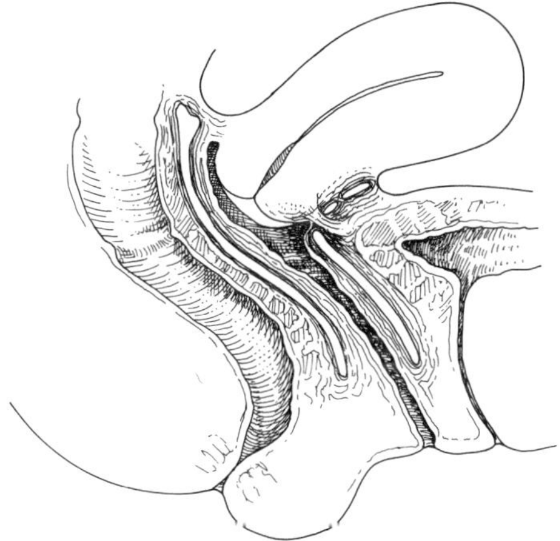

FIG 7–2.
Median sagittal section through the pelvis showing the midline connective tissue spaces between the bladder, vagina, rectum, and cervix. The vesicocervical space is separated from the vesicovaginal space by fusion between the adventitia of the cervix and bladder called the supravaginal septum. The rectovaginal space is shown between the rectum and vagina, extending from the perineal body to the bottom of the cul-de-sac of Douglas. The rectovaginal septum is a condensation of tissue attached to the underside of the posterior vaginal wall along the full length of the rectovaginal space. (Redrawn from Nichols DH, Randall CL: *Vaginal Surgery,* ed 3. Baltimore, Williams & Wilkins Co, 1989.)

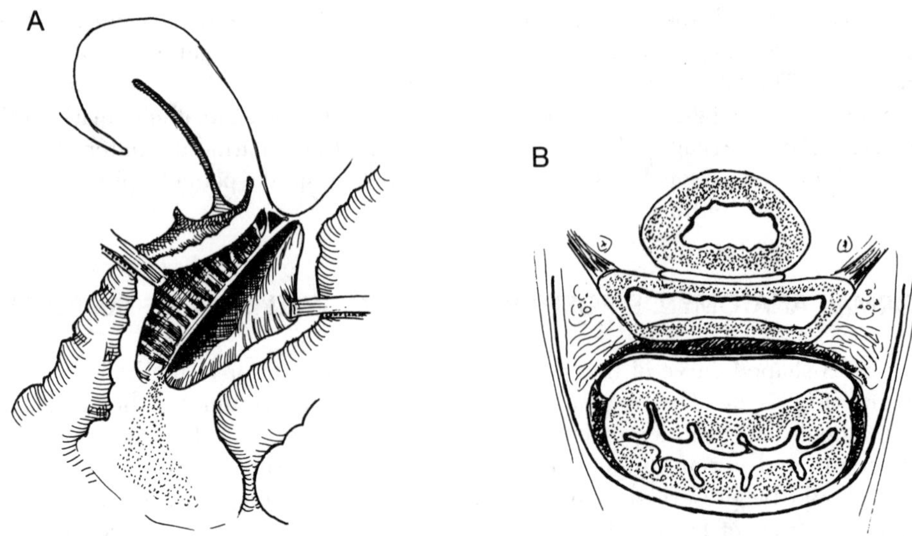

FIG 7–3.
A, rectovaginal septum, which is partly dissected from the undersurface of the vagina. It extends from the pouch of Douglas to the perineal body and forms the anterior surface of the rectovaginal space. Note the attachment of the perineal body to the fascia of Denonvilliers. **B,** its adherence to the posterior vaginal wall along with its posterolateral curve. (Redrawn from Nichols DH, Milley PS: *Am J Obstet Gynecol* 1970; 108:217.)

neum gives rise in adult life to a congenitally deep cul-de-sac of Douglas, and when filled with bowel or omentum, it constitutes congenital enterocele. Failure of fusion weakens this fascia of Denonvilliers and, therefore, its overlying posterior vaginal wall, a deficiency conducive to high rectocele. This weakness accounts in part for the frequent coexistence of high rectocele with the congenital type of enterocele (Fig 7–4). So frequent is this association that when one is found, the other should be sought and usually repaired at the same time before it progresses sufficiently to require subsequent surgery.

The more or less horizontal axis of the upper portion of the vagina is a consequence of its resting on a usually empty rectum, which, in turn, lies more or less passively on the levator plate, formed by the fusion of the right and left pubococcygeus posterior to the rectum.[4] Relatively few muscular fibers of the pubococcygei converge anterior to the rectum. The lateral walls of the midportion of the vagina are attached to the medial borders of the pubococcygei by a connective tissue framework described as the fibers of Luschka. Therefore, techniques of posterior repair that emphasize primarily a bringing together of the levatores ani between the vagina and rectum are essentially unanatomic and can create physically constricting ridges when sutures placed directly in the muscle bellies are later replaced by areas of painful fibrosis. It is these tender ridges that account for most of the postsurgical dyspareunia or apareunia reported by Jeffcoate.[5] So frequently was this seen in his practice (50% incidence of postoperative dyspareunia, 25% incidence of apareunia) that he advised against posterior repair unless significant damage was confirmed by preoperative examination of the unanesthetized patient. Because anesthesia effectively paralyzes the skeletal muscles of the pelvis, an examination under anesthesia provides a false idea of anatomic weakness. Because of this temporary paralysis, the voluntary muscles cannot contract, "fight back," or resist effec-

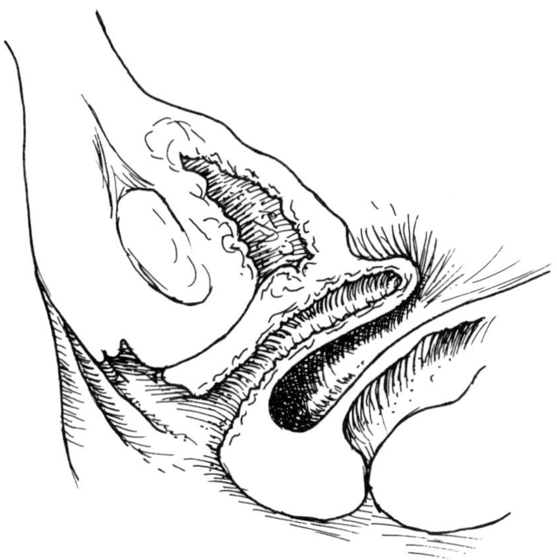

FIG 7–4.
Posterior enterocele without eversion of the vagina in a posthysterectomy patient. (Redrawn from Nichols DH: *Obstet Gynecol* 1972; 40:257–263.)

tively the forces of examination, and it appears as though every anesthetized woman has a rectocele.

In the days before intraperitoneal surgery and hysterectomy became relatively safe means of treating genital prolapse, an alternate treatment was the use of an intravaginal pessary, retained in the upper vagina cranial to the lateral pressures exerted by the levatores ani. With time, pressure against the pelvic diaphragm by the pessary caused the introitus to widen progressively. The patient could then no longer retain a pessary and was more uncomfortable than ever. Around the turn of the century, the introduction of prerectal levator plication as a feature of perineorrhaphy enabled such a patient once again to retain a pessary since the operation narrowed the levator or genital hiatus. Pessary use was gradually supplanted by vaginal hysterectomy and appropriate repair when these procedures became safer, more effective, and more popular for treatment of genital prolapse. Although pessary use has faded into the background, the procedures it helped engender have permitted the evolution of an erroneous concept suggesting that a firm perineum will function as a "cork in the neck of a bottle" and that perineorrhaphy would retard or prevent uterine prolapse. To the contrary, Kelly had previously observed that uterine prolapse was uncommon among the many women who had long before suffered unrepaired complete perineal tear.[6]

Rectocele and perineal defects most commonly develop from rapid overdistention of the vaginal wall during labor, although there may be congenital perineal defects related to underdevelopment of the perineal body. Such obstetric damage is more common in those patients in whom the elastic tissue component is reduced. It is more frequent in the primipara who is more than 25 years old, and may be predicted as more frequent among persons with an abundance of wide abdominal striae, which imply a low elastic index.[7] The risk of subsequent rectocele and perineal defect may be lessened for such a patient by early and adequate episiotomy during labor and delivery, followed by a careful and meticulous repair bringing

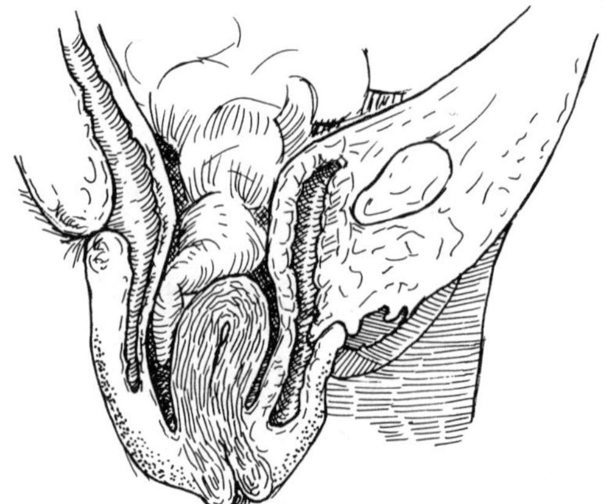

FIG 7–5.
Procidentia may evolve as a result of unrestrained progression of any of the types of prolapse. (Redrawn from Nichols DH: *Postgrad Med* 1969; 46:183–187.)

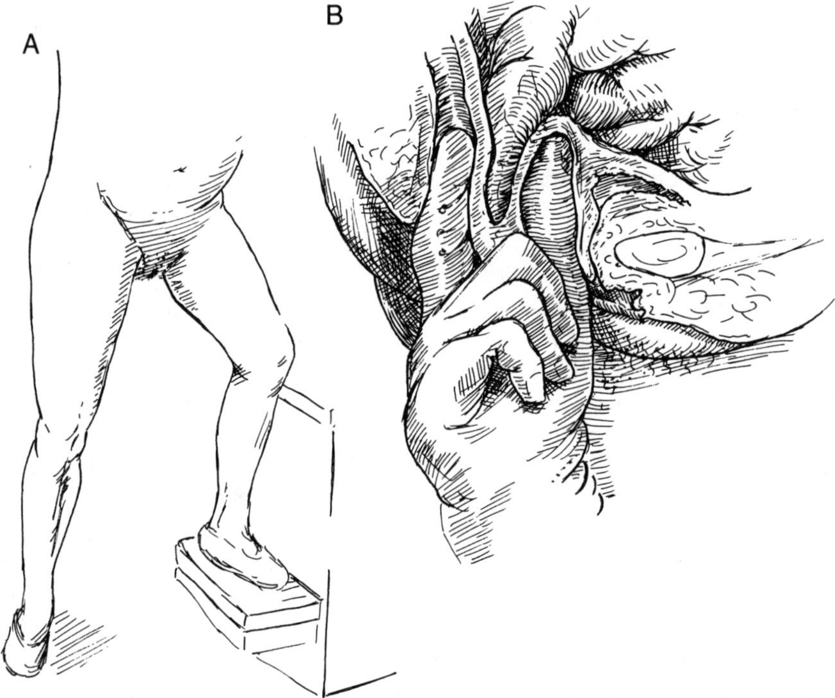

FIG 7–6.
Examination of the patient in a standing position **(A)** permits the thumb in the vagina **(B)** to note and replace any descent of the vaginal vault while the index finger introduced into the rectum permits evaluation of any possible rectocele. When the patient strains, any enterocele present is evidenced by palpation of a bowel-filled sac dissecting the rectovaginal septum. (Redrawn from Nichols DH: Repair of enterocele and prolapse of the vaginal vault, in Barber H [ed]: *Goldsmith's Practice of Surgery*. Philadelphia, JB Lippincott Co, 1981.)

back together those tissues that have been cut. Weakness of the supports of the posterior vaginal wall may also develop coincident with massive eversion of the vagina attended by a shearing or avulsing of the fibers attaching the vagina to the pelvic diaphragm. This displacement of the vagina, another cause of rectocele, creates a large area of weakness into which the anterior rectal wall may expand, sometimes massively (Fig 7–5).

Preliminary pelvic examination of the unanesthetized patient should attempt to correlate the findings with the patient's symptoms. Examination of the patient when she is standing and straining (Fig 7–6) may disclose a coincident and often unsuspected prolapse of the vaginal vault. When found, remedy of this defect should be included as well in the plan for surgical reconstruction.

Because the length of the perineal body approximates that of the female urethra, reconstruction of a damaged perineum will improve urethral support and future function. Curiously, it will also lengthen the vagina.

TECHNIQUE OF REPAIR

The goals of reconstructive surgery are (1) relief of symptoms, (2) restoration of normal anatomic relationships, and (3) restoration of function. Surgical repair of the posterior vaginal wall should endeavor to recreate or duplicate a normal anatomic relationship in which there are an intact and effective perineal body, attachment of the upper margin of the perineal body to the fascia of Denonvilliers, and elimination of the weak spot in the midportion of an overdistended and thus enlarged vagina, but with preservation of the rectovaginal space that will permit continued independent function of the vagina and rectum. Secondary ballooning of the anterior rectal wall can be corrected by plication. If there is eversion of the vaginal vault, this should be corrected by coincident colpopexy, performed either transvaginally as in sacrospinous colpopexy or transabdominally as in sacral colpopexy (see Chapter 5). Any coincident enterocele should be surgically eliminated.

Long-acting but absorbable sutures of the polyglycolic acid type have replaced those of catgut, in our practice, because they provide a longer period of support during wound healing, less edema and discomfort interfering with restoration of function, and elimination of batch-to-batch variability in suture strength. If postmenopausal, the patient is started preoperatively on a course of estrogen replacement using an intravaginal estrogen cream, which is continued for several months postoperatively. It will restore and improve vaginal elasticity and, by increasing the vaginal blood supply and thickening the vaginal wall, promote better wound healing.

Dissection and repair of rectocele should begin above the highest point of weakness. The undersurface of the perineal body is uncovered from beneath a V-shaped skin incision (Fig 7–7), the width of which is determined by the width of the introitus desired at the conclusion of the operation. Care should be taken to leave the introitus somewhat loose for the aging patient so that postoperative coital obstruction does not become a problem.

With the patient for whom perineorrhaphy is not necessary, a midline episiotomy will provide access to the lower portion of the vagina. The dissection is carried beneath the posterior vaginal wall, separating it from the vaginal surface of the perineal body, until the rectovaginal space is identified and opened. An appropriately

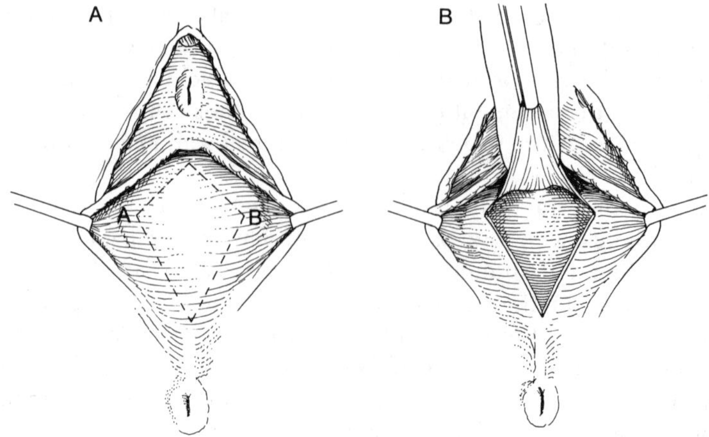

FIG 7–7.
An initial V-shaped incision between points *A* and *B* is indicated by the *dashed line* **(A).** A flap will be mobilized by sharp dissection **(B)** and the incisions carried under and up the posterior vaginal wall to a point cranial to the rectocele. At the conclusion of the repair, the tissue identified by *A* will meet *B,* and the circumference of the introitus will be narrowed by the preselected distance *AB.* (Redrawn from Nichols DH, Randall CL: *Vaginal Surgery,* ed 3. Baltimore, Williams & Wilkins Co, 1989.)

wide strip of the full thickness of the posterior vaginal wall is removed to a point cranial to the rectocele (Fig 7–8). If high rectocele is present, the removal of this strip extends the full length of the vagina to the vault. Failure to correct rectocele for its full depth leaves a residual weakness in the midvagina that superficially resembles enterocele (see Fig 8–12), but careful examination discloses the residual rectocele, which is often still symptomatic. Careful examination of the undersurface of the vagina will identify the fascia of Denonvilliers attached to it. The fascia can

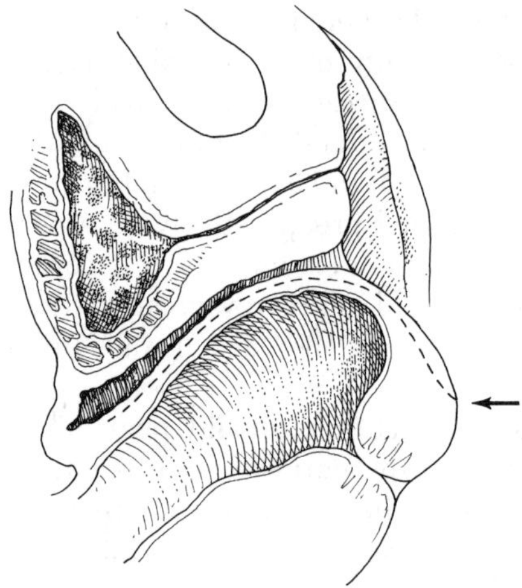

FIG 7–8.
Sagittal section showing the initial line of dissection exposing the full perineum in the rectocele. Above the perineum, the dissection enters the rectovaginal space and continues to a point proximal and above the rectocele. The incision begins at the spot indicated by the *arrow,* and its course follows the *dashed line.* (Redrawn from Nichols DH, Randall CL: *Vaginal Surgery,* ed 3. Baltimore, Williams & Wilkins Co, 1989.)

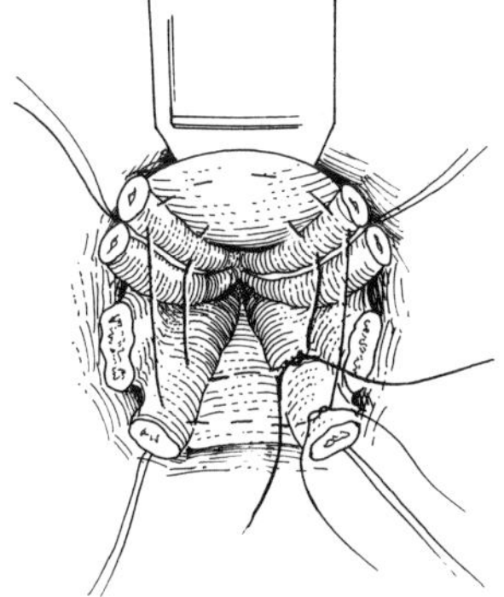

FIG 7–9.
The enterocele sac has been resected and the peritoneal cavity has been closed by a pursestring suture that incorporates the uterosacral and round ligaments. A second purse string stitch, placed 1 cm distal to the first, reinforces the closure. (Redrawn from Nichols DH, Randall CL: *Vaginal Surgery,* ed 3. Baltimore, Williams & Wilkins Co, 1989.)

be identified by touch. It has a smooth peritoneum–like feel. If further dissection reveals the double fold of peritoneum so characteristic of an enterocele, the sac should be opened, the neck closed by high ligation, a second ligation placed 1 cm distal to the first (Fig 7–9), and the excess peritoneum excised.[8] This double ligation of the neck of the sac will not only take the tension from the initial closing stitch of the peritoneum but will increase the thickness of the scar in this area, making it more resistant to recurrence of the enterocele. Closure of the neck of the en-

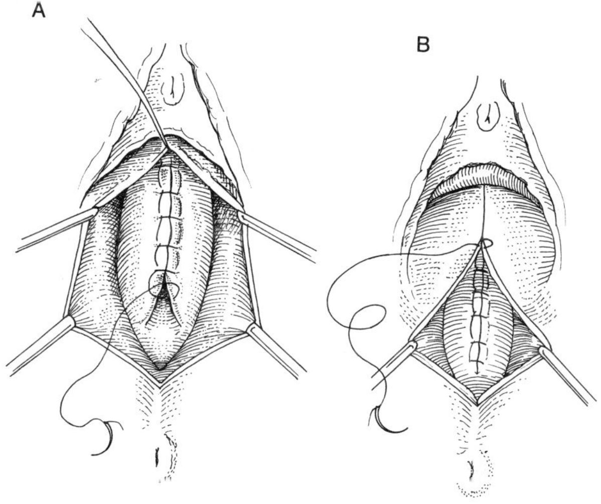

FIG 7–10.
Any ballooning of the anterior rectal wall may be corrected by one or more layers of running, locked, fine absorbable suture commencing proximal to the defect and continuing distally for its full length. Reconstitution may be carried posterior to the site of the new perineal body, not yet restored **(A).** Side-to-side closure of the full thickness of the posterior vaginal wall is accomplished by running, subcuticular sutures **(B).** The cranial margin of the perineal body is reattached to the underside of the vagina at the bottom of the rectovaginal space. The perineal body is reconstructed by a series of interrupted stitches. (Redrawn from Nichols DH, Randall CL: *Vaginal Surgery,* ed 3. Baltimore, Williams & Wilkins Co, 1989.)

terocele sac not only brings together the thin mesothelial epithelium of the peritoneal cavity but also incorporates the rather strong subperitoneal retinaculum of connective tissue to increase the strength of the peritoneal floor. If strong uterosacral ligaments can be identified at the vault of the vagina, they should be sewn together in the midline.

Any ballooning of the anterior rectal wall and its fascia may be reduced by a layer or two of running locked suture continued to the perineum (Fig 7–10).

The cut edges of the vagina are brought together by a running subcuticular suture that goes well back into the fascia of Denonvilliers,[9] thickening the posterior vaginal wall (Fig 7–11). When the subcuticular vaginal wall suture has reached the site of the cranial edge of the perineal body, a stitch should be taken in this cranial edge, reestablishing the attachment that is normally present between perineal body and fascia of Denonvilliers. At the conclusion of the posterior colporrhaphy and before the perineorrhaphy, the operator should be able to insert a finger into the rectovaginal space, demonstrating the freedom of the posterior vaginal wall from the rectum (Fig 7–12).

Some operators prefer to split the rectovaginal septum (including the fascia of Denonvilliers and a few fibers of the fibromuscular wall of the vagina to which the fascia is attached) from the vaginal wall and close this as a separate layer (Fig 7–13). The residual vaginal membrane is then trimmed appropriately and closed by subcuticular suture. This method, particularly in the older patient, not only risks disturbing the vaginal blood supply with some increased postoperative fibrosis and longer wound healing but also renders less precise the amount of vaginal wall that should be removed. The amount of vagina to be excised with posterior colporrhaphy

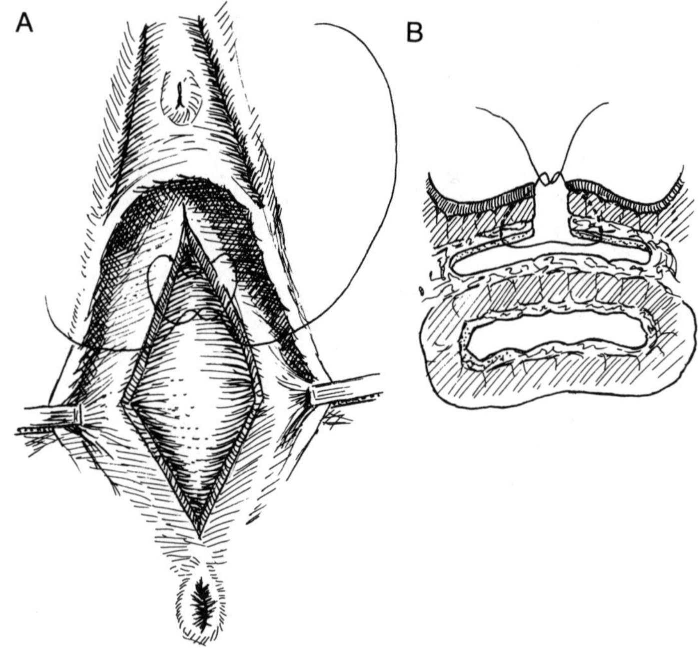

FIG 7–11.
A full-thickness wedge of posterior vaginal wall has been excised, and the tissues, including a fused rectovaginal septum (the fascia of Denonvilliers) are closed from side to side **(A)** using a running, subcuticular suture **(B).**

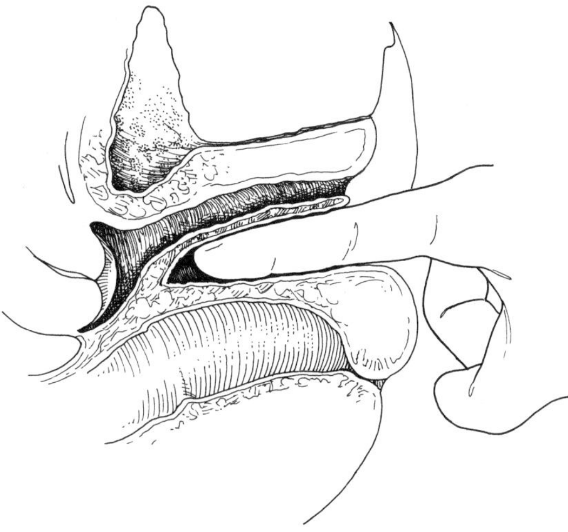

FIG 7–12.
At the completion of the posterior colporrhaphy and before starting the perineorrhaphy, the operator should be able to insert an index finger between the posterior vaginal wall, to which the rectovaginal septum (fascia of Denonvilliers) is attached, and the anterior surface of the rectum, demonstrating the desired freedom of this space. (Redrawn from Nichols DH, Randall CL: *Vaginal Surgery,* ed 3. Baltimore, Williams & Wilkins Co, 1989.)

should be such that at the conclusion of the operation the vagina will admit three fingers, unless preoperative inquiry reveals that the patient's coital partner differs from this size.

During posterior colporrhaphy and reconstruction, the operator at all times should check frequently for the presence of palpable subepithelial ridges, which, if found, should be immediately relieved by cutting the offending suture. Such ridges will invariably remain postoperatively, often becoming symptomatic and tender and forming a coital obstruction. Because of their fibrosis, they can be very difficult to stretch.

The perineal body is reconstructed by a series of horizontal interrupted mattress stitches placed in the soft tissues medial to the pubococcygei and including the smooth muscle of the perineum (Fig 7–14). Although these stitches are not

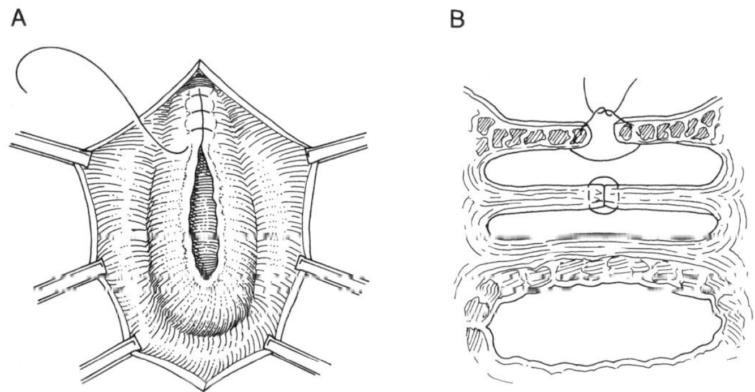

FIG 7–13.
Bullard modification, in which the rectovaginal septum has been dissected from the posterior vaginal wall and closed as a separate layer between the rectum and the vaginal membrane **(A).** The excess vaginal skin is trimmed and the sides brought together by subcuticular suture **(B).** (Redrawn from Nichols DH, Randall CL: *Vaginal Surgery,* ed 3. Baltimore, Williams & Wilkins Co, 1989.)

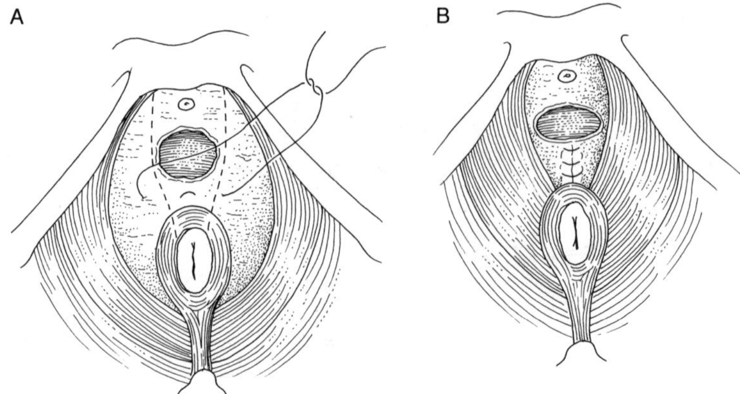

FIG 7–14.
Perineorrhaphy may be accomplished without placement of stitches directly into the muscle bellies of the pubococcygei. The wide genital hiatus is shown in **A** and the normal position of the medial borders of the pubococcygei indicated by the *dashed line.* When the interrupted stitches **(A)** have been tied, the lateral attachments of this tissue to the fascia of the pubococcygei will bring the latter closer together, narrowing the genital hiatus **(B).** No stitches have been placed directly into the muscular substance of the pubococcygei, nor do the muscles cross or come together at the midline of the vagina, which might produce a palpable and painful ridge. (Redrawn from Nichols DH, Randall CL: *Vaginal Surgery,* ed 3. Baltimore, Williams & Wilkins Co, 1989.)

placed in the bellies of the levator muscles themselves, the tissues into which they have been put are attached to the medial borders of the pelvic diaphragm. When these stitches are tied, they will effectively narrow the levator hiatus without the risk of levator spasm, fibrosis, and tenderness.

In an occasional patient, there is a perineal defect for which no soft tissues can be found to be brought together. In such a patient, "levator muscle stitches" can be placed, although the operator should check after each stitch for ridge production. If a ridge is found, the stitch is removed and replaced by one located closer to the rectum. Levator stitches should never be tied tightly, because they may destroy the muscle in which they have been placed and convert it to a tender band of fibrous tissue, which may require future secondary perineotomy for relief.

The perineal skin is reapproximated in the midline by a running subcuticular suture. Finally, the caliber of the vagina is assessed carefully with consideration of future coital satisfaction. If it is unexpectedly constricted, appropriate full-thickness lateral vaginal wall relaxing incisions are made at the 3 or 9 o'clock positions (or both). With relaxing incisions, a vaginal packing or postoperative vaginal obturator must be inserted to prevent postoperative constriction. The obturator is removed frequently for cleaning but is kept in place until a firm bed of granulation tissue has been formed and reepithelialization is underway.

Rectal examination is performed to confirm the integrity of the rectum. If a transgressing stitch is found, it is cut on the rectal side and allowed to retract. Cutting such a stitch lessens postoperative pain and the risk of rectovaginal fistula.

POSTOPERATIVE CARE

The patient is placed on a regular diet but uses stool softeners and gentle laxatives so as to avoid straining against the fresh repair while having a bowel movement. Ascorbic acid is given for 1 month or longer to promote wound healing, and postoperative estrogen supplementation is given if the patient is postmenopausal. Coitus may be resumed after 4 to 6 weeks of healing on the first or second postoperative day. The patient is started on isometric perineal resistive exercises (15 strong voluntary pubococcygeal contractions, each of 3 seconds' duration, 6 times daily) to be continued for at least 3 months. This will aid both in reestablishing perineal circulation and in restoring physiologic bowel function and habits.

When a patient with rectocele and perineal defect receives only a perineorrhaphy as her surgical treatment, the unrepaired rectocele persists as such, and if she was previously symptomatic, the rectal symptoms of incomplete bowel movement and postevacuation pressure and aching, remain. The physical appearance within the vagina masquerades as enterocele (see Fig 8–11), but the true nature of the persistent rectocele is evident by rectovaginal examination, particularly in the standing patient who is bearing down. Failure to carry a rectocele repair high enough to a point beyond the upper limit of the defect produces this clinical and anatomic picture. It is corrected by transvaginal reoperation with more extensive rectocele repair, which is dissected and then repaired starting at the highest point of the rectocele.

SUMMARY

Recurrent rectocele should be approached thoughtfully and evaluated with great care to assure correlation between symptoms and findings. Physical examination should determine all areas of weakness so that their repair may be incorporated in the final surgical plan. A search for unexpected prolapse of the vaginal vault should be made by examination of the patient in a standing position. If found, it should be corrected. Any coincident enterocele should be identified and surgically repaired.

REFERENCES

1. Henry MM, Swash M: *Colpoproctology and the Pelvic Floor*. London, Butterworth, 1985.
2. Nichols DH: Retrorectal levatorplasty with colporrhaphy. *Clin Obstet Gynecol* 1982; 25:939–947.
3. Milley PS, Nichols DH: A correlative investigation of the human rectovaginal septum. *Anat Rec* 1969; 163:443–447.
4. Berglas B, Rubin IC: Study of the supportive structures of the uterus by levator myography. *Surg Gynecol Obstet* 1953; 97:677–692.
5. Jeffcoate TNA: Posterior Colporrhaphy. *Am J Obstet Gynecol* 1959; 77:490.
6. Kelly HA: *Operative Gynecology*, Vol I. New York, Butterworth, 1898, p 506.
7. Magdi I: Obstetric injuries of the perineum. *J Obstet Gynaecol Br Emp* 1942; 49:687–700.
8. Nichols DH, Randall CL: *Vaginal Surgery*, ed 3. Baltimore, Williams & Wilkins Co, 1989, p 406.
9. Harrison JE, McDonagh JE: Hernia of Douglas' pouch and high rectocele. *Am J Obstet Gynecol* 1950; 60:83.

Chapter 8

Recurrent Enterocele

David H. Nichols, M.D.

When a primary repair has unsuccessfully correlated the cause of an enterocele with a technique of repair specifically designed to correct the etiology, recurrence of the enterocele is not only possible, but likely, bringing with it a recurrence of both symptoms and physical findings. This necessitates re-repair, but using a choice of more effective technique. The surgeon must decide whether the enterocele is truly recurrent or is only persistent.

For successful re-repair, it is desirable to determine the correct etiology. This usually may be correlated with the findings on physical examination. These observations correlate, in turn, with the optimal specific surgical treatment.

ETIOLOGY

There are four principal causes of enterocele: (1) congenital, (2) pulsion, (3) traction, and (4) iatrogenic from a change in the vaginal axis.

Congenital Enterocele

Congenital enterocele is identified by a deep cul-de-sac that contains bowel, usually small intestine, and often omentum (Fig 8–1,A).[1] It is a consequence of failure of fusion or defusion of the peritoneal walls of the cul-de-sac, which in fetal life extends all the way to the perineal body. Fusion of the anterior and posterior layers of perineum produces a strong surgically useful layer of the fascia of Denonvilliers. This peritoneal fusion fascia is firmly attached to the underside of the posterior vaginal wall; the very nature of this adherence giving some strength one to the other.

The presence of bowel within this deep cul-de-sac extending between the rectum and vagina is responsible for the symptoms of enterocele (e.g., backache and pulling). The symptoms are worse in the erect position and intensify as the day goes on, the consequence of the pull of gravity on the bowel and its elongated mesentery. Filling of the sac may produce a coincident sensation of vaginal fullness. These

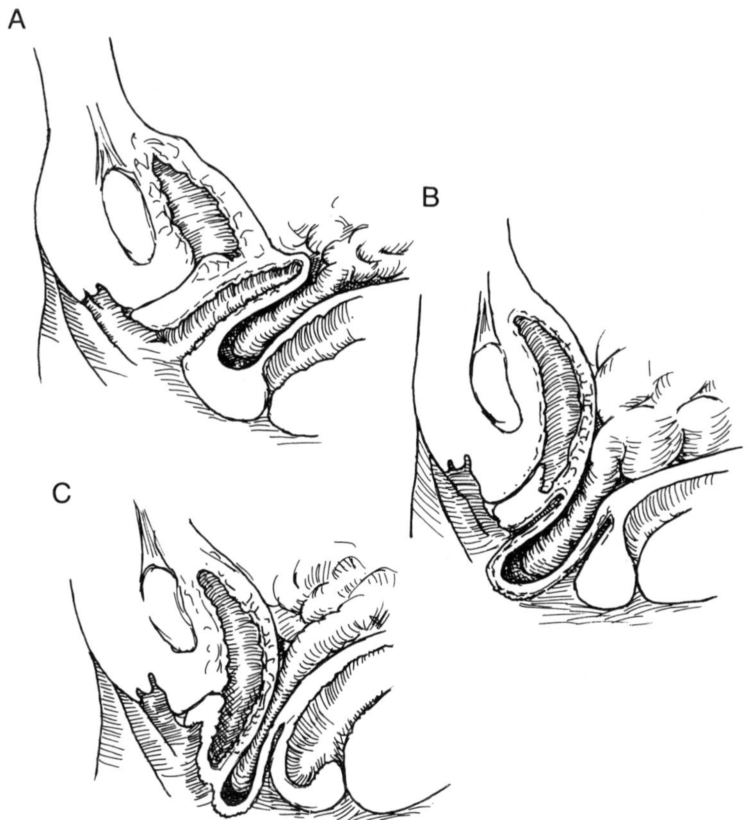

FIG 8–1.
A, congenital-type posterior enterocele without eversion of the vagina in the posthysterectomy patient. **B,** pulsion enterocele in a posthysterectomy patient. The vaginal vault is everted, bringing with it an enterocele, but there is no significant cystocele nor rectocele. **C,** traction enterocele in which there is eversion of the vault and lower portion of the vagina and including enterocele, cystocele, and rectocele. There is a notable change in the urethral axis with descent of the vesicourethral junction. (Redrawn from Nichols DH: *Obstet Gynecol* 1972; 40:257–263.)

symptoms are relieved by lying down, when gravity pulls the intestine and its contents in a different direction, relieving the painful pull on the mesentery. A deep cul-de-sac without bowel content is itself not necessarily an enterocele, but it is a potential one. For there to be bowel within the sac, the intestinal mesentery must be pathologically long. A question might be asked as to whether this mesenteric elongation is the cause or the result of the deep cul-de-sac, and the answer is not clear. It is certain, however, that once this elongation develops, whatever the etiology, it will remain and serve to make persistent pressure against the site in an enterocele repair, often with persistance of symptoms of backache and pressure. It is, therefore, necessary that the repair be firm and strong enough to effectively resist this pressure if the chance of recurrence of enterocele is to be minimized.

Physical findings of the congenital type of enterocele include the presence of a deep cul-de-sac of Douglas and palpation of bowel within the sac, best appreciated when a rectovaginal examination is performed when the patient is standing and bearing down, as by a Valsalva maneuver. There need be no prolapse of the vaginal vault nor coincident cystocele and rectocele.

Spinal anesthesia reduces the postoperative strain against the fresh repair that is more common coincident with nausea and vomiting following recovery from a general anesthetic. Intrathecal or epidural anesthesia further assures surgical success of the reoperation by removing or minimizing this unnecessary postoperative strain.

The surgical treatment is by exposure and opening of the peritoneal sac, high ligation of its neck using a synthetic permanent or long-lasting suture, usually accompanied by a second ligation 1 cm distal to the first (Fig 8–2).[2] This will increase the thickness and firmness of the scar and provide suture reinforcement, one for the other. This is accomplished, alternately in the patient with a very wide enterocele, by obliterating the sac with a series of sagittally placed sutures. After all of the sutures have been tied, a reinforcing purse string suture is placed, the excess peritoneum is excised and the vaginal wall closed, preferably in a vertical direction.

Pulsion Enterocele

Enterocele may exist with or without coincident prolapse of the vaginal vault; just a prolapse of the vault may occur with or without enterocele, though most frequently with. Chronically increased intra-abdominal pressure seems etiologically significant, especially when the vault is poorly supported, is short (ending anterior to the margin of the levator plate), or there is an anteriorly inclined vaginal axis.

The condition, which may produce feelings of pelvic fullness, backache, and falling out, all made worse when the patient is in the erect position, can be best demonstrated when the vagina is examined with the patient is standing and while straining (see Fig 7–6). Because the primary weakness is in the supporting tissues of the upper portion of the vagina, coincident cystocele and rectocele may be absent (see Fig 8–1,B). Treatment requires opening and high ligation of the neck,

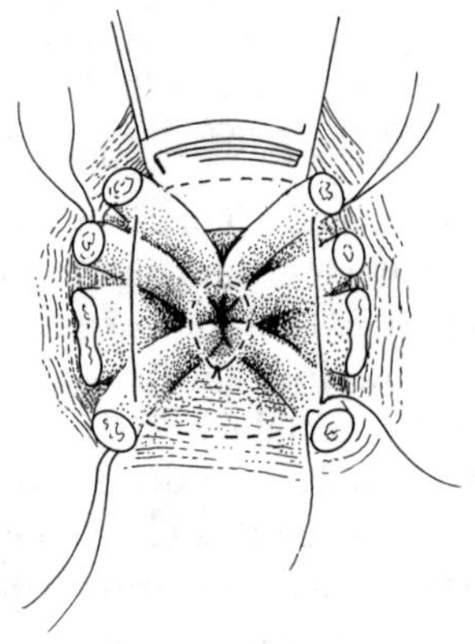

FIG 8–2.
The enterocele has been resected and the peritoneal cavity closed by a pursestring suture that starts on the peritoneal side of the left uterosacral ligament, reefs the posterior peritoneum, the right uterosacral ligament, right round ligament, anterior peritoneum, and left round ligament. After this has been tied, a second pursestring suture is placed 1 cm distal to the first, reinforcing the closure. (Redrawn from Nichols DH, Randall CL: *Vaginal Surgery,* ed 3. Baltimore, Williams & Wilkins Co, 1989.)

then excision of the sac, followed by appropriate colpopexy, which will restore a normal vaginal axis. Colpopexy can be accomplished by either the transvaginal route (sacrospinous ligament fixation) or the transabdominal route (sacral colpopexy). Unless there are coincident cystocele and rectocele, simultaneous colporrhaphy is unnecessary.

Traction Enterocele

Traction enterocele is the consequence of downward pulling of a poorly supported vaginal vault by progressively enlarging cystocele and rectocele, which are invariably present (see Fig 8–1,C), and may or may not be symptomatic. Again, the pathology of pelvic support here is best demonstrated by pelvic examination of the erect patient who is straining. Vault descent with enterocele, cystocele, and rectocele are readily demonstrated. Surgical treatment is by dissection and opening of the enterocele, high double pursestring ligation of its neck, excision of the redundant peritoneum, colpopexy, and colporrhaphy, restoring both vaginal depth and caliber, and axis. This combination of procedures will not only relieve the patient's symptoms but also aid in restoring the normal anatomic relationships and organ functions.

Iatrogenic Enterocele

Iatrogenic enterocele is the consequence of a surgical change in the normal vaginal axis, thus leaving the cul-de-sac of Douglas unprotected and exposing it to the full range of changes in intra-abdominal pressure that occur daily. The most common surgery that produces this change in vaginal axis is the Marshall-Marchetti-Krantz[3] or the Burch[4] procedure, each of which pulls the vagina in an abnormal anterior direction, exposing the cul-de-sac, unless specific intraperitoneal surgical steps are taken to obliterate the cul-de-sac.

Ventral suspension of the vagina or the uterus incurs the same risk, in addition to limiting the volume of bladder filling, which may give rise to overflow incontinence (Fig 8–3). A pathologically wide vaginal vault is especially vulnerable to future prolapse and enterocele formation. Intraperitoneal obliteration may be produced by the sagittally placed sutures (Fig 8–4) described by Halban,[5] which cannot pull on the path of the ureter as might happen occasionally when sequential pursestring obliterative Moschcowitz sutures[6] are used, originally but ineffectually introduced to treat rectal prolapse.

This postsurgical abnormal vaginal axis is readily demonstrable during pelvic examination.

Treatment includes high ligation of the neck of the sac, with resection of excess peritoneum, and restoration of a normal horizontally inclined vaginal axis. If there is coincident vault prolapse, colpopexy is required, and if there are strong but long uterosacral ligaments, the New Orleans or McCall[7] type of culdeplasty may be used effectively (Figs 8–5 to 8–7). If strong and surgically useful ligaments are absent, transvaginal sacrospinous or transabdominal sacral colpopexy are useful (see Chapter 5). Correction of an abnormal pelvic tilt from a patient's poor posture is helpful.

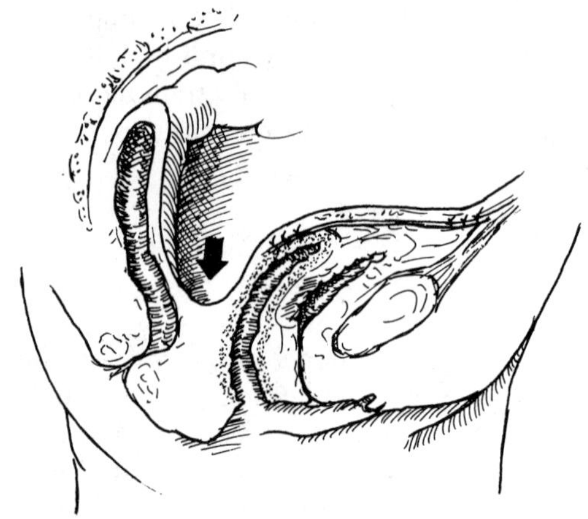

FIG 8–3.
Change in the vaginal axis, as by ventral fixation, will expose an otherwise unprotected cul-de-sac *(arrow)*, risking progressive enterocele and prolapse of the posterior vaginal vault. (Redrawn from Nichols DH: Repair of enterocele and prolapse of the vaginal vault, in Barber H [ed]: *Goldsmith's Practice of Surgery*. Philadelphia, JB Lippincott Co, 1981.)

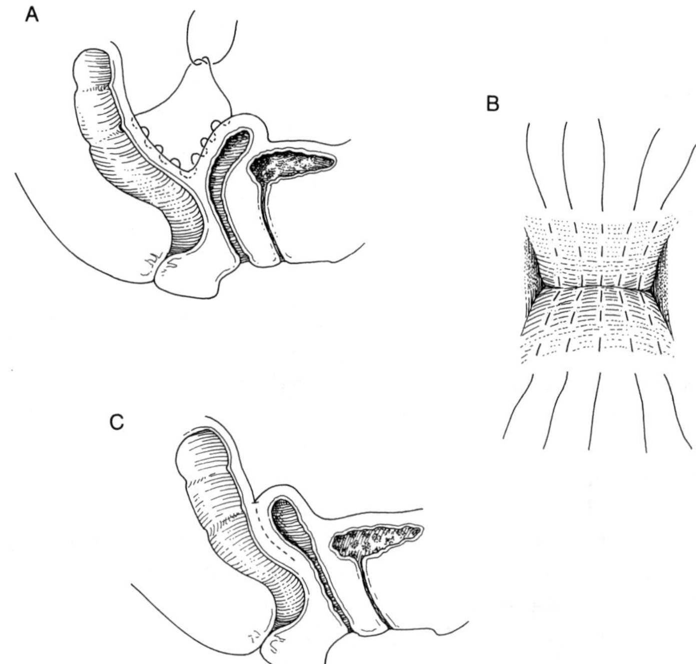

FIG 8–4.
The cul-de-sac of Douglas may be obliterated by a series of sutures placed in the sagittal plane. After all of them have been placed, they are tied sequentially, fusing the posterior vaginal wall and vaginal vault to the anterior surface of the rectum. Stitches placed in this sagittal fashion do not disturb the course of the ureter. (Redrawn from Nichols DH, Randall CL: *Vaginal Surgery*, ed 3. Baltimore, Williams & Wilkins Co, 1989.)

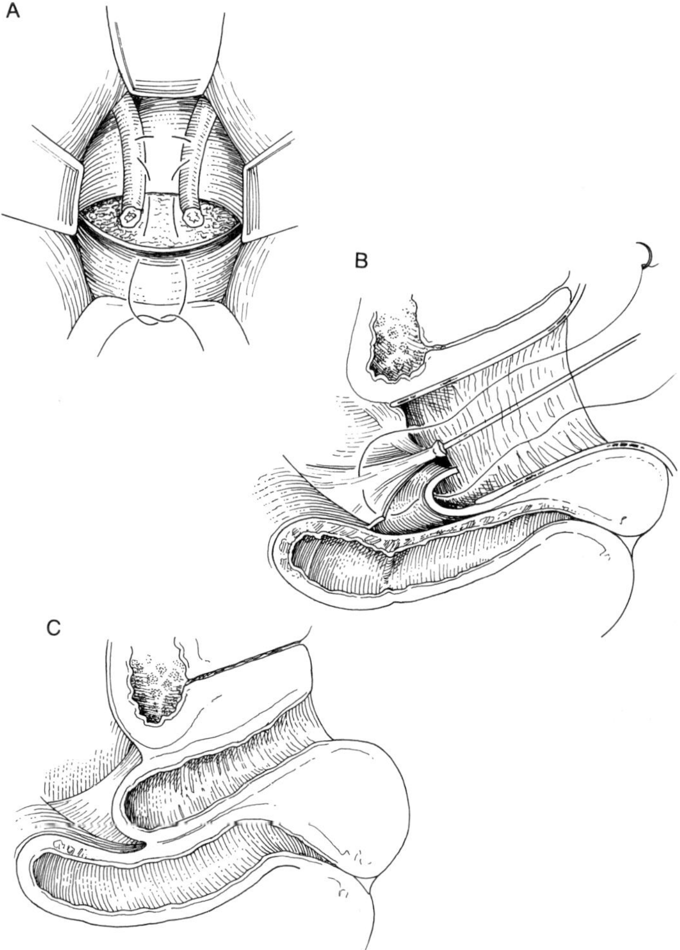

FIG 8–5.
Modified cul-de-plasty. **A,** the enterocele sac has been resected, and a long-lasting synthetic absorbable suture has been placed through the vault of the vagina and cut edge of peritoneum. Traction on the stumps of the strong but long uterosacral ligaments *(arrows)* permits a deep bite into the substance of the left uterosacral ligament, then through the peritoneum covering the anterior surface of the rectum and the same structures on the opposite side. **B,** suture placement in the sagittal section. **C,** effects of tying and subsequent closure of the peritoneal cavity. The apex of the vagina is now cranial and posterior to the new peritoneal closure. (Redrawn from Nichols DH, Randall CL: *Vaginal Surgery,* ed 3. Baltimore, Williams & Wilkins Co, 1989.)

ANTERIOR ENTEROCELE

When a surgeon has experienced difficulty finding the anterior peritoneal fold during vaginal hysterectomy and has dissected for some distance beneath the uterine peritoneum before opening it (Fig 8–8), an excess of anterior peritoneal flap remains that should be removed before peritonealization. Failure to recognize this redundancy in the anterior peritoneum is as troublesome as it is in the posterior peritoneum. The redundant peritoneum is not always obvious during hysterectomy when the patient is anesthetized and in the usual Trendelenberg position. Failure

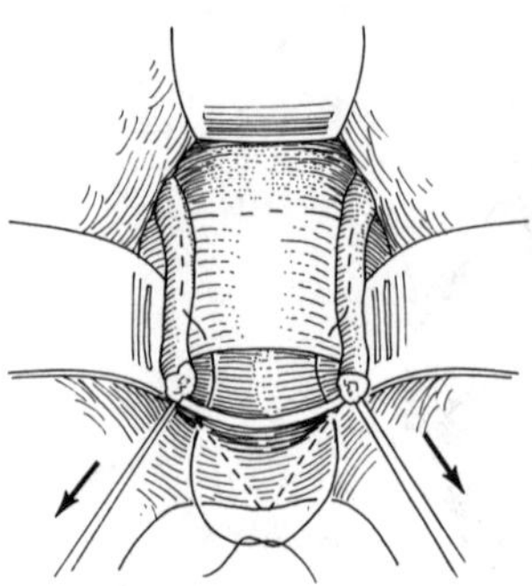

FIG 8–6.
A pathologically wide vaginal vault should be narrowed by excision of a V-shaped wedge *(dashed line)*. (Redrawn from Nichols DH, Randall CL: *Vaginal Surgery,* ed 3. Baltimore, Williams & Wilkins Co, 1989.)

to recognize and resect to this redundant peritoneum is invariably followed by enterocele, in the former instance, anterior to the vagina (Fig 8–9). Preoperatively, it resembles the appearance of recurrent cystocele, but the distinction becomes obvious during reoperation when the peritoneum lined sac is opened. Treatment is by high ligation and excision of the sac.

MISCELLANEOUS TYPES OF ENTEROCELE

Obturator Hernia

Recurrent obturator hernia is a rare occurrence. The hernia is one in which the sac penetrates the pelvic diaphragm (Fig 8–10) and may recur if the suture line holding the neck shut becomes disrupted. The pain, often a sudden onset, may be bizarre. It may run down the leg, particularly when the patient is standing. More

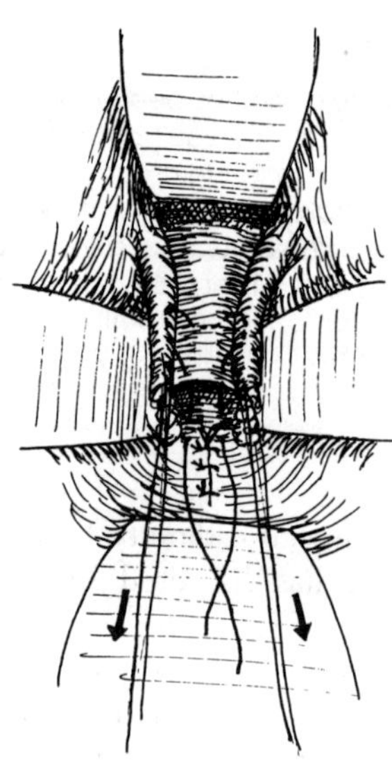

FIG 8–7.
The edges of the V are sewn together, thus narrowing a pathologically wide vaginal vault.

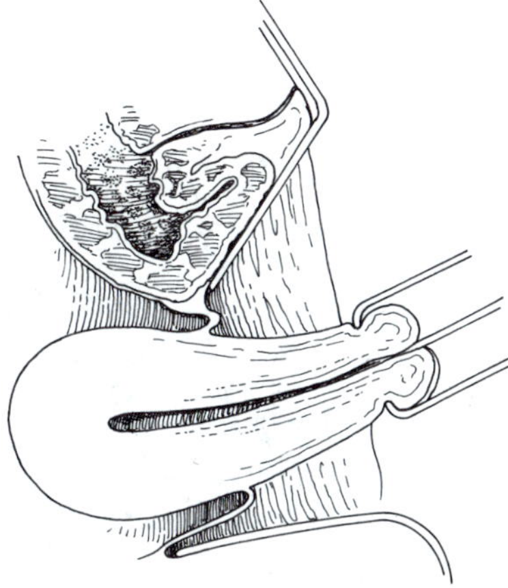

FIG 8–8.
During vaginal hysterectomy, the bladder has been separated by sharp dissection from the lower uterine segment and held out of the way by an appropriate retractor. If the anterior peritoneum is dissected and opened far cranially, failure to resect this redundant peritoneum before peritonealization will risk subsequent anterior enterocele. (Redrawn from Nichols DH, Randall CL: *Vaginal Surgery,* ed 3. Baltimore, Williams & Wilkins Co, 1989.)

commonly, there is an acute intestinal obstruction, partial or complete, manifested by the usual nausea, vomiting, and abdominal distention, because a loop of small bowel becomes trapped in the neck of the sac. The diagnosis is suspected by a history of previous obturator hernia. There may or may not be a precipitating incidence of sudden increase in intraperitoneal pressure, as during a fit of coughing, which disrupts the previous repair. Examination of a flat plate or gastrointestinal series may show a loop of bowel identified as outside the pelvis. It will, of course, be in the hernial sac. The patient has lower abdominal tenderness and distention, and if the hernia extends low in the pelvis, it may occasionally be palpated as a tender mass beneath the lateral wall of the vagina. If it should follow the canal of Nuck, it may be palpable within a labium majora.

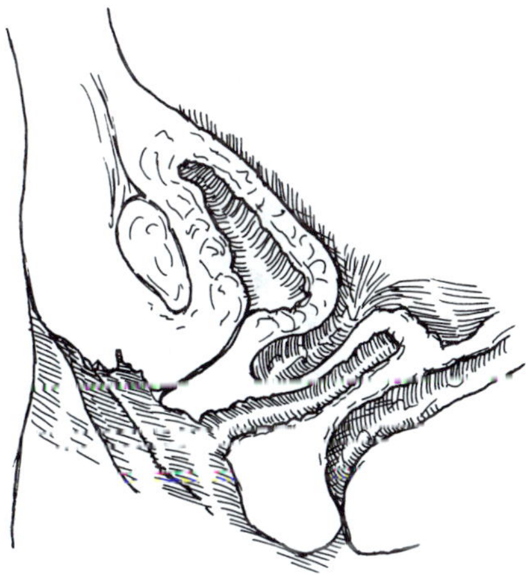

FIG 8–9.
Sagittal view of an anterior enterocele located between the bladder and the anterior vaginal wall of a posthysterectomy patient. (Redrawn from Nichols DH: *Obstet Gynecol* 1972; 40:257–263.)

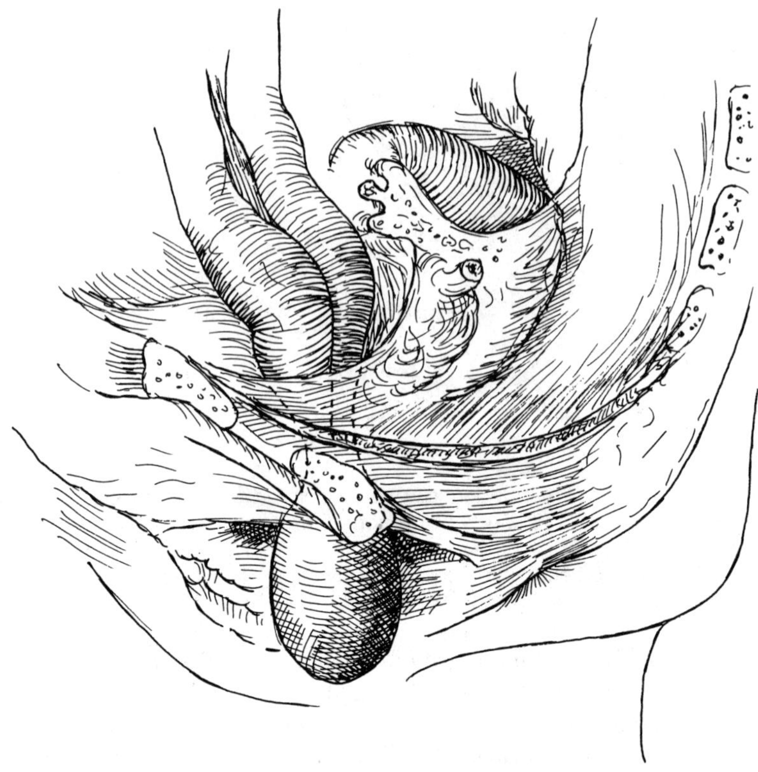

FIG 8–10.
Lateral or pudendal enterocele projecting through a pathologic opening in the pelvic diaphragm or into the obturator canal. Notice the constriction of the bowel that may favor intestinal obstruction. (Redrawn from Nichols DH: *Obstet Gynecol* 1972; 40:257–263.)

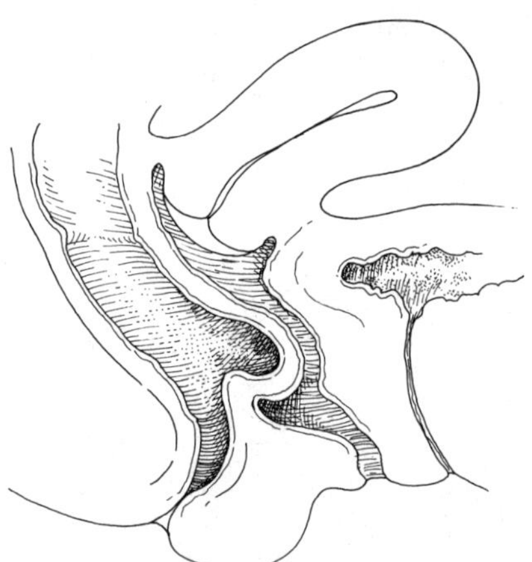

FIG 8–11.
Perineorrhaphy may hide an unrepaired midvaginal rectocele, which may masquerade as a pseudoenterocele. Effective repair must always begin proximal to the weakness. (Redrawn from Nichols DH, Randall CL: *Vaginal Surgery,* ed 3. Baltimore, Williams & Wilkins Co, 1989.)

Abdominal Hernias

Recurrent umbilical, femoral, or inguinal hernia is in a sense enterocele. The latter usually refers generically to pudendal hernia, but it is a cumbersome term not often used. These miscellaneous hernias are represented by the reappearance of a soft mass at the site of the previous herniation and repair. The content of the sac is usually reducible. However, if it becomes incarcerated, edema, swelling, and pain supervene, and an emergency re-repair often using a layer or two of permanent-type suture material is necessary (see Chapter 3).

Pseudoenterocele

Persistent unrepaired rectocele, as may be seen in a patient with rectocele who has received only a perineorrhaphy for repair, looks very much like an enterocele on superficial examination (Fig 8–11), but its true nature is revealed by vaginal examination, particularly in the standing patient. It may have all the symptoms of the original rectocele, incomplete bowel movements and postevacuation aching, and is treated by reoperation and more extensive posterior colporrhaphy to repair the entire rectocele.

SUMMARY

We have seen how the cause of a specific enterocele can be correlated with its location, which, in turn, correlates with the recommended surgical treatment (Table 8–1). This can apply to both the common and the rare type of enterocele. Appropriate choice of suture and surgical operation, correctly performed, and usually using synthetic long-acting or permanent suture material, will result in effective relief of symptoms and restoration of normal anatomic relationships and function. Appropriate choice of specific treatment reducing the chance for reoccurrence and its attendant risks, discomforts, and expense, are well worth the trouble.

TABLE 8–1.
Enterocele Correlation

Type and Cause	Location	Treatment
Congenital	Posterior to vagina	Excision of the sac with high ligation of its neck
Pulsion (pushed)	With eversion of vaginal vault	Restoration of vault depth by transvaginal sacrospinous fixation, or transabdominal sacropexy if cardinal and uterosacral strength is poor or culdeplasty if strong; coincident hysterectomy often desirable
Traction (pulled)	Lower vaginal eversion (cystocele and rectocele) pulling vault into descent and upper vaginal eversion	Same for pulsion plus anterior and posterior colporrhaphy
Iatrogenic	Anterior to vagina, or posterior from change in vaginal axis	Excision or obliteration of sac and restoration of normal vaginal axis, if defective

REFERENCES

1. Nichols DH: Types of enterocele and principles underlying the choice of operation for repair. *Obstet Gynecol* 1972; 40:257–263.
2. Nichols DH, Randall CL: *Vaginal Surgery.* ed 3. Baltimore, Williams & Wilkins Co, 1989.
3. Marshall VF, Marchetti AA, Krantz KE: The correction of stress incontinence by simple vesicourethral suspension. *Surg Gynecol Obstet* 1949; 88:509–518.
4. Burch JC: Urethrovaginal fixation to Cooper's ligament for correction of stress incontinence, cystocele, and prolapse. *Am Obstet Gynecol* 1961; 81:281–290.
5. Halban J: Gynäkologische Operationslehre. Berlin, Urban and Schwarzenberg, 1932, pp 171–172.
6. Moschcowitz AV: The pathogenesis anatomy and cure of prolapse of the rectum. *Surg Gynecol Obstet* 1912; 15:7–21.
7. McCall ML: Posterior culdeplasty: Surgical correction of enterocele during vaginal hysterectomy, a preliminary report. *Obstet Gynecol* 1957; 10:595–602.

BIBLIOGRAPHY

Anderson WR: Pudendal hernia. *Obstet Gynecol* 1968; 32:802–804.

Torpin R: Excision of the cul-de-sac of Douglas for the surgical cure of hernias through the female caudal wall: Including prolapse of the uterus. *J Med Assoc Ga* 1947; 36:396–406.

Waters EG: Vaginal prolapse. *Obstet Gynecol* 1956; 8:432–436.

Weed JC, Tyrone C: Enterocele. *Am J Obstet Gynecol* 1950; 60:324–332.

Zacharin RF: *Pelvic Floor Anatomy and the Surgery of Pulsion Enterocele.* New York, Springer-Verlag New York, 1985.

Chapter 9

Reoperation of the Tubes and Ovaries

Tiffany J. Williams, M.D.

Operative procedures carried out to restore fertility generally have not had enthusiastic endorsement because of their poor results. An overall success rate of about 5% was prevalent in the 1930s.[1] Improved patient selection allowed an increase to about 15% over the next 20 years.[2] It was only with the use of the operating microscope that any substantial improvement was achieved[3–6]; the success rates increased nearly twofold. Despite this change in the results, a live-birth rate of approximately 30% cannot be considered good. Progress continues in attempts at assisted reproduction, but as yet, the results are no better than what can be achieved by an operative procedure upon the patient's own tissues, even though damaged. Because these results are so poor, it is thought that the initial microsurgical tuboplasty will provide the patient with her best chance for conception.

Restoration of fertility shall be considered only from the standpoint of surgical procedures, specifically, repeat operation. It is meant, therefore, to consider the advisability of a reoperation to restore fertility on those patients who have had an initial operative procedure because of infertility that was unsuccessful.

It has generally been accepted, from both experience as well as reports in the gynecologic literature, that initial operative procedures have the best chance of curing the disease or correcting the problem for which the operation was performed.[7, 8] Although the results may be very good in some situations and in the hands of master surgeons, generally the success rates of second procedures, whether done for urinary incontinence, pelvic relaxation, or gynecologic neoplasm, are not as likely to be as successful as the initial surgical attempt. Therefore, it would seem logical to assume that this same tenet would apply to infertility surgery.

It has been evident that some of the operative failures encountered in gynecologic surgery may be more likely the fault of the execution of the procedure than of the procedure itself. It is immaterial whether this is due to surgical inadequacy on the part of the operator from the technical standpoint or from an incorrect perception of the appropriate method by which to perform the operation in question.

Specific consideration shall be given to the surgical procedures carried out as second attempts to restore fertility because of tubo-ovarian adhesive disease. Avoidance of a problem will be better than attempts to correct one. An inappropriate tuboplasty poorly executed not only will have decreased chance of success but also will compromise the chances that a proper operation later will succeed, even in the very best of surgical hands.

MICROSURGERY IN TUBAL RECONSTRUCTIVE SURGERY

The use of the operating microscope in performing tubal reconstructive surgery has won wide acceptance, particularly for reversal of sterilization. Acceptable rates for reestablishment of patency of at least one tube would seem to lie between 70% and 90% for procedures by competent microsurgeons, depending on the method of sterilization that had been performed.

The microsurgeon should have not only the appropriate equipment, which requires constant inspection and care, but a skilled team as well. The procedure is difficult and tedious, and an assistant as well as a scrub nurse or technician should be trained components of the team. Dual operating microscope heads allow not only assistance but also participation and training. Videotaping allows the rest of the scrub team to see the procedure and anticipate the needs of the surgeon.

A matter of paramount importance is adequate cleansing of the gloves of the operating team. A brief pass through the splash basin is inadequate in removing powder from gloves. After thorough washing, every member of the team should have the gloves thoroughly rinsed with a sterile solution. The same procedure should be followed by all parties after any glove change, and new solution should be placed in a fresh splash basin.

Anastomosis is accomplished using 8-0 coated polyglactin 910 (Vicryl) sutures, which are dyed for better visualization. The sutures are placed through the lumen and are mucomuscular, aiming for a patent and watertight approximation. These are supported with 7-0 Vicryl as a musculoserosal layer interdigitating with the mucomuscular sutures. Permanent sutures are recommended for mesosalpingeal approximation, and 6-0 polypropylene (Prolene) is satisfactory, any defects being closed with the same suture or 5-0 Vicryl. Placement should allow luminal approximation without tension or distortion.

The choice of abdominal incision must be such that the microscope can not only be adequately focused but worked around with delicate tissue manipulation. A longitudinal incision can always be extended and is required if there is an adnexal mass present. Transverse incisions are more cosmetic, bloodier, more uncomfortable, and stronger but may not allow easy access to the pelvic organs. The four-bladed retractor such as the O'Connor-O'Sullivan may allow better exposure, but surgery may be hampered by the ring of the retractor on which the hands will rest. There is the increased risk of nerve damage, particularly with prolonged procedures such as microsurgery. The selection of the incision is generally made at the time of examination under anesthesia and following the patient's desires if such is appropriate. Because of the optics of the microscope, obesity is a contraindication to tubo-ovarian microsurgery.

The documentation of patency is a necessary part of the operative procedure. Intratubal manipulations should be avoided at all costs and, if required, should be minimized as much as possible. The use of a probe is the most traumatic but should be used if it is the only method by which patency can be assured.

In the days before the use of the operating microscope, there seemed to be a small degree of improvement in pregnancy results when splints were used. These were usually left through the anastomotic or implantation site, with a loop lying within the uterine cavity. They could then be removed after about 3 months as an outpatient procedure, healing generally by secondary intention. Today there is practically no place for the use of such intratubal stents except for the possibility of a soft polymeric silicone (Silastic) tube to assure alignment and approximation during the anastomosis itself.

Postoperative hysterosalpingograms are recommended 1 year postoperatively if intrauterine pregnancy has not ensued. Analysis of the results of microsurgery for tubal disease reveals that the curve for conceptions does not start to flatten until 2 years following the operation. It is believed that any unnecessary manipulation should be avoided, and infection is a recognized risk of hysterosalpingogram. However, since many patients are older and may have other parameters for infertility, a complete reevaluation is recommended at 1 year if the patient has not conceived. If pregnancy has occurred, neither x-ray nor laparoscopy may be needed.

Some concern has been expressed as to whether or not the use of such microsurgical techniques on diseased tubes (usually secondary to an inflammatory condition) will achieve enough benefit to justify the time and expense of the operative procedure itself. Comparisons of macrosurgery and microsurgery for tubal reconstruction reported by competent surgeons generally show an improvement in both patency and delivery rates among those women in whom an operating microscope and microsurgical techniques were used.[4, 5] This improvement in the success rate appears to apply to all of the different operative procedures accomplished on the tubes: neosalpingostomy, fimbrioplasty, salpingolysis, or anastomosis.

RESTORATION OF FERTILITY

Tubal reoperation to restore fertility may be divided into two groups on the basis of the cause of the infertility: reversal of a sterilization procedure and an operative attempt to correct occlusion subsequent to tubal disease. These two groups represent two entirely different situations and must be considered separately.

Reversal of Sterilization

Reversal of a sterilizing operation should be accomplished with some degree of technical ease, particularly when anastomosis is required. The fact that in most instances these women have documented previous fertility should be a factor in achieving good success rates.

Tubal length, as an expression of the amount of tubal destruction, may have a bearing on this success rate. Although the length of reconstructed tube may be relevant, there is no information as to the minimum amount of tube required for conception. No good data indicate that one portion of the tube is more important than another (i.e., fimbria, ampulla, ampullary-isthmic junction, isthmus, or cornu). Success rates are reported to be nearly 50% after fimbriectomy. Although fimbria are important, they are not a sine qua non for pregnancy.

Because anastomosis is the most common operative procedure required for reversal of a sterilization, failure of an anastomotic procedure should be uncommon. This should be true regardless of the portions of tube that are approximated (i.e., ampullary-ampullary, ampullary-isthmic, isthmic-interstitial, or ampullary-interstitial). When a well-apposed and patent anastomosis has failed, I have found that there is separation of the anastomosed segments. They present an appearance very similar to that noted before the initial anastomosis. Accordingly, I believe that should such occur, reanastomosis of the separated segments is an entirely reasonable procedure. In my experience, it has been accompanied by a high success rate not only in anatomic apposition but also in subsequent conception and birth. This situation is one of the rare instances in which the success rate of a second operation should approach that of a first operation.

Repeat Operation for Tubal Disease

If an appropriate operation has been selected and satisfactorily executed by a competent microsurgeon, there would seem to be little reason to believe that a second operation would be likely to have much benefit. However, a second procedure would be reasonable if something different could be accomplished by it that might improve the chances of success. If the initial operation had not been accomplished with appropriate magnification, microsurgical techniques, and minimally reactive fine suture materials, it would be reasonable to consider a second procedure appropriately performed. It is mandatory that microsurgical techniques be used. Optical augmentation is of paramount importance, and there is strong preference for the use of the operating microscope with its versatility and magnification as opposed to what can be obtained with loupes alone.

Failure of a tubal reconstruction procedure that was accomplished by macroscopic techniques would appear to leave a situation in which there might be some chance of success with an appropriate microscopic procedure. The additional delicacy of tissue handling as afforded with proper visualization through the microscope should improve the chances of success, as would the use of fine minimally reactive suture materials.

Several factors must be considered before a decision regarding repeat operation is made. The first consideration would be: Can something different be accomplished at the time of the second procedure that was not available or not provided at the initial operation? Should such be the case, reoperation by a skilled microsurgeon is reasonable.

The second consideration would be: Are there other alternatives that might accomplish the desired goal, which is birth of a living child? Assisted reproductive technology such as in vitro fertilization–embryo transfer (IVF-ET) has not met this need except in the most experienced hands. Should such an alternative be available, it would appear that the success rates of reoperation and of IVF-ET are nearly comparable. It is important that the patient be aware of this option. One must remember, however, that a successful IVF is successful for just that one pregnancy; subsequent attempts at pregnancy each require a separate in vitro attempt. Successful tubal anastomosis, on the other hand, may affect an unlimited number of opportunities for future pregnancies. It is even more important for the patient and her family to understand that not all IVF programs have good results, nor do all surgeons who use a microscope perform good surgery and have results comparable with those recorded in the literature.

Regardless of the decision reached, it is imperative that a complete infertility evaluation be accomplished before any operative procedure, whether it be the first or the second. The status and efficacy of ovulation must be established as well as the normality of the spouse's semen. If abnormalities are noted, correction should be planned or accomplished before a reoperative procedure. Otherwise, such recognized abnormalities may be remedied in the immediate postoperative period so there will be no delay in attempts at conception once healing has been completed.

It is believed very strongly that all conditions encountered that might have any adverse effect on accomplishment or maintenance of conception should be treated at the time of microsurgery. All adhesions involving the tube and ovary must be excised, particularly because they may affect ovum pickup and tubal motility.

Myomata uteri or endometriosis, if encountered, should be cared for as well. Excision and verification by histology is recommended, but the use of electrocauterization or laser ablation will accomplish the same end. If bowel endometriosis is suspected, preoperative bowel preparation is indicated. However, if encountered unexpectedly, it should still be treated even if resection is required. The surgical procedure should completely eradicate the disease process. Despite the previous recommendation concerning possible bowel resection, the intestinal lumen should be avoided if at all possible. Spill, contamination, and subsequent infection and adhesions can only negate an appropriately performed and meticulous operation. The use of routine appendectomy would appear illogical, therefore, and unless the appendix is diseased, an appendectomy is contraindicated during infertility surgery.

Adjunctive techniques to improve results of infertility surgery are commonly utilized. However, there are no statistical data to document improvement in live-birth rates, regardless of the method. This applies to the dexamethasone-promethazine regimen, the use of dextran, and postoperative hydrotubations. The preoperative and intraoperative use of antibiotics, however, is recommended in any patient undergoing tubal surgery who is known or suspected to have a history of inflammatory disease.

Adherence to microsurgical principles is mandatory. The use of the operating microscope with its advantage of improved magnification is strongly recommended. Atraumatic tissue technique with delicate manipulation is required. Fine suture material that is nonreactive is a necessary item. Permanent sutures, such as 8-0 nylon, are recommended for neosalpingostomy and mesosalpingeal approximation. Resorbable sutures such as Vicryl are preferred for the tubal anastomosis itself, but the results seem to show little difference in respect to suture type—polyglycolic acid (Vicryl or Dexon) vs. nylon.

Use of fine permanent sutures provides better success rates than does use of highly reactive sutures or resorbable sutures in certain parts of the tube. A micro-unipolar cautery is used for adhesiolysis, and a fine bipolar cautery is used to accomplish meticulous hemostasis. The operative procedure is accomplished under continuous irrigation with a physiologic solution with added heparin (3,000 units per 1,000 mL). Occasionally, ovarian suspension or uterine suspension is used when there is extensive cul-de-sac disease. This will allow one to avoid readherence to the back of the broad ligaments or cul de sac until reperitonization has occurred. Minimally reactive resorbable sutures are recommended for this. Pelvic lavage at the completion of the procedure is accomplished, and exact and complete hemostasis is required.

RESULTS

Four articles in the literature allude to repeat tuboplasty accomplished to restore fertility. The data from those articles confirm the premise that a second operative procedure does not have the benefit for restoration of fertility that the primary operation does. Chartier and associates reported on 15 patients, 3 (20%) of whom had term pregnancies after reoperation[9]; these operations were not performed with magnification (Table 9–1). The cases reported included four patients in whom three operations were carried out but none became pregnant. Table 8–1 also gives the results of this group's overall tubal procedures.

Two articles from the University of Düsseldorf also mentioned reoperation. These two articles appear to be subsets of the same group of patients. The first report was by Frantzen and Schlösser and analyzed data on 234 patients.[10] This group had a 30% intrauterine pregnancy rate and a term pregnancy rate of 27%. The results by type of operative procedure are given in Table 9–2. In the group of patients undergoing repeat operation, 11 (19%) of 58 conceived, and 9 had live births, for a 16% overall success rate. They did not separate these reoperative procedures according to the type of operation performed.

Verhoeven and colleagues reported on surgical procedures for distal tubal occlusion.[11] Unfortunately, they referred to different numbers of patients, stating that there were 33 with previous tuboplasty, of whom 27 had had previous salpingostomy. Apparently, there were 23 who underwent repeat salpingostomy. Their data can be calculated from these numbers. In the entire group having previous tuboplasty, there were three pregnancies (9%) that did go to delivery. When they reconsidered only repeat salpingostomy, the results were 3 of 23, for a 13% delivery rate (Table 9–3).

In Copenhagen, Lauritsen and associates reported a conception rate of 5 (16%) of 31 repeat tuboplasties and 3 (10%) of 31 live births (see Table 9–2).[7] They thought that the poor results most likely were due to mucosal damage, which they thought to be irreversible. Their group of operations included bilateral salpingostomy, unilateral salpingostomy, contralateral salpingectomy, bilateral fimbriolysis, bilateral implantation, and bilateral lysis of adhesions.

Thie and colleagues reported on 21 patients who had had a previous macrosurgical procedure.[8] Four (19%) of these patients conceived and delivered. These patients likewise included distal, proximal, and combined occlusion as well as readhesive disease in the presence of patency, as did the other combined series. When only repeat salpingostomy was considered, there was a 22% delivery rate among nine patients (see Table 9–3). They reported a very small group, three patients,

TABLE 9–1.
Tuboplasty by Macrosurgery*

	Cases, No.	Pregnancy, %	IUP,† %	Birth, %
Primary operation	138	36	28	25
Repeat operation	15‡	47§	33‖	27¶

*Data from Chartier M, Dubost M, Cornu C: *Rev Fr Gynecol Obstet* 1972; 67:209–215.
†IUP = intrauterine pregnancy.
‡Four operated on three times, no pregnancies.
§One patient had two ectopic pregnancies and one delivery.
‖One patient with tuberculosis and abortion at 2 mo.
¶Two deliveries and two ongoing late pregnancies.

TABLE 9–2.
Tuboplasty

Author	Primary Operation				Repeat Operation			
	Cases, No.	Pregnancy, %	IUP,* %	Birth, %	Cases, No.	Pregnancy, %	IUP,* %	Birth,%
Lauritsen et al.[7]	71	34	30	27	31	16	13	10
Frantzen & Schlösser[10]	234	59	51	44	58	?	19	16
Thie et al.[3–]	161	51	46	38	21	19	19	19
Total	466	48	42	36	110	18	17	15

*IUP = intrauterine pregnancy.
†First events.

TABLE 9–3.
Distal Salpingostomy

	Primary Operation				Repeat Operation			
Author	Cases, No.	Pregnancy, %	IUP,* %	Birth, %	Cases, No.	Pregnancy, %	IUP,* %	Birth, %
Chartier et al.[9†]	81	27	20	17	4	0	0	0
Lauritsen et al.[7]	39	43	36	23	23	17	13	9
Verhoeven et al.[11]	82	34	30	24	23	17	17	13
Thie et al.[8‡]	71	47	41	32	9	22	22	22
Total	192	41	35	27	55	19	17	15

*IUP = intrauterine pregnancy.
†Macroscopic; data not included in totals.
‡First events only.

who had undergone a previous microsurgical procedure. There were no conceptions, although patency was documented in two of the patients. In the third having reocclusion, IVF-ET failed because of maternal antisperm antibodies.

These results may be compared with the overall group of patients operated on during the same time period (see Tables 9–2 and 9–3). There was no selection among the patients reported by Thie and co-workers.[8] No other adjuvants had been used other than the antibiotics. (These adjuvants, commonly used by many surgeons, include dexamethasone and promethazine or dextran instillation.)

Postoperative hydrotubations have been accomplished in some individuals. However, it has not been possible to demonstrate improved results. The data from Thie and associates are inconclusive,[8] although data reported by others seem to show that there is no benefit. These results (see Table 9–2) show a 51% conception rate and a 38% live-birth rate.

DISCUSSION

From the literature and my own experience, it appears that microsurgical capabilities and techniques have improved the success in restoration of fertility nearly twofold compared with macroscopic procedures, even with diseased tubes. This is true even for those patients for whom there was no selection relative to type or extent of disease. When a second operation was performed because of failure of the first operation, the success rate for delivery decreased by nearly 50%.

It is readily apparent, therefore, that the first operation is the one with the best chance of success in fertility surgery (as well as in other gynecologic operations). It is of paramount importance that this first operation be well conceived and meticulously executed. I believe that any good surgeon is capable of operating through the microscope. The converse, however, is not true. A microscope will not make just anyone a good microsurgeon.

Aside from the principles mentioned earlier, a compulsive dedication to completion of the procedure is required. All disease processes that are present must be treated, in case they have an effect on conception or maintenance of a pregnancy. Even if there is patency, disease processes are best treated, as in the case of salpingitis isthmica nodosa. When they are left untreated, subsequent obstruction is to be anticipated; this would be less likely if the total diseased area were excised. Similar views are presented by Frantzen and Schlösser as well.[10] Moreover, if both tubes are present, both should be repaired. Failure to repair part of a tube or to extirpate it in a young woman may compromise her future with an incomplete operation or leave a castrate if disease were to occur in the remaining adnexa. Even though results may be poor when there is double obstruction, salpingostomy with anastomosis is indeed the appropriate treatment. Even though the success rate of such combined procedures may be lower than for each procedure alone, conception and delivery may be achieved in some instances.

Although it has been stressed that reoperation is an appropriate alternative when there has been a failed primary procedure, as stated earlier, the initial operation is the important one. The mere availability of an operating microscope has not guaranteed to the patient that she has had a good operation. Attendance at a weekend continuing medical education course does not provide an adequate experience to make a surgeon a competent microsurgeon. Not all gynecologic surgeons are trained to do exenterations, and neither are they truly trained to accomplish microsurgery. Intellectual honesty on the part of the surgeon is a requirement in delivering the appropriate surgical care.

After training in the microsurgical laboratory, I have found that about 25 procedures are required before the assistant becomes adept and knowledgeable concerning the microsurgical operation. Recognition of tissue planes and hand-eye coordination are variables that most surgeons can develop once competency has been achieved, the third dimension being an additional variable from other pelvic operations. Two or three procedures per month are probably adequate to maintain the technical expertise.

SUMMARY

Reoperations may be accomplished for tubal disease with success rates that may be better than those attainable by the assisted reproduction technologist. Such procedures require appropriate evaluation preoperatively and the full use of microsurgical techniques and equipment. The operator must be a trained and experienced microsurgeon. This tenet is just as important for the initial operative procedure, which should be accomplished completely.

The patient deserves the right to know whether her surgeon is so experienced and accomplished. She should require from the surgeon the results of his or her own personal experience in such surgery. It is morally reprehensible for a surgeon to quote to a patient the results recorded in the literature as one's own unless such is indeed the truth.

REFERENCES

1. Greenhill JP: Evaluation of salpingostomy and tubal implantation for the treatment of sterility. *Am J Obstet Gynecol* 1937; 33:39–51.
2. Siegler AM, Hellman LM: Tubal plastic surgery: Report of a survey. *Fertil Steril* 1956; 7:170–177.
3. Betz G, Engle T, Penney LL: Tuboplasty—comparison of the methodology. *Fertil Steril* 1980; 34:534–536.
4. Diamond E: A comparison of gross and microsurgical techniques for repair of cornual occlusion in infertility: A retrospective study, 1968–1978. *Fertil Steril* 1979; 32:370–376.
5. Fayez JA, Suliman SO: Infertility surgery of the oviduct: Comparison between macrosurgery and microsurgery. *Fertil Steril* 1982; 37:73–78.
6. Gomel V: Surgical correction of sequelae of pelvic inflammatory disease. *J Reprod Med* 1983; 28(suppl):718–726.
7. Lauritsen JG, Pagel JD, Vangsted P, et al: Results of repeated tuboplasties. *Fertil Steril* 1982; 37:68–72.
8. Thie JL, Williams TJ, Coulam CB: Repeat tuboplasty compared with primary microsurgery for postinflammatory tubal disease. *Fertil Steril* 1986; 45:784–787.
9. Chartier M, Dubost M, Cornu C: Notre expérience des interventions itératives dans la chirurgie tubulaire: A propos de 15 observations. *Rev Fr Gynecol Obstet* 1972; 67:209–215.
10. Frantzen C, Schlösser H-W: Microsurgery and postinfectious tubal infertility. *Fertil Steril* 1982; 38:397–402.
11. Verhoeven HC, Berry H, Frantzen C, et al: Surgical treatment for distal tubal occlusion: A review of 167 cases. *J Reprod Med* 1983; 28:293–303.

Chapter 10

Resterilization After Tubal Sterilization Failure

Jaroslav Fabian Hulka, M.D.

Linda Mitchell

In the United States, more than 6 million women have undergone tubal sterilization and are continuing to be sterilized at the rate of about 500,000 per year. The incidence of failure of these sterilizations is low, estimated to be between 2 to 12 per 1,000 sterilizations, or less than 1% per year. Thus, every year, out of 500,000 women, 1% (5,000) will experience a pregnancy after sterilization. These events can bring personal distress to the couple and can raise medicolegal problems in this litigious era. In addition, the physician managing the pregnancy is eventually faced with the problem of how to deal with the sterilization failure to prevent reoccurrence, or how to resterilize the patient. This chapter will review the known causes for these pregnancies and suggest management based on these causes.

ANATOMY AND PHYSIOLOGY OF TUBAL DIVISION

Both the uterus and ampulla secrete fluid, mostly during the follicular phase. This fluid is constantly exchanged in minute amounts as a result of the pumping action of uterine contractions throughout the cycle. Both the amount of fluid and the pressure of the contractions vary considerably from individual to individual. When tubes are occluded in some women, the pressure and amount of fluid normally generated by the uterus will be sufficient to pump fluid by force through the healing process at the occlusive site, with resultant fistula formation. In 1973 Courey and associates demonstrated these uteroperitoneal fistulas by performing hysterosalpingograms in women 3 or more months after unipolar electrocoagulation.[1] More than 10% of these sterilized women had demonstrable fistulas. Histologically, these fistulas were carefully documented by Stock in 1983 in both proximal and distal segments with tubal endothelium everted at the peritoneal surface of the fistula.[2] These fistulas allow the passage of sperm from the uterine cavity (where they are normally distributed after unprotected intercourse) into the peritoneal cavity. Some sperm will be swept in peritoneal fluid into the distal ampullary

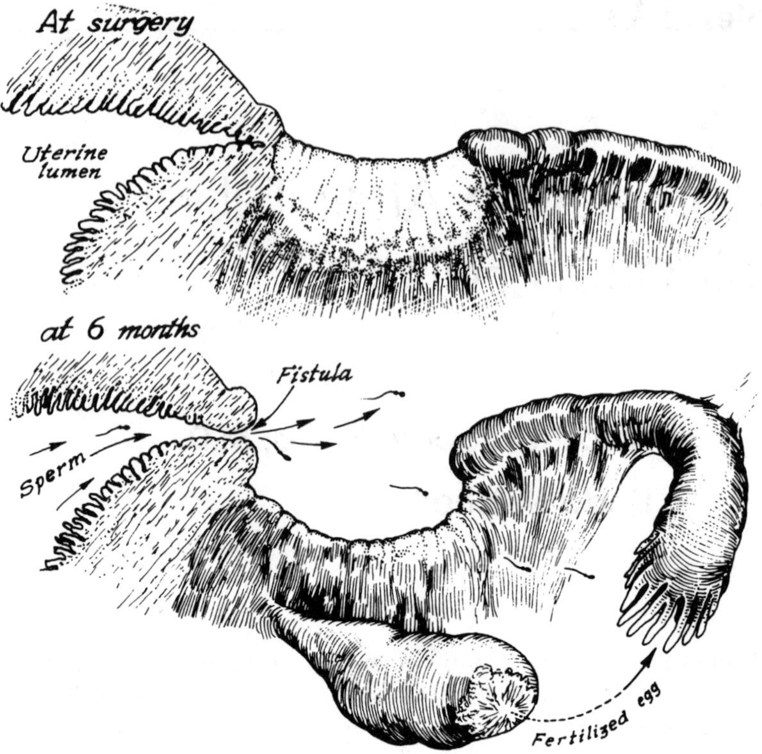

FIG 10–1.
After electrocoagulation near the uterus, the isthmic segment is aborbed, allowing uterine fluid under pressure from uterine contractions to create a fistula to the peritoneum. Subsequent unprotected intercourse allows sperm to enter the peritoneum, reach the fimbria, and fertilize an egg. (From Hulka J: *Textbook of Laparoscopy*. Orlando, Fla, Grune & Stratton, 1985. Used by permission.)

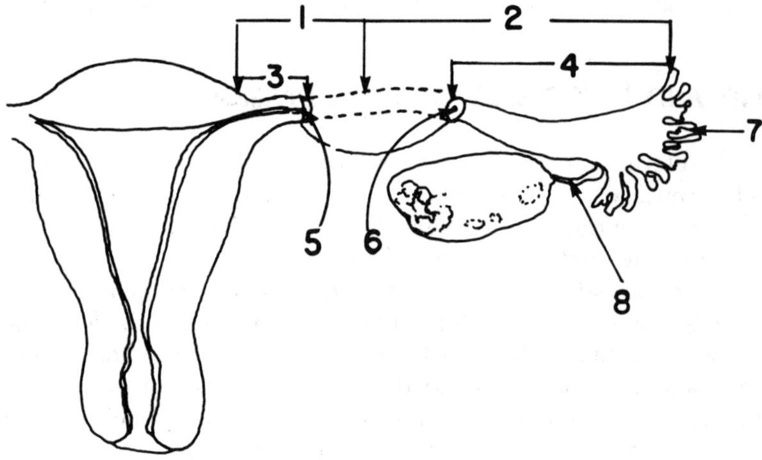

FIG 10–2.
1, isthmus; *2,* ampulla; *3,* proximal segment; *4,* distal segment; *5,* proximal (tuboperitoneal, uteroperitoneal) fistula; *6,* distal fistula; *7,* fimbria; and *8,* fimbrica ovarica.

stump by fimbria, where they can fertilize an egg brought into the ampulla during normal ovulation. Metz and Mastroianni[3] and Stock and Nelson[4] hypothesize that a fertilized egg can then implant in the ampulla and present itself clinically as an ectopic pregnancy (Fig 10–1). More remarkably, the fertilized egg can pass through a fistula in the ampullary stump, back into the uteroperitoneal fistula, and present itself clinically as a normal intrauterine pregnancy. These are rare events, but they do occur and account for some pregnancies occurring after properly occluded tubes.

In the description of the different techniques of sterilization and the subsequent healing process, a number of anatomic terms will be used and are summarized for clarity in Figure 10–2.

TECHNIQUES OF STERILIZATION

The Pomeroy Procedure

This procedure is the most common operation in the United States, performed postpartum or at the time of cesarean section. A knuckle of tube is brought up by a Babcock clamp, an O plain catgut ligature occludes the base of the loop, the loop is excised, and the specimen is sent to the pathology laboratory for confirmation of the correct structure being occluded. Six months after the procedure, the necrotic stumps have been absorbed, and the patient is left with a proximal segment (usually >2 cm) consisting of isthmus next to the uterus, a gap of about 3 cm where the loop of tube had been excised, and a distal segment consisting of varying lengths of ampulla. Sutures tight enough to achieve hemostasis may still allow fistula formation and recanalization of both segments.[2] After Pomeroy ligation, pregnancies are estimated to occur in 2 to 8 of 1,000 sterilizations, primarily intrauterine.

Bipolar Coagulation

Electrocoagulation with bipolar forceps is the most common method of laparoscopic tubal sterilization in the United States. The fallopian tube is grasped by a forceps and an electric current passed between the prongs of the forceps through the tube. In serial laparoscopies following bipolar coagulation, Fishburne and Hulka observed that hypervascularization occurs around the dead coagulated tissue, which then is slowly reabsorbed.[5] When the absorption is complete 6 months later, the remaining segments fall apart, and the end stage of healing is similar to that seen after a Pomeroy: a segment of isthmus next to the uterus, a gap of varying length depending on the extent of coagulation, and a distal ampullary segment with varying incidence of fistula.

The incidence of pregnancy subsequent to properly performed bipolar sterilization techniques is about 2 to 4 of 1,000 sterilizations, with pregnancies tending to be ectopic as well as intrauterine. Pregnancy is believed to result from a short proximal segment leading to a uteroperitoneal fistula. Pregnancies associated with operator error often involve a mismatch between forceps and the electrocoagulation current designed for that forcep, with the result that tubes are incompletely coagulated.[6] Pregnancy rates with incomplete coagulation have been as high as 20 of 1,000, the majority intrauterine.

Unipolar Elecrocoagulation

In the 1970s, the most popular method of laparoscopic sterilization was unipolar; a current flowed from a metal forcep on the tube to a ground plate on the patient's body. The end result was variable, from damage similar to that after Pomeroy to extensive destruction of the tube, with no proximal segment, and with minimal ampulla and fimbria remaining. Pregnancies are both ectopic and intrauterine after this procedure, with an incidence of 2 to 4 of 1,000 sterilizations.

As concern about the immediate and late complication (ectopic pregnancy) of electrocoagulation emerges, the mechanical methods of laparoscopic tubal occlusion are steadily increasing in popularity. Both mechanical techniques were introduced in the 1970s as alternatives to electrocoagulation.

The Band Procedure

The band is essentially a type of Pomeroy procedure, where a knuckle of tube is lifted up and constricted by an elastic band at its base and the loop allowed to necrose. The healing process is also similar to the Pomeroy; about 6 months later, the segments have been separated, and the band is enclosed in the peritoneum of one of the segments. A 3- to 4-cm segment of tube is missing with a fairly healthy proximal isthmic portion and a variable distal ampullary segment. Subsequent pregnancies occur after this operation at a rate of 2 to 8 of 1,000 sterilizations; the majority of these pregnancies are intrauterine. Pregnancies attributable to operator error result from failure to completely occlude the lumen with the band, from incorrect application of the band onto the wrong structure, and even from slippage of the band off the tube.

The Spring Clip

The spring clip is designed to go across the isthmic portion of the tube. At the end of the healing process, in about 6 weeks, the clip remains where it was placed and is covered by epithelium. Both proximal and distal segments of the endothelium of the tube form blind pouches, and about 0.5 cm of tube is destroyed. Incidence of proximal or distal fistula after this procedure is quite rare. Pregnancies occurring after this procedure are in the 2 to 8 of 1,000 range, and most are intrauterine. Pregnancies result almost entirely from operator error in applying the clip incompletely across the isthmus or onto the ampullary segment.[6, 7]

The Irving Procedure

The isthmus of a tube is divided and the proximal isthmic segment buried into the peritoneum of the uterus so that a proximal uteroperitoneal fistula is prevented. This procedure is usually done for sterilization at the time of elective cesarean section, when the tube and entire fundus can be easily visualized. An extensive review of the literature by Garb failed to reveal any pregnancies reported after this procedure.[8]

Cornual Resection

Excising the tube and performing a cornual resection were occasionally recommended as part of the management of ectopic pregnancy. A critical review of its efficacy revealed a variable incidence of ectopic and interstitial pregnancies subsequent to cornual resection.[8] In 1955, Rotten reported 5 such pregnancies after 105 cornual resections, for a subsequent pregnancy rate of 4.7%,[9] probably resulting from the formation of uteroperitoneal fistula.

Fimbriectomy

In 1969, Kroener described his father's successful technique of bilateral fimbriectomy by culpotomy.[10] He emphasized the importance of recognizing the fimbrica ovarica, a variable structure connecting the ovary and the fimbria. Although he described separate ligation of the structure to remove the fimbria completely, subsequent reports of failures did not mention this important detail; this omission led to remnants of fimbria[2] when clamps and sutures did not get completely between the fimbria and the ovary. Though the vaginal approach has been abandoned, some physicians do fimbriectomies postpartum or at cesarean section. Pregnancies following fimbriectomies are usually intrauterine, because the egg is brought into a normal tube through a remnant of fimbrial opening.

Summary

Most techniques of sterilization have their failures. Failures can result from technical error at the time of sterilization or from the normal healing process after sterilization. It is mandatory for the total management of a pregnancy after sterilization to determine the exact anatomic cause of the pregnancy to choose the most effective technique of resterilization.

MANAGEMENT OF SUBSEQUENT PREGNANCY

Intrauterine Pregnancy

Although the majority of patients will be upset or distraught by a pregnancy after sterilization, some patients will consider the event a gift or a blessing. Depending on the patient's reaction, a therapeutic abortion or a term delivery will be chosen.

If abortion is chosen, the patient should be urged to consider laparoscopy during the procedure or soon after the procedure to determine the cause of failure and to allow resterilization. At the time of resterilization, careful note should be made as to whether or not both tubes are, in fact, properly divided or occluded or whether an operator error had occurred. Sensitivity to the medicolegal implications of operator error while dictating operative notes and while describing to the patient the findings is urged in the spirit of "There, but by the grace of God, go I." It is my (J.F.H.) experience and that of others[6,7] that many intrauterine pregnancies result from technical errors. The proper management of this situation is to perform a correct sterilization at the time of laparoscopy by electrocoagulation, clip, or band as the patient and physician feel appropriate. If both tubes are properly occluded or divided but the intrauterine pregnancy has occurred anyway, the procedure should be a diagnostic laparoscopy only, and the patient should be involved in the next step of management. Vasectomy for the husband is a simple solution in a monogamous marriage. Resterilization of a technically successful sterilization would involve a laparotomy and an Irving procedure to bury the proximal isthmic stumps (if isthmic stumps are available). A hysterectomy may be an option if the patient feels it is worth the freedom from concern over subsequent pregnancy.

If the pregnancy goes to term, the patient should again be offered a postpartum tubal ligation with a larger incision to evaluate the cause of the pregnancy. If at this point a technical error is discovered, a repeat standard Pomeroy procedure (using a strongly ligated O plain catgut suture) could be carried out. If the tubes were properly divided or occluded and intrauterine pregnancy nevertheless occurred, an Irving procedure should be performed at this time. If there are insufficient tubal stumps to bury the tube, the patient should be so advised and should consider vasectomy of the husband or hysterectomy.

Ectopic Pregnancy

Ectopic pregnancy is a moderate to acute emergency where cool decisions and informed consent may not be reasonably expected. If the situation is elective (vasomotor stability, 1 or 2 days of observation of β–human chorionic gonadotropin titers, or ultrasound changes), the patient may have had an adequate chance to consider alternatives. The physician should use judgment to determine if the patient can make an informed consent as to the alternatives of management available.

Early Unruptured Pregnancy

Early unruptured pregnancies in the ampulla are increasingly managed by laparoscopy. In this technique, a salpingostomy is performed, and the ampullary ectopic pregnancy is aspirated. A laparoscopy then gives the opportunity to review the cause of the ectopic pregnancy. A judgment can be made whether the ampullary stumps could be excised by laparoscopic coagulation and excision of the base. If this is judged not to be feasible, a laparotomy can be performed and bilateral ampullary removal performed. Some physicians may not be comfortable with the laparoscopic management of ectopic pregnancy. A patient with an unruptured ectopic pregnancy who agrees to bilateral ampullary excision should be managed directly with a laparotomy for a standard bilateral partial salpingectomy. There are no animal or human data to suggest that such surgery has any effect on subsequent endocrine function such as menstrual regularity.

Acute Ectopic Pregnancy

In the acute ectopic pregnancy with vasomotor instability, an emergency laparotomy is the usual method of management. After the ectopic pregnancy is excised and bleeding is controlled, a decision can be made, based on the patient's degree of informed consent, as to whether the remaining distal ampullae should be removed as well.

Cornual Resection

Although cornual resection has been recommended by some as an additional step in the management of ectopic pregnancies, the rather high incidence of intrauterine or interstitial pregnancy after cornual resection[8, 9] would seem to make this approach inappropriate. If no proximal fistula is found and a proximal isthmic stump is present, a performance of a cornual resection rather than an Irving procedure may actually increase the risk of a repeat ectopic pregnancy.

PREVENTION OF THE NEED FOR RESTERILIZATION

The choice of techniques in the performance of sterilizations should reflect the lessons learned in management of pregnancies subsequent to sterilization failures. As this chapter indicates, uteroperitoneal fistulas are a common factor in pregnancies after sterilization procedures where a segment of tube is destroyed or excised (see Fig 10–1). Current recommendations at the time of the initial sterilization are to leave at least 1 or 2 cm of isthmic tube as a stump at the uterine end (Fig 10–3).[7] The musculature of the isthmus will then absorb the pressure of a uterine contraction expelling fluid into the tube and will minimize the risk of fistula formation. This principle can be put into practice by the following recommendations to minimize the need for resterilization.

The Irving Procedure

The Irving Procedure is to be recommended at elective cesarean section. This technique has good reversal potential in that no tubal tissue is destroyed. It is relatively easy to perform when the uterus is exposed after cesarean delivery. Since the proximal stump is buried in the myometrium, fistula formation is not a problem.

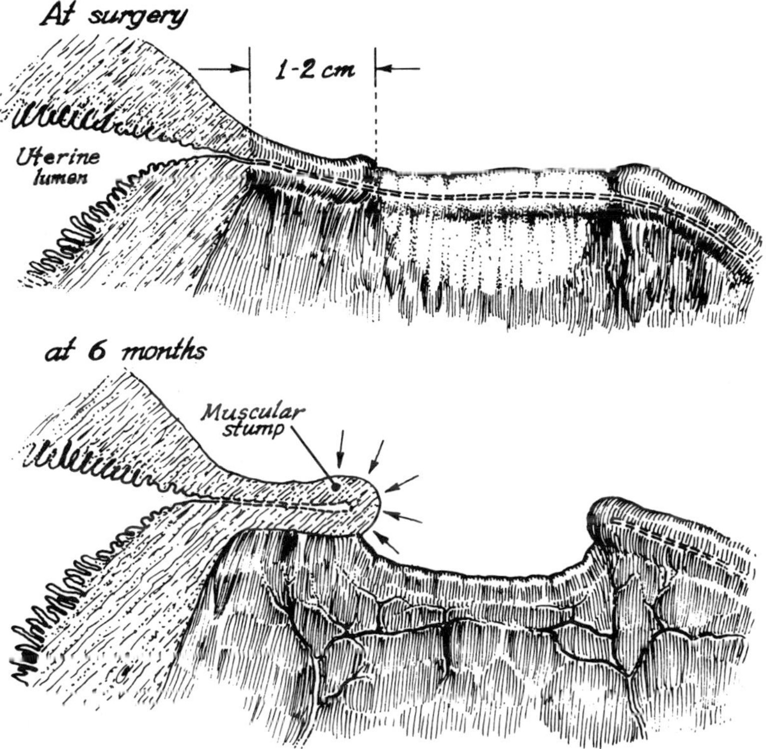

FIG 10–3.
Electrocoagulation of a tube at least 2 cm from the uterus allows an isthmic segment to remain, which should minimize the chance of fistula formation by allowing a greater distribution and absorbtion of the pressure of uterine fluid. (From Hulka J: *Textbook of Laparoscopy*. Orlando, Fla, Grune & Stratton 1985. Used by permission.)

The Pomeroy Procedure

The Pomeroy procedure is a good technique in the early postpartum period after spontaneous vaginal delivery. Pomeroy used one O plain catgut suture tied strongly. A good portion (1–2 cm) of proximal isthmic stump should be left to minimize the chance of proximal fistula and subsequent ectopic pregnancy.

Bipolar Coagulation

Bipolar coagulation should be performed at laparoscopy by starting at least 2 cm away from the uterus and coagulating three times, going distally along the tube.[7] In addition, proper matching of forceps and generator had been stressed by Kleppinger,[11] Soderstrom,[6] and Hulka.[7] The end point for bipolar coagulation should be the disappearance of electric flow (as measured by a flowmeter) between the tips of the forceps during the process. Other clinical end points such as "turning white" or "popping" may represent superficial coagulation that allows lumen between the forceps to remain viable.

Bands and Clips

Bands and clips should be meticulously placed on the structures with correct technique: the band on the isthmic-ampullary junction where the tube is most mobile and clips completely across the isthmus about 2 to 3 cm away from the uterus. Mechanical laparoscopic techniques require strict attention to surgical detail.

REFERENCES

1. Courey NG, Cunanan RG Jr, Taefi P: Sterilization via laparoscopy *NY State J Med* 1973; 73:539–561.
2. Stock RJ. Histopathologic changes in fallopian tubes subsequent to sterilization procedures. *Int J Gynecol Pathol* 1983; 2:13–27.
3. Metz KGP, Mastroianni L: Tubal pregnancy subsequent to transperitoneal migration of spermatozoa. *Obstet Gynecol Surv* 1979; 34:554–560.
4. Stock RJ, Nelson KJ: Ectopic pregnancy subsequent to sterilization: Histologic evaluation and clinical implications. *Fertil Steril* 1984; 42:211–215.
5. Fishburne JI, Hulka JF: Tubal healing following laparoscopic electrocoagulation. *J Reprod Med* 1976; 16:129–134.
6. Soderstrom RM: Sterilization failures and their causes. *Am J Obstet Gynecol* 1985; 152:395–400.
7. Hulka JF: *Textbook of Laparoscopy*. Orlando, Fla, Grune & Stratton 1985, p 152.
8. Garb AE. A review of tubal sterilization failures. *Obstet Gynecol Surv* 1979; 34:554–560.
9. Rotten GN: Failure in sterilization. *West J Surg* 1955; 63:146–150.
10. Kroener WF Jr: Surgical sterilization by fimbriectomy. *Am J Obstet Gynecol* 1969; 104:247–254.
11. Kleppinger RK: Female outpatient sterilization using bipolar coagulation. *Bull Postgrad Comm Med Univ Sydney* November 1977, pp 144–154.

Chapter 11

Recurrent Endometriosis

James M. Wheeler, M.D., M.P.H.

L. Russell Malinak, M.D.

Endometriosis is the common name of a disease with a wide clinical spectrum. The mild form of superficial peritoneal implants is so common, and often asymptomatic, that it may not actually represent disease but a normal variation in pelvic anatomy. The more severe forms of endometriosis are unquestionably pathologic, distorting anatomy with fibrosis and adhesions and usually causing pain and perhaps infertility. To borrow an infectious disease model, mild endometriosis behaves like microbial colonization, living symbiotically with the host tissues, whereas severe endometriosis is akin to infection with its destruction of normal tissue structure and function. Unfortunately, the natural history of endometriosis is yet to be clearly understood, and clinicians cannot yet predict which women will have the mild forms of endometriosis and which will have the destructive forms. Until the natural history of endometriosis is better defined, clinicians must rely on their observations in the treatment of this disease.

INCIDENCE

One aspect of the natural history of endometriosis is clear: both medical and surgical treatments are associated with all too frequent cases of recurrent disease. Danazol is the drug with the most information available regarding recurrence; following danazol treatment, 5% to 15% of patients per year develop symptomatic recurrence. After 3 years, 40% of women treated with Danazol alone had recurrent endometriosis.[1] Little long-term information as to recurrence following treatment with gonadotropin-releasing hormone (GnRH) agonists is yet available, but one would expect similar recurrence rates as other drugs with similar modes of action.[2]

For several years, we have reported the incidence of recurrence following conservative surgery for endometriosis.[3–5] Of 423 women treated for endometriosis by conservative laparotomy, 20% of women followed for 5 years had recurrent endometriosis diagnosed by repeat surgery (Fig 11–1). One obvious difficulty with the current methods of diagnosing recurrent endometriosis is the reliance on reoperation; only those women with persistent infertility or recurrent symptoms will likely accept the risks and discomforts of repeat operation. Therefore, the incidence of re-

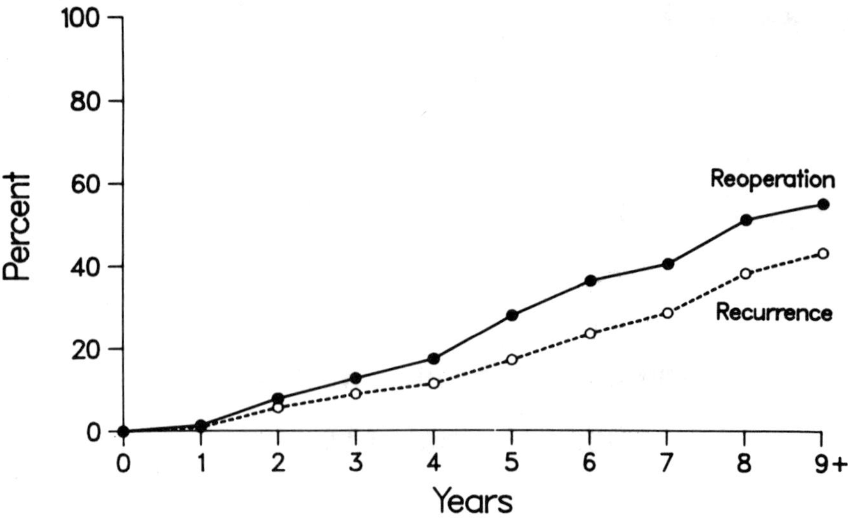

FIG 11–1.
Cumulative rates of reoperation and recurrent endometriosis in 423 infertile women treated by conservative laparotomy. (From Olive D, in Schenken RB [ed]: *Endometriosis, Contemporary Concepts in Clinical Management,* Philadelphia, JB Lippincott Co, 1989, p 235. Used by permission.)

currence after surgery may indeed be higher than that reported from clinical case series. Until noninvasive techniques allow us to diagnose recurrence without resorting to surgery, we will never accurately estimate the incidence of recurrent endometriosis.[6]

"Recurrence" Versus "Persistence" Following Surgical Treatment

One of the inherent problems with estimating the incidence of recurrent endometriosis after surgery is distinguishing recurrence, the growth of new lesions, from persistence, the growth of lesions inadequately treated at initial surgery. We have previously reported the use of a schematic representation of the pelvis, which allowed recurrent lesions to be distinguished from persistent endometriosis lesions.[7] At short-interval second-look laparoscopy, one half of the patients with implants had persistent disease (i.e., lesions at a site of dissection at primary surgery). Only by adopting this sort of accurate record keeping (Fig 11–2) will we be able to map out the course of endometriosis following surgical treatment.

MORPHOLOGY OF ENDOMETRIOSIS IMPLANTS

The many visual appearances of endometriosis presents another problem for surgical treatment and estimating recurrence. In addition to the classic blue or blue-black blebs, endometriosis was histologically confirmed in lesions that were flat, red to pink, subperitoneal, or even clear and vesicular.[8] As described by Stripling and colleagues[8] and then Batt and Smith,[9] peritoneal pockets as those depicted in Figure 11–3 may often contain endometriosis implants; these pockets may be everted and excised either laparoscopically or at laparotomy. The surgeon must be alert to the many visual appearances of endometriosis at the time of surgery; aware-

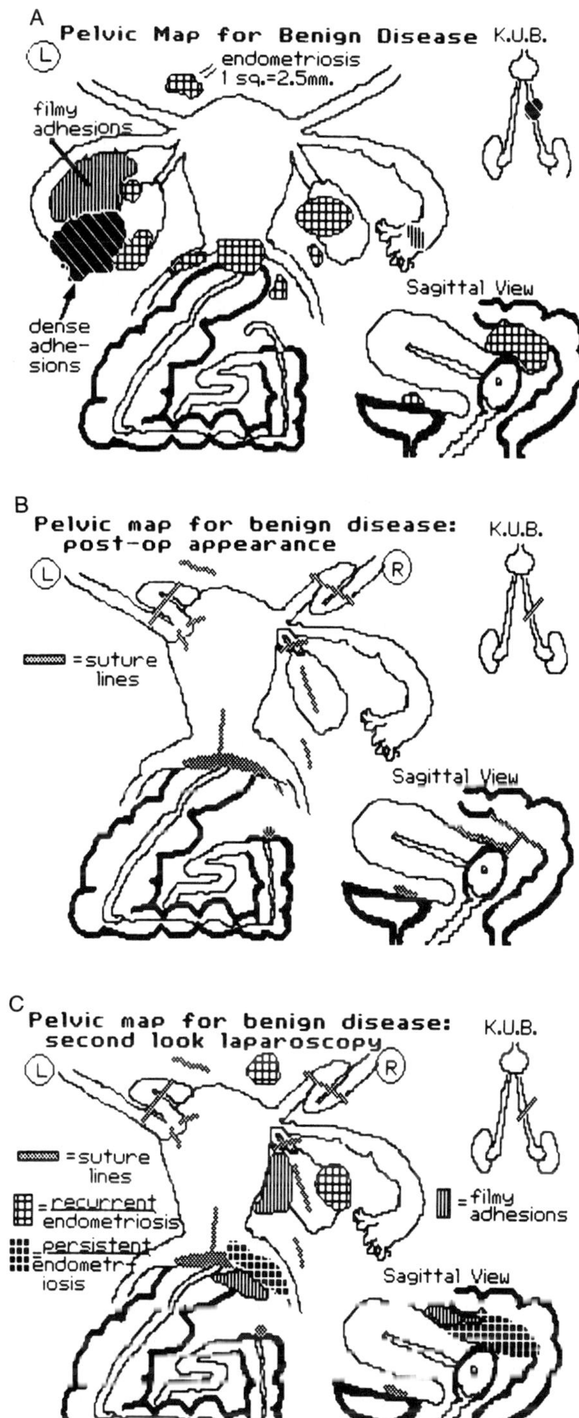

FIG 11–2.

Pelvic mapping to distinguish recurrent from persistent endometriosis after conservative laparotomy. **A,** extent and size (each square = 0.25 cm) of endometriosis and adhesions found at laparotomy. **B,** postoperative appearance of the pelvic, including suture lines. **C,** appearance of second-look laparoscopy 4 weeks after laparotomy. *Recurrent* lesions are de novo implants, whereas *persistent* lesions are at sites of previous dissection and represent incomplete excision.

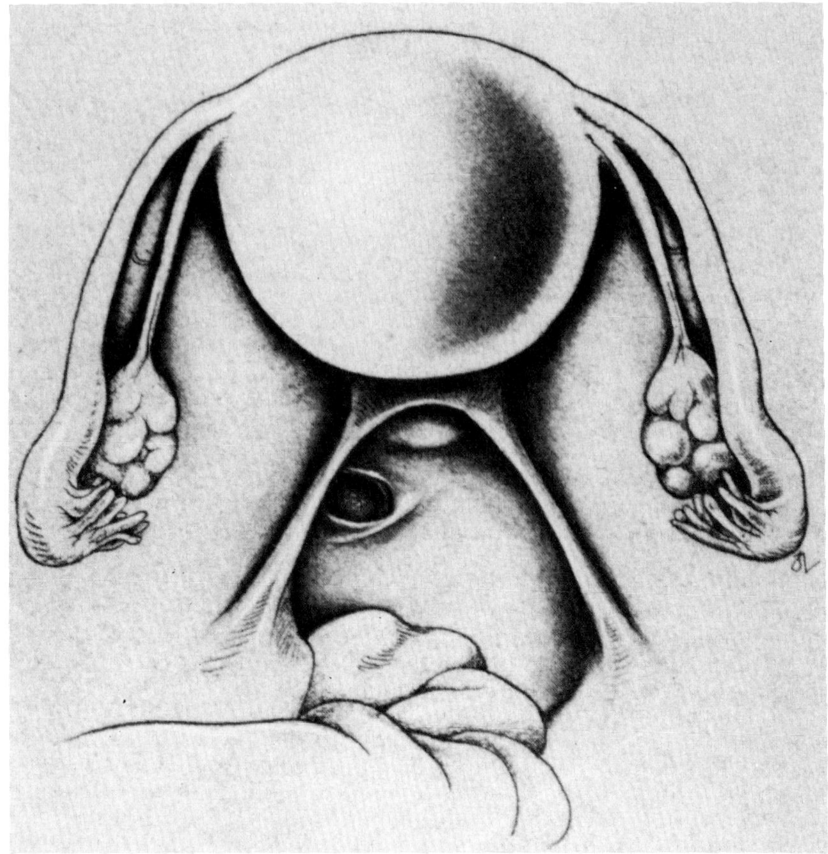

FIG 11–3.
Posterior cul-de-sac peritoneal pocket under left uterosacral ligament; excision demonstrated endometriosis foci. (From Batt RE, Smith RA: *Obstet Gynecol Clin North Am* 1989; 16:15–28. Used by permission.)

ness combined with magnification will likely improve the completeness of removing subtle forms of the disease. Unfortunately, microscopic endometriosis cannot be identified by the surgeon's eye; 20% of biopsy specimens of grossly normal peritoneum were found to harbor endometriosis using electron microscopy.[10] Again, our failure to understand the natural history of endometriosis prevents us from determining whether "microscopic endometriosis," whether defined by light or electron microscopic criteria, is at all clinically relevant to the treatment of women with endometriosis.[11]

The problem of persistent microscopic endometriosis prompted several investigators to study combination medical and surgical therapy.[12] The concept inspiring combination therapy was adapted from the treatment of epithelial tumors of the ovary: initial surgery should be debulking, removing as much disease as possible, with postoperative chemotherapy used to treat residual implants. In women with moderate and severe endometriosis, 3 to 6 months of postoperative Danazol produced lower long-term recurrence rates than those patients treated by surgery alone.[13] This study still needs to be confirmed with the experience of other authors and, preferably, a longitudinal prospective comparative trial. Until then, many clinicians use adjunctive postoperative medical treatment in more severe cases of endometriosis.

WHY DOES RECURRENCE OCCUR AFTER "COMPLETE" OPERATIONS?

The most obvious answer to this question is the multifocal nature of endometriosis and the likely possibility of missing a lesion or two during surgery. More than 20 years ago, Rogers and Jacobs at our institution emphasized the importance of en bloc dissection of juxtaposed endometriosis implants.[14] As shown in Figure 11–4, the many implants in the posterior cul de sac were considered a "field," and the entire field was completely removed. In those days, 2-0 chromic sutures were used to close the peritoneum. Many of us have wondered if those days of sharp dissection of multiple implants were associated with lower recurrence rates. One could safely assume that complete removal of the involved peritoneum, including the entire depth of the lesions, would certainly not increase the risk of recurrence.

Because the depth of infiltration of endometriosis implants is so variable, more superficial treatments might well fail to treat deeper depths of disease. Martin and co-workers found that one fourth of patients had lesions that penetrated the peritoneum greater than 5 mm.[15] Because one pass of the CO_2 laser will vaporize tissue to a depth of 0.1 to 0.5 mm, even several passes of the laser could leave disease behind. Endometriosis has been histologically confirmed immediately juxtaposed to carbon particles from previous laser surgery, suggesting incomplete treatment.[16] Whenever possible, fields of endometriosis should be excised, whether the surgeon is using knife, scissors, or laser, to incise peritoneum. Figure 11–5 depicts this principle using laser as the instrument for peritoneal incision; note the peritoneum is removed completely to the depth of retroperitoneal fat. Whether surgery is performed by laparoscopy or laparotomy, the ureter must be clearly identified throughout the case to avoid injury.

REPEAT CONSERVATIVE SURGERY

When persistent infertility or recurrent somatic symptoms warrant evaluation for recurrent endometriosis, laparoscopy is performed. The pelvis is systematically inspected for implants of endometriosis; care must be taken not to confuse suture materials previously used for uterine suspension, presacral neurectomy, or peritoneal closure with implants of endometriosis. Many cases can be performed laparoscopically, adapting the same microsurgical principles used during laparotomy. Tissues are manipulated bluntly to provide traction and countertraction for lysis of adhesions. If grasping instruments are used, the adnexa are manipulated only by the utero-ovarian ligament; the tube and ovarian cortex are not grasped. Adhesions are excised rather than incised; all visible endometriosis is excised or completely vaporized. Ample irrigation and meticulous hemostasis complete the laparoscopic procedure. In most cases, 100 mL of dextran 70 (Hyskon) is instilled as an attempt to inhibit adhesion formation.

If the disease is not amenable to laparoscopic treatment, the patient is prepared

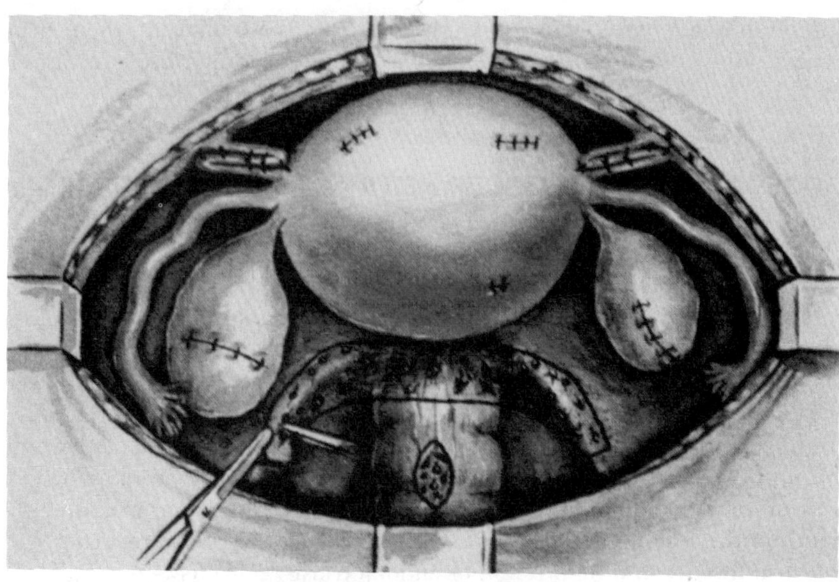

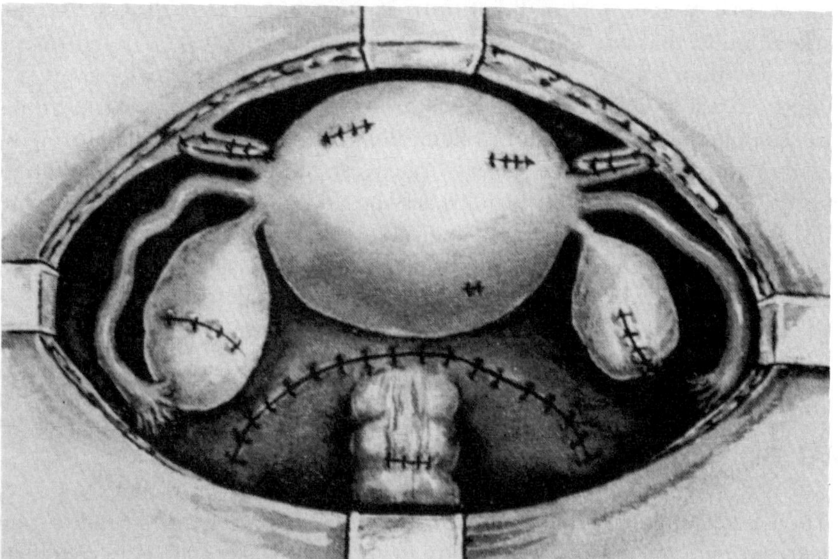

FIG 11–4.
Management of posterior cul-de-sac with numerous endometriosis implants after closure of ovarian and uterine lesions. The entire field is excised en bloc and the peritoneum closed with continuous absorbable suture. (From Rogers SF, Jacobs WM: *Fertil Steril* 1968; 19:529–536. Used by permission.)

for repeat laparotomy. The previous scar is usually excised in elliptiform fashion, wedging the subcutaneous fat down to the anterior rectus fascia. Care is taken on incising the peritoneum because omentum or bowel may adhere to the previous anterior abdominal wall incision. Once moistened laparotomy sponges are placed around the wound edges and self-retaining retractor is positioned, the procedure is performed very much like primary conservative surgery for endometriosis.[17] However, repeat presacral neurectomy is usually not attempted due to difficulty in dissection and bleeding caused by retroperitoneal scarring.[18] Magnification in the form

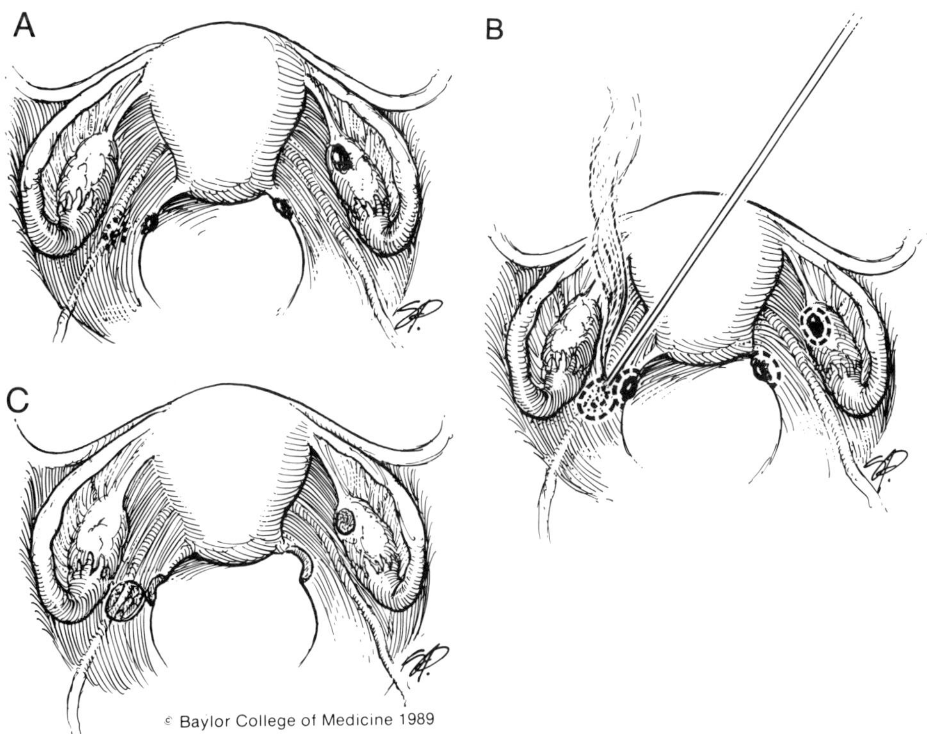

FIG 11–5.
Management of diffuse endometriosis lesions with laser. **A,** group of lesions, removed with 2- to 4-mm margins of normal margins, through the full thickness of the peritoneum. **B,** lesions are circumscribed with CO_2 laser highly focused with 16 to 20 W of power, preferably with superpulse mode. Once the lesion is circumscribed, the edge is lifted, and the laser is passed to and fro under the peritoneum to separate it from underlying adventitia and fat. Carbonization is minimized. **C,** retroperitoneal fat as it appears after excision of the lesion; the same effect is possible with sharp dissection. The position of the ureter must be known to the surgeon operating via laparoscopy or laparotomy. (Copyright © Baylor College of Medicine.)

of 2.5 or 4 × loupes, or microscope, is useful in removing as much disease as possible. Tissues are handled minimally and kept continually moistened with a solution of warmed lactated Ringer's with 20 mg of dexamethasone and 5,000 units of heparin/L. The procedure is anatomically orchestrated to effect complete removal of disease. Special attention is paid to the gastrointestinal (GI) tract, including the appendix, which may have been previously incompletely treated.[19]

Once all areas of endometriosis and adhesions are excised, there are several options in the managment of the peritoneal defects. If the peritoneum can be reapproximated with 4–0 or 5–0 absorbable suture without tension, primary closure is our usual first choice. Peritoneal defects may be left open if underlying tissue is vital and clean. Free peritoneal grafts have been useful in some of our cases with large, raw areas; these areas have been remarkably free of adhesions at short-interval, second-look laparoscopy. Free omental grafts have been abandoned, whereas fashioning a large omental carpet may be used on huge peritoneal defects. Also, new barriers such as Interceed (TC7) will help prevent adhesions of deperitonealized areas.[20] If Interceed is not available, many surgeons use 100 to 200 mL of intraperitoneal dextran 70 following conservative laparotomy for endometriosis.

The role of second-look laparoscopy 2 to 12 weeks after conservative laparotomy is useful in lysing new adhesions but has unknown effect on recurrence of endometriosis.

"COMPLETE" OPERATIONS

All treatises on surgical management of endometriosis include a section on so-called complete, or definitively curative, operations.[17] Unfortunately, endometriosis may recur following hysterectomy and oophorectomy if special care is not taken to completely remove all areas involved with disease.[21]

If a woman has completed her childbearing, and recurrent endometriosis is suspected of causing pelvic pain, laparoscopic examination may demonstrate only mild to moderate extent of disease. If the woman is otherwise a good candidate anatomically for vaginal hysterectomy, operative laparoscopic techniques may be used to vaporize or coagulate adhesions or endometriosis inaccessable to the vaginal surgeon. Certainly, vaginal hysterectomy should be undertaken only if the goal of complete removal of disease, including ovarian endometriosis, is attainable. Thus, most hysterectomies for endometriosis, especially more severe forms of the disease, are better treated by total abdominal hysterectomy.

Abdominal hysterectomy is usually performed via the previous incision, unless a separate indication warrants a midline incision. We maintain careful tissue handling at hysterectomy quite similar to that of conservative laparotomy; the only tissues clamped or grasped are those that will be ultimately removed. Remaining tissues are kept moist and not abraded with sponges. As depicted in Figure 11–6, an en bloc incision is made, and all contiguously involved peritoneal surfaces are removed. All lesions of endometriosis are removed with 2- to 4-mm circumferential margins and to the depth of retroperitoneal fat. In more cases than not, the ureter has to be identified high on the pelvic brim and dissected free of diseased peritoneum, especially if a severely diseased adnexa is being removed. If the posterior cul-de-sac is obliterated, the rectum must be dissected free, leaving as much disease on the uterus and as little residua on the colon as possible. If dissection is not possible, segmental resection and anastomosis of prepared bowel probably decrease the likelihood of future long-term recurrence of endometriosis. Dissection of the pararectal spaces in cases of endometriosis, leaving only healthy uninvolved tissues behind, is likely to lessen recurrence.[22] Following definition of these margins for hysterectomy, a standard *extrafascial* hysterectomy is performed.[23] If cervical or vaginal endometriosis is suspected from preoperative speculum examination, the involved portion of the posterior vagina is included with the hysterectomy specimen. Otherwise, the cervix is completely removed, and the vaginal length is maximized.

In the most severe cases of endometriosis, the margins for dissection between the uterus, rectum, and bladder can be obliterated by active disease and fibrosis. Intrafascial hysterectomy is appropriate in these circumstances to avoid ureteric injury if they cannot be dissected free of disease. If fibrosis prevents safe intrafascial hysterectomy, we will still occasionally perform supracervical hysterectomy in particularly severe cases.

Ovarian preservation at the time of hysterectomy for endometriosis is controversial. Each ovary should be removed if it is seriously involved with endometriosis

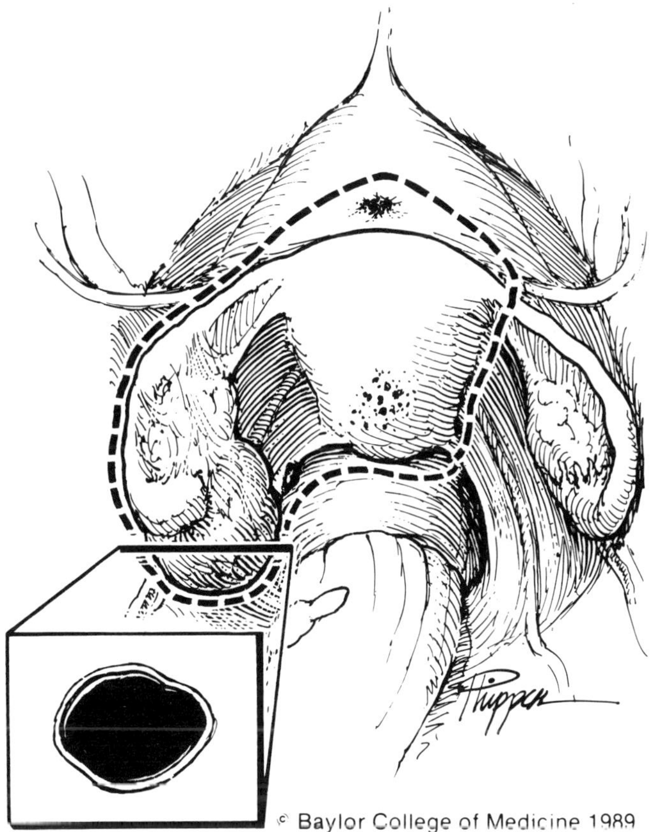

FIG 11–6.
Hysterectomy for endometriosis. All endometriosis lesions are removed, preferably as an en bloc dissection *(dashed line)*. Any residual implants are removed or destroyed with laser or cautery. The left ovary containing a large endometrioma *(inset)* is removed. The normal right ovary can be preserved if the patient has no symptoms referrable to that adnexa. (Copyright © Baylor College of Medicine.)

or compromised by adhesions. An ovary with only a superficial implant or two may be preserved. Also, if the woman gives a history more of adnexal pain rather than the more classic central pain, removal of the ovaries is more likely to give complete pain relief. In our experience, if the ovaries are suitable for preservation at the time of hysterectomy and are suspended away from the vaginal cuff, the chances of subsequent need for reoperation is 5% or less. One technique of ovarian suspension after hysterectomy is depicted in Figure 11–7. The interrupted round and utero-ovarian ligaments are sutured to the high lateral abdominal wall, without kinking the infundibulopelvic ligament and without the ovaries resting on the vaginal cuff.

Following hysterectomy, all areas are carefully checked for hemostasis; the cuff can be safely closed if hemostasis is complete. The abdomen and pelvis are copiously irrigated. Reperitonealization is performed only with fine sutures and only if it can be done without tension. If a large raw bed of deperitonealized tissue remains, and if hemostasis was complete enough to permit closure of the cuff, several techniques may lessen adhesion formation: a vascularized omental carpet or a particularly redundant rectosigmoid colon can cover most of the pelvis, and Interceed can be applied to the suture lines, or intraperitoneal dextran 70 can be instilled. If

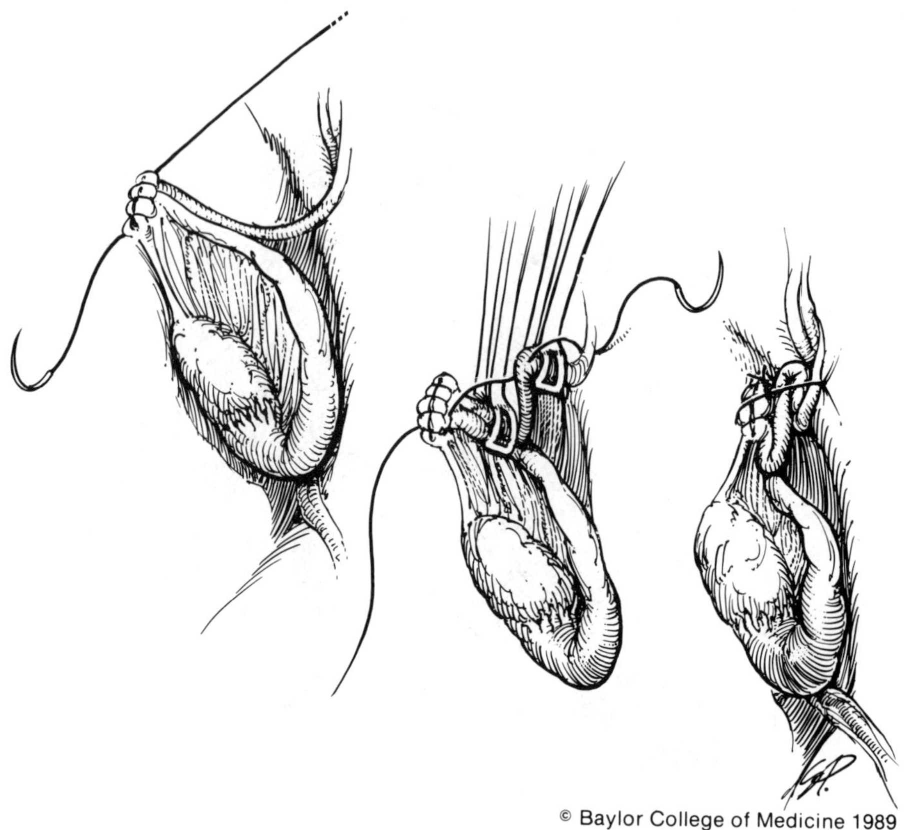

FIG 11–7.
Management of the uninvolved adnexa at hysterectomy. The ovary is suspended from the proximal round ligament/utero-ovarian ligament stump high on the lateral abdominal wall. Care is taken not to distort the infundibulopelvic ligament with the suspension. (Copyright © Baylor College of Medicine.)

the adnexa are preserved, they must not be near any raw areas because they adhere and cause pain.

The appendix is removed if it is involved with endometriosis or if the cecum is redundant enough to allow the appendix to reach the pelvis and possible adhere postoperatively. Cecopexy may be used to prevent descent of the cecum into the true pelvis.

Recurrence After Hysterectomy and Bilateral Oophorectomy

Occasionally, a patient who has had hysterectomy and bilateral salpingo-oophorectomy will present with symptoms and signs suggestive of ovarian remnant syndrome (see Chapter 23). Laboratory findings of high-normal levels of follicle-stimulating hormone, or nearly normal estradiol levels suggest the presence of ovaries. However, ovarian remnants can cause pain and masses even without biochemical evidence of ovarian function. These cases are managed surgically by careful dissection of the ureters and pararectal spaces, followed by removal of large areas of peritoneum containing the residual ovarian tissue.[24] In these cases, postoperative treatment with Danazol or GnRH agonist may be warranted due to the possibility of residual disease.

COMPLICATIONS

If the endometriosis is amenable to laparoscopic surgery, care must be taken to avoid injury to the ureters and GI tract. The largest blood vessels encountered by the careful operative laparoscopist are usually branches of the uterine artery during uterosacral ligament dissection, which can bleed severely unless grasped and coagulated or ligated. Reports of laser laparoscopic injury to the ureters are only now starting to be publicly discussed but are likely to occur in 1% or 2% of cases. Although the GI tract may be treated laparoscopically, the same precautions are taken as at laparotomy: prepared bowel, intrarectal finger to assess mural depth of dissection, and endosuturing of large areas of excision.

Repeat conservative laparotomy is associated with rare complications. Ureteric injuries may be largely prevented if the ureter is identified high on the pelvic brim and the overlying peritoneum is dissected free. The ureter itself should never be stripped of its adventitial tissue, because vascular compromise may occur, promoting fistula formation. If the ureter is denuded due to direct invasion of endometriosis, a cystoscopically placed diversionary stent should be used until healing can be assured.

If endometriosis is mild enough to permit vaginal hysterectomy, no additional complications over the ordinary are likely. However, severe endometriosis treated by abdominal hysterectomy can be as difficult as cases of severe tubo-ovarian abscess or ovarian carcinoma. Again, the ureters must be identified and dissected free under direct vision. The integrity of the bowel must also be protected; a preoperative mechanical and antibiotic prep is sorely missed should the colon be inadvertently entered.

If the blood supply to the adnexa (even if visually normal) is compromised by the surgery, oophorectomy is indicated. Otherwise, the adnexa are surgically suspended to the high lateral abdominal wall above the iliac vessels and far above the ureters and vaginal cuff.

RESULTS

Virtually no data are available on recurrence of endometriosis after a second procedure. We have reported a 47% (7/15) pregnancy rate in infertile women treated with a second conservative laparotomy and followed at least 18 months.[4] We have performed a third conservative operation only rarely; this is usually in the form of an operative laparoscopy. If, on the third operation, the endometriosis is severe beyond laparoscopic surgical bounds, hysterectomy is advocated. In consultation, we have seen a single woman with endometriosis and pelvic pain operated on six times in 18 months (three laparoscopies, three conservative laparotomies); she had never had a trial of any medical treatment. The conscientious pelvic surgeon should be well versed in medical treatment of endometriosis, including perioperative adjunctive use. We use postoperative medical treatment for 3 months in women with severe endometriosis and those with known residua that could not be dissected free at surgery.

HORMONAL REPLACEMENT IN THE WOMAN WITH RECURRENT ENDOMETRIOSIS

Women undergoing hysterectomy with bilateral salpingo-oophorectomy for endometriosis are often young and would benefit from estrogen replacement therapy. However, there is some concern that exogenous estrogens might stimulate endometriosis regrowth. If macroscopic disease is left behind, 3 to 6 months of postoperative Danazol or GnRH agonist treatment may decrease further recurrence. Medroxyprogesterone acetate in doses of 20 to 30 mg daily may treat both residual endometriosis and some symptoms of surgical menopause.

If there is no macroscopic residual disease, many clinicians wait 6 weeks or so before starting hormone replacement. Then, the lowest dose possible that will control symptoms is prescribed, typically beginning with 0.625 mg of conjugated estrogens daily. Due to the concern of unopposed estrogens encouraging recurrence of endometriosis, 2.5 to 5 mg of medroxyprogesterone daily is usually added.

SUMMARY

Many of the principles for treating endometriosis at initial operation hold true for treating recurrent disease. Surgical success is dependent on excision or vaporization of all gross disease; postoperative medical treatment may then help with microscopic lesions or lesions incompletely removed at initial surgery. The infertile woman with endometriosis may be counseled that a second conservative laparotomy (and probably operative laparoscopy) has a reasonable chance of success; alternatives are in vitro fertilization or hysterectomy. For the woman with pelvic pain, preferably having completed her family, hysterectomy offers the greatest chance of long-term freedom from the pain of her disease. At hysterectomy, the ovaries may be preserved if normal, and oophoropexy away from the cuff will lessen the chance for deep dyspareunia that otherwise would be attributed to recurrent disease.

The frequent recurrence of endometriosis, like its ability to invade contiguous structures and metastasize to distant sites, is another example of the malignant nature of this histologically benign disease. To the woman with endometriosis, risk of recurrence is a concern second only to likelihood of relief of pain or success of conception. More research is needed as to what factors and surgical techniques promote recurrence, as well as improved noninvasive methods of screening for recurrence, such as the antibody CA 125.[25] Until then, the most complete operation that is also the least damaging to remaining tissues is the method of choice, requiring case-by-case individualization by the gynecologic surgeon.

Acknowledgment

The editorial assistance of Lisa H. Wheeler is appreciated.

REFERENCES

1. Buttram VC: Surgical treatment of endometriosis in the infertile female: A modified approach. *Fertil Steril* 1979; 32:635–640.
2. Metzger DA, Luciano AA: Hormonal therapy of endometriosis. *Obstet Gynecol Clin North Am* 1989; 16:105–122.
3. Schenken RS, Malinak LR: Reoperation after initial treatment of endometriosis with conservative surgery. *Am J Obstet Gynecol* 1978; 131:416–424.
4. Wheeler JM, Malinak LR: Recurrent endometriosis: Incidence, management and prognosis. *Am J Obstet Gynecol* 1983; 146:247–253.
5. Wheeler JM, Malinak LR: Recurrent endometriosis. *Contrib Gynecol Obstet* 1987; 16:13–21.
6. Redwine DB: Incidence of recurrent endometriosis remains unknown [letter]. *Am J Obstet Gynecol* 1984; 149:804.
7. Wheeler JM: The epidemiology of endometriosis-associated infertility. *J Reprod Med* 1989; 31:41–46.
8. Stripling MC, Martin DC, Chatman DL, et al: Subtle appearance of pelvic endometriosis. *Fertil Steril* 1988; 49:427.
9. Batt RE, Smith RA: Embryologic theory of histogenesis of endometriosis in peritoneal pockets. *Obstet Gynecol Clin North Am* 1989; 16:15–28.
10. Murphy AA, Green WR, Bobbie D, et al: Unsuspected endometriosis documented by scanning electron microscopy in visually normal peritoneum. *Fertil Steril* 1986; 46:522.
11. Dmowski WP: Visual assessment of peritoneal implants for staging endometriosis: Do number and cumulative size of lesions reflect the severity of a systemic disease? *Fertil Steril* 1987; 47:382–384.
12. Wheeler JM, Malinak LR: Postoperative danazol therapy in infertility patients with severe endometriosis. *Fertil Steril* 1981; 36:460.
13. Wheeler JM, Malinak LR. Danazol following conservative surgery for endometriosis at laparotomy significantly improves term pregnancy and recurrence rates in infertile women with moderate and severe endometriosis. Paper presented at the American Fertility Society Annual Meeting, Chicago, October 1985.
14. Rogers SF, Jacobs WM: Infertility and endometriosis: Conservative surgical approach. *Fertil Steril* 1968; 19:529–536.
15. Martin DC, Hubert GD, Levy BS: Depth of infiltration of endometriosis. *J Gynecol Surg* 1989; 5:55–60.
16. Martin DC, Hubert GD, Zwaag RV, El-Zeky FA: Laparoscopic appearances of peritoneal endometriosis. *Fertil Steril* 1989; 51:63–67.
17. Wheeler JM, Malinak LR: The surgical management of endometriosis. *Obstet Gynecol Clin North Am* 1989; 16:147–156.
18. Malinak LR, Wheeler JM: Presacral neurectomy, in Garcia C-R, et al (eds): *Current Therapy in Surgical Gynecology*. Philadelphia, BC Decker, 1987, pp 70–71.
19. Prystowsky JB, Stryker SJ, Vjiki GT, et al: Gastrointestinal endometriosis: Incidence and indications for resection. *Arch Surg* 1988; 123:855–858.
20. Interceed (TC7) Adhesion Barrier Study Group: Prevention of postsurgical adhesions by Interceed (TC7), an absorbable adhesion barrier: A prospective, randomized multicenter clinical study. *Fertil Steril* 1989; 51:933–938.
21. Dmowski WP, Radwanska E, Rana N: Recurrent endometriosis following hysterectomy and oophorectomy: The role of residual ovarian fragments. *Int J Gynaecol Obstet* 1988; 26:93–103.
22. Knapp RC, Donahue VC, Friedman EA: Dissection of paravesical and pararectal spaces in pelvic operations. *Surg Gynecol Obstet* 1973; 13:758–762.
23. Malinak LR, Wheeler JM: Therapeutic gynecologic procedures, in Pernoll, Benson

(eds): *Current Obstetric and Gynecologic Diagnosis and Treatment*. Norwalk, Conn, Appleton & Lange, 1987, pp 822–840.
24. Pettit PD, Lee RA: Ovarian remnant syndrome: Diagnostic dilemma and surgical challenge. *Obstet Gynecol* 1988; 71:580–583.
25. Fedele L, Arcaini L, Vercellini P, et al: Serum CA 125 measurements in the diagnosis of endometriosis recurrence. *Obstet Gynecol* 1988; 72:19–22.

Chapter 12

Myomectomy

Celso-Ramón García, M.D.

Uterine myomas are among the most common tumors encountered in women. They are particularly confusing since they can produce a variety of symptoms depending on the number, size, and location, as well as any associated pathologic condition that may accompany their presence. This wide array of symptoms includes abnormal menstrual bleeding, abdominal and pelvic pain, abdominal enlargement, gastrointestinal (GI) pressure symptoms related to the impingement of the tumor, and distortions related to this pressure, which can also produce dysfunctions of the urinary bladder, or in rare occasions, even obstruction of the ureter. Myomas are also associated with infertility although pregnancy can and does occur in their presence. Moreover, the basis by which myomas interfere with achieving pregnancy, while not clearly understood, is due to their effects on the endometrium, which may lead to hypermenorrhea, vascular changes, problems that might affect ovarian function, including anovulation through adnexal distortion, as well as alterations of gamete transport. Moreover, distortions of the cavity by intramural and submucus myomas could affect the pregnancy, causing pregnancy losses. The submucus myomas also could produce an intrauterine device–like effect and prevent pregnancy. The association of myomas and endometriosis to infertility is noted.

Generally, myomas are simple insignificant pathologic tumors of the female reproductive system that have exceedingly low malignant potential. When the myomas are asymptomatic, and particularly if they are 3 months gestational size or less, most physicians concur that nothing need be done. Multiple myomectomy may often be advised for young infertile women who are symptomatic and in whom the uterine mass is comparable to the size of a 12-week pregnancy. The procedure may be less appropriate for women who have reached an age of decreasing fertility. However, when the myomas are symptomatic, and particularly if they are over 3 gestational months in size, hysterectomy can often be advocated. The latter procedure is frequently advised for the patient with multiple myomas, some of which may be pedunculated, raising confusion as to whether these masses might represent an ovarian tumor. Hysterectomy also is considered because myomas can and do recur after myomectomy. To some extent the recurrence can depend on how successfully all of the myomas have been totally eliminated.

Management of a myomatous uterus has been modified greatly through the advent of laparoscopy and imaging technology such as hysterosalpingography, ultrasonography, and magnetic resonance imaging (MRI). Laparoscopy may prove difficult or even be contraindicated when the myomatous uterus reaches the region of the umbilicus. Hysterosalpingography is of particular pertinence since it may diagnose an intracavitary myoma that could be overlooked at laparotomy. Ultrasonography and MRI are of more recent utility and seem to give increasing promise as noninvasive techniques. Magnetic resonance imaging gives increasingly fine images with good resolution. In addition to these advances, the availability of gonadotrophic-releasing hormone (GnRH) analogs has offered great promise in the management of myomas although they have certain drawbacks that will be discussed later. As a result of these technologies, there has been a greater precise appreciation of assessment of uterine growth. Moreover, since the advent of acquired immunodeficiency syndrome (AIDS) as a general public health problem, society has a greater awareness of the dangers of blood transfusion. Thus, the importance of improved awareness of surgical hemostasis and improved cardiovascular dynamics has been stressed in patients undergoing surgical procedures. Transfusions are used truly as a last resort, and judicious intravenous hydration is used prophylactically.

Myomectomy for infertility or a symptomatic myomatous distortion are the most compelling reasons to perform multiple myomectomy when the woman wants to preserve her reproductive function. However, the recurrence of myomas raises concerns regarding the appropriateness of myomectomy since under these circumstances the new tumor growth may lead to possible reoperation. The malignant transformation of myomas are of less concern since they occur in less than one tenth of 1% of cases; solitary or rapidly enlarging myomas, however, are more suspect. Nonetheless, this remote possibility must always be discussed with the patient. When encountered, these tumors also require surgical attention and treatment.

Kelly[1] warned readers about the performance of myomectomies less they recur; however, he acquiesced when reflecting on the successful preservation of reproductive function with the intent borne thereof. The feminist community argues for preservation of the reproductive organs and prefers myomectomy rather than hysterectomy at any age. They believe not only that it is a reproductive loss but that it seriously affects sexual feelings because of the loss of deep orgasm and can also bring about premature estrogen deficiency secondary to ovarian failure. Much disagreement still exists regarding the advisability of performing a myomectomy, especially in older women, where the reproductive needs may be unrealistic. It may severely affect some women who perceive it as a loss of their femininity. When discussing hysterectomy they challenge the male surgeon by asking whether he would be willing to have his reproductive organs removed. Aside from the psychosexual social considerations and the concern of not being able to preserve reproductive function, there still exists in many women the fear of blood loss and the recurrence of myomas. This procedure is categorized as having an increased risk of complications and the possible need for a future reoperation. The difficulties associated with making the diagnosis of a leiomyosarcoma is another contributing factor of concern. The presence of coexisting pathology may make the surgery more prolonged and tedious. With the perception of so many confounding factors, many are less inclined to perform a myomectomy and advise hysterectomy instead.

GENERAL CONSIDERATIONS

Since there is such pleuralism regarding this procedure, it is well to discuss the general and specific aspects of myomectomy as well as the potential need for reoperation for the recurrence of myomas and the specific features that affect good outcome. Prior to myomectomy, patients should have a preoperative screening that includes laparoscopy, hysterosalpingography (perhaps hysteroscopy), dilatation and curettage (D & C), and an excretory urogram. Thus, the extent of the myomas and the relationship to the total clinical features can be detailed and a truly informed consent can be obtained from the patient. Asymptomatic myomas allow for more of an attitude of watchful expectancy. However, the more symptomatic, the more pressing the need for intervention. Endotracheal controlled general inhalation anesthesia supplemented by relaxing agents and analgesics allows for excellent relaxation, which affords better exposure. A Foley catheter, placed in the bladder, assures an empty viscus and monitors urinary output. Control of blood loss should start with the initial skin incision. A transverse lower abdominal modified Pfannenstiel incision in which a dissection carried out with the Shaw hemostatic scalpel (Oximetric) assures careful hemostasis and good exposure even with a myoma extending to the umbilicus. When in doubt the larger myomas may be better addressed by a midline incision. When reoperating on a patient who has recurrent myomas, it is important to relate their present role to the present clinical picture. Moreover, the abdominal incision probably should follow that of the prior surgery. If a repeat transverse lower abdominal modified Pfannenstiel incision is to be carried out, the Shaw scalpel with its thermal-hemostatic capability is exceedingly valuable in dissecting the tissues. Careful, meticulous hemostasis can be supplemented with bipolar forceps for the larger vessels. Such careful hemostasis must be assured with each step. The midline incision is less time-consuming but it leaves the patient with a visible scar that constantly reminds her of the operation.

Good exposure, good assistance, and careful isolation of the tumor or tumors are essential to reduce blood loss. It is also important to be experienced in the effective modes of achieving hemostasis. Hemostasis can be assured with myometrial injection of vasoconstrictors such as dilute epinephrine, oxytocin (Pitocin) or vasopressin (Pitressin) (I prefer the latter), and/or tourniquet application. When using the tourniquet placed around the cervicouterine junction, I prefer to include the oviducts and ovaries as well. This will constrict not only uterine vessels but also the infundibulopelvic vessels. I like to inject the Pitressin into the myometrium a few minutes before applying the tourniquet. This causes a vasoconstriction of the uterine corpus, reducing the blood volume within the organ. While some report a histamine reaction, I have never seen it. No serious untoward effects of curtailing uterine and ovarian blood supply for up to 3 to 4 hours have been noted. Nonetheless, it is preferable to aim to complete the myomectomy in under 2 hours. This gives optimal time for most dissections and repair. Although the crop of ovarian follicles in the current cycle are lost, the subsequent cycle awaits the new crop generated from the primordial germ cells, which tolerate this ischemia well.

MYOMECTOMY TECHNIQUE

The technique of myomectomy is illustrated in Plates 1 through 8.

Dissection of myomas should be carried out by incising the uterine wall starting at the thinnest locus over the myomas and by aiming to least disrupt the myometrial blood supply. After enucleation of the myoma through dissection in the pseudocapsule, permanent hemostasis can be assured by using a concentric spiraling stitch that obliterates the defect or defects while assuring anatomic restitution. This applies not only to an initial myomectomy but also to repeat surgery.

Many patients may not be safe candidates for surgery and may need preoperative management. Such is the case for those women with myomas who also are severely anemic secondary to hypermenorrhea. These anemic patients need aggressive management of their anemia. Some surgeons recommend having the patient donate 2 units of her blood before surgery for autologus use, but I have never been totally convinced that this approach is truly physiologically sound for anemic women. Truly severely anemic patients need all the blood they have since their menses are usually profuse and often even aggressive hematinic therapy may not be adequate. Most patients respond well to aggressive hematinic therapy. Although autologous blood may have been made available, it should be discarded if not needed. Transfusing patients with their own autologous blood when not needed may not be so innocuous. The risk of giving a patient the blood collected before surgery when she does not need it could produce cardiac overload as well as other risks. These risks have been appreciated and addressed by plaintiffs and their attorneys. Preoperative collection of blood to replace the blood loss at surgery may still not be adequate where there is severe blood loss at myomectomy. Since 2 units of blood may not be enough, the situation may warrant more blood from the blood bank. Upward of 7 or 8 units may be needed when there is significant bleeding. The careful surgeon, who is constantly aware of the need to use every technique to attain meticulous hemostasis and who is continually alert for bleeding can avoid excessive blood loss. With such care and by using speed without compromising the woman's tissues, the need for transfusion will be virtually eliminated. Indeed, in well over 20 years, in hundreds of multiple myomectomies, I have never needed to transfuse a patient *during* myomectomy because of the blood loss.

A preoperative alternative may be the use of a short-term continued estrogen and progestogen therapy to induce amenorrhea. Alternatively, GnRH therapy might be used to down-regulate the pituitary and create a pseudomenopause. Although the Food and Drug Administration has not yet approved the use of these agents for this indication, such an approach may nonetheless be useful to stop the hypermenorrhea, and one can manage anemia with iron replacement during the menopause-like amenorrhea. By contrast, those studies advocating GnRH to simplify the myomectomy as well as reduce the mean blood loss report saving about 200 mL of blood. One can well imagine what the total blood loss represents. In my experience in the last 200 multiple myomectomies over a period of almost 20 years, I did not have to give a single transfusion, but the average blood loss was 150 mL. Rarely was the blood loss greater than 1 L. Most often, the blood loss was less than 100 cc even with the dissection of multiple large myoma.

Despite such concerns, it must be pointed out that the control of bleeding at myomectomy is easier than when a pedicle gets loose at the time of hysterectomy. Similarly, there should be a continued awareness of the need for possible changing the compression and for replacement of the tourniquet application. Continual hemostasis can be maintained through appropriate compression, appropriate suture, or other variation. Repeat injection of dilute vasopressin may be needed.

GnRH AND OVARIAN SUPPRESSION IN MYOMECTOMY

Treatment of myomas with antiestrogens or ovarian suppression with GnRH has been hailed as a promising alternative to surgery. Myomas thus treated do regress a reported 20% in uterine volume. However, this reduction is maintained for only a limited duration after cessation of the use of these pseudomenopausal agents. Data support that the bone mineral content loss is significantly affected by GnRH. While the mean values of bone mineral content in patients studied are believed to revert to normal levels of their bone mineral content after cessation of the GnRH suppression, it must be emphasized that these are mean values and that some of these patients *did not* have a return to normal levels. It is of concern that use of these GnRH analogs may sustain and aggravate this undesirable adverse effect. Thus, repeated courses of GnRH for reduction of uterine volume do not constitute an acceptable approach. The addition of estrogen and progestogen in a concomitant manner with the GnRH is limited to one ongoing study. An alternate use of the GnRH as a medical management to obviate surgery has been the preoperative use of GnRH to reduce the size of myomas before myomectomy. Because of the formula for volume of a sphere or a spheroid, the reduction in volume in large myomas represents proportionately an exceedingly small reduction in the diameter of the myoma, since a 10-cm myoma will be temporarily reduced by about 1.7 cm in diameter. However, the reduction in volume represents a greater proportionate reduction in diameter in the smaller myomas or the seedlings. A 2-cm myoma may undergo a temporary 50% reduction in diameter. Thus, the effect of the GnRH ovarian suppression effects on small seedlings might reduce the very small myoma to an unrecognizable size at the time of surgery. These can grow again after suppression and may lead to the need for future reoperation.

Even before the use of GnRH, 10% to 35% of postmyomectomy patients have required subsequent surgery because of myoma recurrence. Malone and Ingersol[2] in 1975, reporting on 75 cases, indicated a 29% recurrence. Babaknia and associates[3] in 1978, reporting on 46 cases, indicated a 28% recurrence. Buttram and Reiter[4] in 1981, reporting on 42 cases, indicated a 14% recurrence. Garcia[5] in 1988, reporting on 150 cases, indicated a 12% recurrence. While some advocate that one should avoid removing the myomas that are close to the uterotubal junction or other areas and to leave some myomas behind, this is not a wise approach. Meticulous resection of all myomas without preoperative ovarian estrogen suppression should provide a better long-term cure rate. Microsurgical techniques may be required for these areas.

It is well to remember that myomas arise from myometrial cells. Although these cells are somewhat responsive to the GnRH down-regulation of the gonadotropins, the interstitial cells can also proliferate through perhaps other influences. In some areas these fibrous elements can exceed the myometrial ones. The interstitial elements do not follow the same response to GnRH as the myometrial ones. Thus, the reduction in size of many myomas is not always as dramatic as what the GnRH in theory should lead us to expect. Moreover, the exact mechanism of the growth of myomas is not related solely to estrogens but also to other factors such as platelet-derived growth factor, insulin-like growth factor, and epidermal growth factor.[6, 7] Indeed serial ultrasonographic monitoring of myomas during pregnancy does not support the level of myomatous growth that is generally believed to occur.[8]

SURGICAL APPROACHES

Meticulous technique is absolutely necessary if one is to perform myomectomy without significant blood loss. Appropriate site selection for the incision and dissection of the pseudocapsule is needed in addition to the appropriate assurance of hemostasis. Uterine incisions should be placed parallel to the arterial supply and not across it.

After each myoma is dissected, it is essential that its vascular pedicle be ligated and that reconstruction progress rapidly. Although speed in enucleation, vascular pedicle ligation, and reconstruction of the uterine defects are essential, common sense in understanding the distorted vascular anatomy in the control of bleeding is paramount. Although myomectomy is based on simple surgical principles, the variations in location and size of the tumors require the ingenuity of an experienced gynecologist.

Once the myoma is extirpated and its vascular pedicle ligated, the dissection should be turned to any adjacent myoma, which can be extirpated in a similar fashion from its locus. As many myomas as feasible should be excised through the same incision. Experience supports the view that it is not advisable to dissect through the endometrial cavity to excise myomas from the opposite wall. Repair of all defects created should reapproximate the tissues preferably with a continuous spiraling stitch of no. 3-0 polyglactin suture material. Catgut should be avoided because of its reactivity and lower tensile strength. Posterior uterine wall approaches should be of concern because of the potential for postoperative adhesions. Meticulous hemostasis and a subserosal approximation of the uterine wall with no. 6-0 polyglycolic acid-type suture (Vicryl or Dexon) have reduced the occurrence of adhesions as in cesarean sections. The site of the prior surgery is often difficult to find later. Pedunculated submucous or intracavity myomas are very difficult to assess at the time of abdominal surgery. These tumors should have been assessed during preoperative hysterosalpingography or hysteroscopy even before the surgery was scheduled. Opening the endometrial cavity may be essential in eliminating the possibility of a myoma that is pedunculated and has not been diagnosed beforehand by hysterosalpingogram or hysteroscopy. Such prior review allows the surgeon to discuss with the patient the option of hysteroscopic resection of small submucous intrauterine myomas. Although hysteroscopic resection, including the application of laser and other techniques, has been used for the smaller submucous myomas, the laser approach is preferable in hysteroscopically skilled hands for the submucosal or intracavitary myomas. These resections should be limited to the myomas of less than 3 × 3 cm with at least 50% of the myoma projecting into the cavity, which itself should not be greater than 10 cm in length. Moreover, the myomas should not impinge on the tubal ostia and if multiple, should not be at the same level as one on the opposing wall that tends to produce "kissing" adhesions. Laparoscopic resection has been advocated and is often used for pedunculated subserous myomas with small pedicles. Morcellation may be needed to remove the myoma through the operative laparoscopy portals or through a culdotomy incision through the pouch of Douglas. Broad myometrial defects following laparoscopic myomectomy lead to adhesions, whereas meticulous repair of defects with microsurgical techniques more often avoids adhesions. It should be recalled that macrosurgical myomectomies without microsurgical techniques risk the significant serious complications of adhesions and intestinal obstruction. Microsurgical techniques tend to obviate these.

Myomas even when multiple and of sizes of 10- to 14-cm in diameter do not, per se, dictate hysterectomy. Meticulous conservational uterine surgery does allow for extirpation and reconstruction of large myomas while preserving the uterine function. Well-controlled studies (hopefully appropriately randomized) comparing surgical myomectomy vs. other forms of therapy for enlarging symptomatic uterine myomas are very much needed. With recurrent myomas, the technique of myomectomy is similar to that described earlier.

In a woman with recurrent symptomatic myomas the probability of successfully achieving pregnancy is less favorable than the 40% to 50% pregnancy rate seen with primary multiple myomectomy. The thought of a repeat myomectomy thus is less appealing. Although complications of myomectomy are infrequent, the overall risk is probably greater than that of supracervical hysterectomy with ovarian preservation when justified. The risks of myomectomy including bleeding, infection, phlebitis, as well as the recurrence of myomas, are greater than those of supracervical hysterectomy; thus, the need and desire for preservation of the uterus has to be great enough to overcome the obvious disadvantages. Using a nondirective approach, one can usually guide the 40- to 45-year-old woman away from myomectomy. Preservation of the cervix with a program of periodic future Papanicolaou smears reduces the risk of cervical carcinoma from what it was years ago. Supracervical hysterectomy takes less operative time than either multiple myomectomy or total hysterectomy and also avoids shortening and scarring of the vaginal apex. Preservation of the cervix seems to be an acceptable alternative to total hysterectomy to the feminists who believe that Kilkku's[9] studies of total vs. supracervical abdominal hysterectomy retain a higher incidence of patient acceptance than total hysterectomy from the standpoint of sexuality.

Following postoperative recovery from multiple myomectomy, women who had hypermenorrhea before the surgery report dramatic improved bleeding patterns, as well as diminution of dysmenorrhea reported before surgery. Moreover, of those women with associated infertility, more than 40% and as high as 87.5% have reported successful term pregnancies among those individuals exposed to the possibility of pregnancy during the first 18 months after surgery. Entering the uterine cavity during myomectomy supports a recommendation for subsequent cesarean section when pregnancy occurs. Generally speaking, there is less need for delay of attempted conception since the risk of potential immediate pregnancy is less following myomectomy than following other infertility procedures. By the time that the earliest pregnancy occurs, which is not any sooner than 2 to 3 months after surgery and more often 6 months to 1 year, these patients experience no difficulty in safely carrying the pregnancy to term.

CONCLUSIONS

Reoperation for recurrence of myomas does not occur with frequency, and repeat myomectomy occurs even less frequently since hysterectomy is accepted by a preponderent number of women requiring reoperation. The surgical ingenuity of the gynecologist is of paramount importance in choosing the incisional site, the persistent retrieval of all the myomas, the meticulous achievement of hemostasis, and one's mastery in the reconstruction of the dissected uterus.

REFERENCES

1. Kelly HA: Benign tumors of the uterus, in *Gynecology*. New York, D Appleton and Co, 1928, p 522.
2. Malone LJ, Ingersoll FM: Myomectomy in infertility, in Behrman SJ, Kistner RW (eds): *Progress in Infertility*. Boston, Little, Brown, & Co, 1975, p 85.
3. Babaknia A, Rock JA, Jones HW, Jr: Pregnancy success following abdominal myomectomy for infertility. *Steril Fertil* 1978; 30:644.
4. Buttram VC, Jr, Reiter RC: Uterine leiomyomata: Etiology, symptomatology, and management. *Fertil Steril* 1981; 36:433.
5. Garcia C-R: The Role of Myomectomy in Infertility and Pelvic Pain. Presented at FIGO Meeting, Rio de Janeiro, Brazil, 1988.
6. Fayed YM, et al: Human uterine leiomyoma cells binding and growth response to epidermoid growth factor, platelet derived growth factor and insulin. *Lab Invest* 1989; 60:30–37.
7. Tonmala P: Binding of epidermoidal growth factor in human myometrium and leiomyomata. *Obstet Gynecol* 1989; 74:658–662.
8. Ahroni A, et al: Patterns of growth of uterine leiomyomas during pregnancy: A longitudinal study. *Br J Obstet Gynaecol* 1988; 95:52.
9. Kilkku PO: Total versus subtotal abdominal hysterectomy, in Garcia C-R, Mikuta J, Rosenblum N (eds): *Current Therapy in Surgical Gynecology*. Toronto, BC Decker, 1987, p 58.

Chapter 13

Operative Injuries to the Urinary Tract

John D. Thompson, M.D.

The bladder and pelvic ureters are directly adjacent to the reproductive tract. They may be involved in gynecologic disease and are always at risk of injury when gynecologic surgery is performed. In spite of this, injuries to the urinary tract are uncommon. This is testimony to the technical skill of gynecologic surgeons, the attention given to understanding the close relationship between the two organ systems, and the pride in doing surgery correctly to avoid injuries to adjacent organs and structures whenever possible. However, in spite of technical skill, pride in one's work, and attention to details, injuries to the urinary tract do still occur. They can cause enormous disability in patients and are the leading cause of malpractice suits against gynecologic surgeons.

In this chapter, the measures to prevent urinary tract injuries as well as their early recognition will be emphasized. Some operative procedures to correct injuries when they occur will be discussed.

OPERATIVE INJURIES TO THE URETER

Injury to the ureter is one of the most serious complications of gynecologic surgery. Ureteral injuries are far more serious and troublesome than injury to either the bladder or rectum. Delay in the diagnosis is often associated with postoperative morbidity, ureterovaginal fistulas, and the potential loss of kidney function. For example, Lee and Symmonds reviewed 68 patients referred to the Mayo Clinic with a diagnosis of ureterovaginal fistula. In 34 (50%), a nephrectomy was necessary because delay in the diagnosis of ureteral injury had resulted in loss of kidney function.

Fortunately, ureteral injury is uncommon. Its prevalence varies between 0.1% to 1.5%, depending on a variety of factors, including the number of extensive hysterectomies and other difficult operations included in the series. However, ureteral injury may also occur unexpectedly even in the course of uncomplicated operations, clearly indicating the need to adopt a routine procedure to confirm ureteral integrity at the end of each major gynecologic operation, vaginal and abdominal.

This discussion will emphasize the prevention and early recognition of ureteral injury, hopefully at the operation of injury. Management of simple injuries by gynecologic surgeons will be discussed. More complicated injuries that require special skill and experience in pelvic surgery will be mentioned.

Anatomy

The reproductive tract and urinary tract develop embryologically in close proximity. Because of this close proximity, alterations in anatomy and physiology may occur in one system in the presence of disease in the other system. Diseases of the reproductive system may cause urinary tract signs or symptoms, and the opposite may also occur. Congenital anomalies of one system may be associated with anomalous development in the other system. When significant parts of the Müllerian duct system are congenitally absent or obstructed, major anomalies of the upper urinary tract will be found in 35% to 40% of patients. Approximately 1% of females will have duplication of the ureters, more common unilaterally than bilaterally. Especially when difficult gynecologic surgery is performed, it is extremely helpful to know if ureteral duplication is present. If a ureteral catheter has been placed preoperatively in only one ureter of the duplicated system, the ureter without the catheter is more likely to be injured. The course of the ureter of a pelvic kidney may be tortuous and difficult to dissect. The commonly accepted explanation for duplication and other anomalies of the ureters is a variation in the origin of the ureteral bud or buds from the posterolateral wall of the mesonephric ducts at the fifth week of embryonic development.

The wall of the ureter is composed of smooth muscle with longitudinal, circular, and spiral fibers to produce regular peristaltic waves several times each minute. The lumen is lined with transitional epithelium. A condensation of connective tissue forms a pseudosheath that surrounds and protects the plexus of freely anastomosing vessels that course longitudinally up and down the ureter. Just before its entrance into the bladder, the lower ureter is surrounded by a layer of smooth muscle that extends a short distance upward from the bladder. This layer is called *Waldeyer's sheath.*

The ureter measures approximately 25 to 30 cm, depending on the person's height. The abdominal and pelvic components are approximately equal in length. In its course from the kidney to the bladder, the abdominal ureter rests on the medial border of the psoas muscle close to the vena cava on the right and the aorta on the left. The ureters enter the pelvis by crossing over the lower common iliac artery just at its point of bifurcation. At this point it is easily identified on the right beneath a thin peritoneal covering. Its entry into the pelvis on the left may be obscured by the sigmoid colon. The pelvic ureter courses beneath the peritoneum on the posterolateral pelvic wall, just above and lateral to the ureterosacral ligaments and anterior and medial to the hypogastric artery. When the anatomy is normal and the peritoneum is not involved or thickened by disease, the ureter can usually be followed visually from the pelvic brim throughout its course beneath the peritoneum along the lateral wall of the pelvis until it disappears beneath the uterine vessels (Fig 13–1). Peristalsis can be seen in the ureter beneath the peritoneum on the lateral pelvic sidewall. Peristalsis can be stimulated by simply stroking the ureter through the peritoneum.

After crossing under the uterine vessels, the ureter enters a tunnel through the

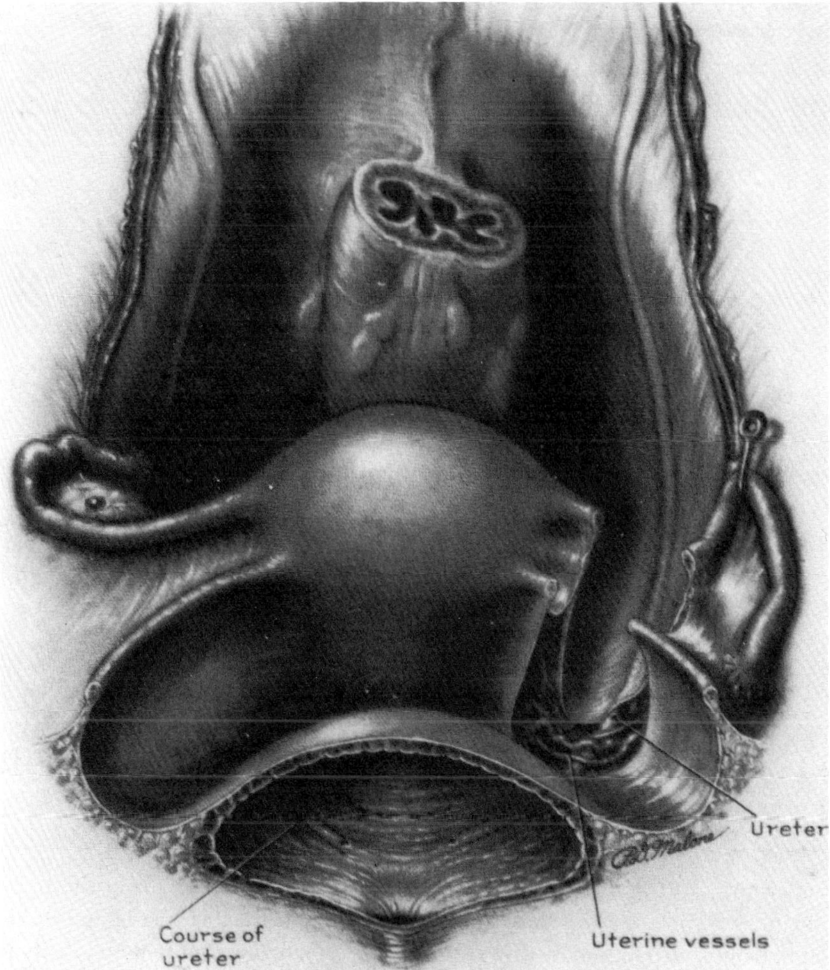

FIG 13–1.
Dissection showing relation of ureters to pelvic viscera. (From Mattingly RF, Thompson JD: *TeLinde's Operative Gynecology,* ed 7. Philadelphia, JB Lippincott Co, 1990. Used by permission.)

cardinal ligament. It is approximately 1 to 1.5 cm lateral to the cervix at the level of the internal cervical os. Just before entering the bladder wall, the ureter turns medially and anteriorly over the lateral vaginal fornix, where it can sometimes be palpated through the vaginal mucosa. It enters the bladder wall just above and lateral to the trigone. This angulation of the lower ureter is sometimes called the "knee" of the ureter.

It is important for gynecologic surgeons to realize that the course of the ureters may not be symmetric in their relation to the cervix. The left ureter is frequently closer to the cervix than the right. As shown by the classic studies of Sampson, the proximity of either ureter to the cervix may vary according to the position of the uterus in the pelvis even in the absence of pathology (Fig 13–2).

The ureter has the advantage of a rich blood supply from multiple sources along its course. The upper ureter receives blood supply from branches of the renal and ovarian arteries, the midureter receives arterial branches from the aorta and com-

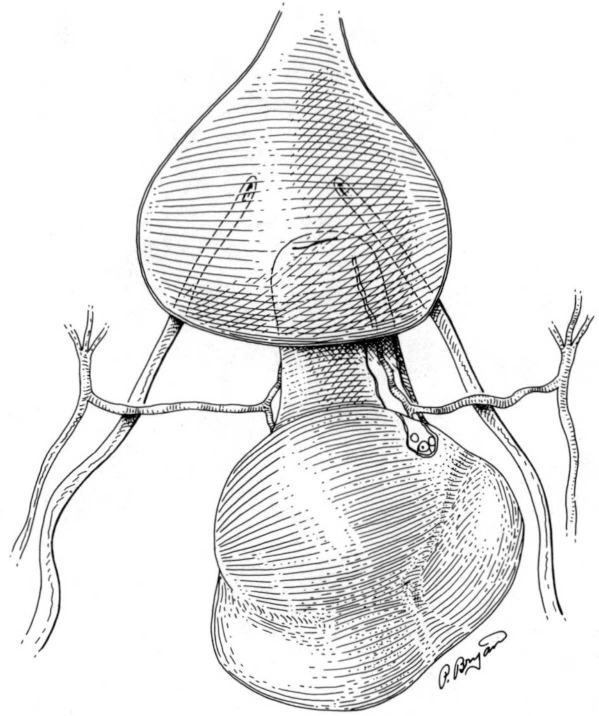

FIG 13–2.
The cervix is closer to the right than left ureter. During total abdominal hysterectomy, the right ureter is at greater risk of injury. (From Mattingly RF, Thompson JD: *TeLinde's Operative Gynecology,* ed 6. Philadelphia, JB Lippincott Co, 1985. Used by permission.)

mon iliac artery; and the pelvic ureter receives arterial branches from the hypogastric, uterine, vaginal, middle hemorrhoidal, and vesical arteries (Fig 13–3). There is a rich collateral anastomosis of vessels up and down the ureter beneath its pseudosheath. In mobilization of the ureter, these vessels will not be damaged as long as the dissection preserves the periureteral pseudosheath. This interconnecting network of vessels gives the ureter preferential healing capabilities in case of injury. Sampson described the importance of preservation of the periureteral arterial plexus, especially in extensive operations for gynecologic cancer. If these vessels are damaged by trauma or by skeletonization of the ureter by removing its sheath, local ischemia of a segment of the ureter may be followed by necrosis and rupture of the ureteral wall. In addition, there may be fibrosis and scarring of the ureteral wall and periureteral tissues with subsequent stenosis of the lumen and hydroureter.

Ureteral Involvement by Gynecologic Diseases, Operations, and Other Conditions

In its course through the pelvis, the ureter is susceptible to involvement, distortion, and/or compression by a variety of normal and pathologic conditions of other pelvic organs and structures. Such involvement may place the one or both ureters at greater risk of injury. These include the following.

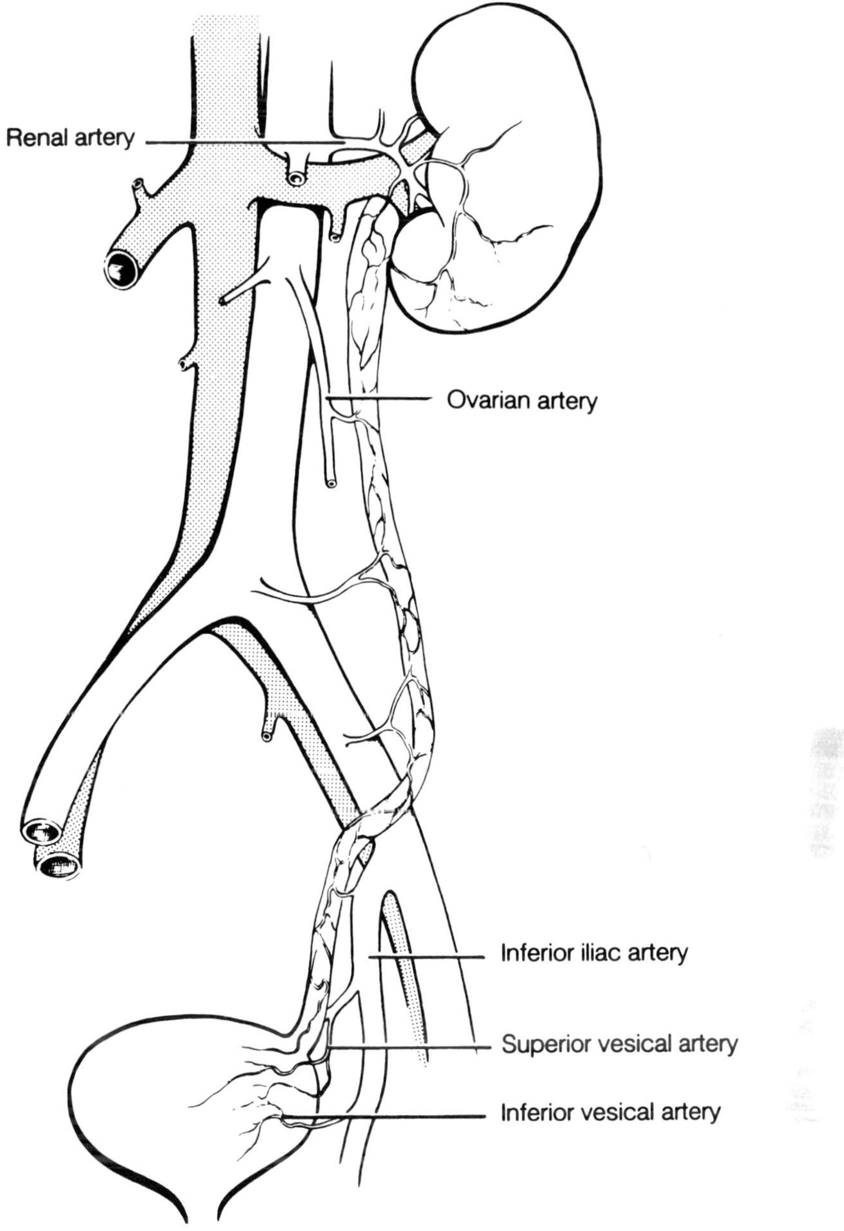

FIG 13–3.
Blood supply of the ureter. (From Mattingly RF, Thompson JD: *TeLinde's Operative Gynecology*, ed 7. Philadelphia, JB Lippincott Co, 1990. Used by permission.)

Intrauterine Pregnancy

An enlarging and dextrorotated gravid uterus and distended vessels in the right infundibulopelvic ligament may compress the right ureter at the pelvic brim causing ureteral dilatation above, whereas the sigmoid colon protects the left ureter against compression. High levels of progesterone in pregnancy also may cause ureteral ectasia, which promptly disappears following delivery. This physiologic dilata tion of the ureters will be impressive but should not be troublesome should pelvic operations be required during pregnancy.

Large Pelvic Tumors

Large solid or cystic ovarian tumors or large uterine leiomyomas may compress the ureters against the pelvic brim. Ordinarily, simply lifting the tumor off the ureter will relieve the compression. Leiomyomas can also cause compression of the lower ureter or ureters if they arise from the cervix or lower uterine segment.

Gynecologic Malignancies

Invasive carcinoma of the cervix may extend laterally into parametrial tissues and obstruct one or both ureters. Endometrial adenocarcinoma, uterine sarcomas, and ovarian malignancies can also involve the ureters but not as commonly as cervical cancer.

Endometriosis

In the presence of extensive endometriosis involving the ovaries, uterosacral ligaments, cul-de-sac, and/or rectosigmoid colon, the ureters may also be involved and obstructed. Involvement of the ureters may not be suspected by clinically specific signs or symptoms.

Pelvic Infection

Although patients with acute and chronic pelvic inflammatory disease usually will show no evidence of ureteral involvement, hydroureteronephrosis may be found in association with acute exacerbations of chronic pelvic inflammatory disease with tubo-ovarian abscess or abscesses. The obstruction may be unilateral or bilateral. If the infection extends to retroperitoneal planes and spaces, ligneous pelvic cellulitis with ureteral obstruction may result. The obstruction will usually be relieved by antibiotic therapy plus removal of the abscess or abscesses when necessary. Skillful dissection will be required to prevent ureteral injury.

Retroperitoneal Tumors

Usually anterior and medial deviation of the ureter will be caused by a retroperitoneal tumor growing beneath the ureter and lifting it away from the pelvic sidewall. Smaller retroperitoneal masses, such as retroperitoneal lymph nodes containing metastatic tumor, will cause less dramatic deviation in the normal course of the ureter. If an excretory urogram is done to detect ureteral displacement, it is helpful to have oblique and lateral views of the abdomen and pelvis. Straight anteroposterior views may not show the displacement.

Uterine Procedentia

Hydroureter and even hydronephrosis may be marked and bilateral when complete uterine procidentia has been present over many months or years. The ureters are caught beneath the uterine arteries and surrounded by the parametrial tissues that compose the tunnel. As these structures descend, the ureters are brought with them to a location outside the body. The so-called knee of the ureter is exaggerated and acutely angulated, causing obstruction above. The obstruction is promptly relieved when the procidentia is relieved.

Miscellaneous Conditions

A variety of other conditions may involve the ureter. An ovarian remnant may cause hydroureter. A pelvic hematoma developing after delivery or after operation or a pelvic lymphocyst developing after pelvic lymphadenectomy may cause deviation obstruction, or both of the ureter. Again, skillful dissection, possibly with the aid of surgical loupe magnification, will be needed to avoid injury. When a postpartum or postabortion patient develops septic pelvic thrombophlebitis that involves the ovarian vein with thrombophlebitis, the inflammatory process may extend to periureteral tissues and cause obstruction. However, the normal ovarian vessels in the infundibulopelvic ligament rarely, if ever, cause clinically significant symptoms from ureteral compression, and operations for the ovarian vein syndrome are rarely, if ever, justified.

Operative Procedures Involved in Ureteral Injury

About 75% of operative injuries to the ureter result from gynecologic operations. The remainder are the result of urologic, general surgical, and vascular surgical procedures. When only gynecologic procedures are considered, about 75% result from abdominal operations and about 25% from vaginal operations.

Almost all gynecologic operations have been implicated in ureteral injury. The incidence is highest with extensive abdominal hysterectomy and pelvic lymphadenectomy (1.0%–2.0%). The incidence is higher for abdominal hysterectomy (0.4%–0.6%) than for vaginal hysterectomy (0.1%–0.3%), although Nichols states that the risk of ureteral injury is greater during a vaginal hysterectomy. I believe the risk is greater during abdominal operations since patients with extensive disease possibly involving the ureters are more likely to have abdominal operations. The incidence of ureteral injury with adnexal surgery or with suprapubic urethropexy is approximately 0.1%. A partial vaginectomy done with either abdominal or vaginal hysterectomy is associated with a higher risk of injury, as is the extrafascial technique of abdominal hysterectomy. The posterior cul-de-plasty technique using the uterosacral ligament to support the posterior vaginal fornix and obliterate the cul-de-sac must be done carefully to avoid ureteral injury. The ureters are located just above and lateral to the uterosacral ligaments. If not done carefully, the Moschcowitz technique of closing the cul-de-sac can cause the same problem. The ureter can be damaged during laser operations done through the laparoscope. Use of laser or electrocoagulation for ablation or removal of endometriosis, lysis of adhesions, transection of ureterosacral ligaments, or tubal sterilization can cause ureteral injury.

Ureteral injuries are possible with obstetric operations. If deep lacerations of the lateral vaginal fornicies are caused by difficult forceps operations for obstetric delivery, the ureter may be involved. Plauche reports that the incidence of ureteral injuries was 0.44% and the incidence of ureterovaginal fistulas was 0.1% among the 5,220 cesarean hysterectomies. The incidence may be higher if the cesarean hysterectomy is done as an emergency in the peripartum period.

Unfortunately, the incidence of ureteral injury has not changed in several decades. However, the fact that injury to the ureter occurs infrequently is a credit to the attention given the ureter by gynecologic surgeons and their technical skill at the operating table. Although ureteral injury may be almost unavoidable in some situations, even in the hands of the most skillful and experienced gynecologic surgeons, a continuing effort must be made to reduce the incidence of ureteral injury even further.

Measures to Prevent Ureteral Injury With Gynecologic Surgery

Preoperative Evaluation and Preparation

Primary prevention of ureteral injuries begins with a careful evaluation of the patient's gynecologic disease and recognition of the likelihood of ureteral involvement either by the disease or by the operative procedure planned. An experienced pelvic examiner will be able to tell whether or not the disease in the pelvis encroaches on the course of the ureter. In complicated cases, special imaging diagnostic imaging techniques (ultrasonography, computed tomography, and/or magnetic resonance imaging) may be useful. Excretory urography has been the most useful special diagnostic procedure but certainly is not needed in the preoperative workup of every patient. It is possible to be selective and avoid unnecessary, expensive, time-consuming, and potentially hazardous preoperative studies by using sound clinical judgment. If disease in the pelvis is strategically located in an area that is likely to involve the ureter, preoperative excretory urography may be helpful. It should also be considered an appropriate part of the preoperative workup when disease is located in strategic parts of the pelvis that may involve the ureter or ureters, when an extensive operation is planned for benign or malignant disease (cancer of the uterus, endometriosis, etc.), when anomalous development of the müllerian ducts are present, and when there is a history of previous pelvic surgery (for medicolegal as well as other reasons). Although there is no proof that preoperative excretory urography can reduce the incidence of ureteral injury, many gynecologic surgeons do believe that prior knowledge of the anatomy of the lower urinary tract may help avoid such injury. When the films show an abnormality, they are likely to be displayed on the x-ray viewbox in the operating room to provide easy access should intraoperative review be needed.

Most experienced gynecologic surgeons prefer not to place ureteral catheters preoperatively, believing that they cause unnecessary trauma to the ureteral wall. In my experience, ureteral catheters have been helpful in only a small number of cases, perhaps 5% of pelvic laparotomies. They may be useful in operations for cervical leiomyomas, for ovarian remnant syndrome, when retroperitoneal fibrosis from endometriosis or infection is present, when one is dissecting around a retroperitoneal tumor, or when one is debulking an extensive ovarian malignancy. They are not used in extensive abdominal hysterectomy and bilateral pelvic lymphadenectomy. If a ureteral catheter is needed during the course of the operation and has not been placed preoperatively, it can always be placed intraoperatively through a cystotomy incision or through a cystoscope. Cystoscopy is more easily accomplished intraoperatively if the patient has been positioned for operation in Allen Universal stirrups.

Exposure

It is necessary to have proper exposure to prevent injury to important structures and organs in the field of operation. This is a basic principle in all of surgery. Certainly proper exposure is necessary to avoid injury to the ureter during gynecologic surgery. Proper exposure begins with an adequate incision. I believe that a

Pfannenstiel incision usually does not provide enough exposure for a safe abdominal hysterectomy or other major abdominal gynecologic procedures. The transverse Maylard incision is preferred because the structures on the lateral pelvic sidewalls are more easily visualized. Good illumination of the operative field, strategically placed retractors, willing assistants, and anesthesia sufficient for good muscle relaxation are also essential elements to provide proper exposure. But most important, the gynecologic surgeon must not allow exposure of important structures in the pelvis to be limited by a limited incision.

It is another cardinal axiom in surgery that the important structures in the operative field at risk of injury should be identified and visualized and, if necessary, dissected and mobilized to allow retraction out of harm's way throughout the procedure. This axiom has no better example than the ureter in gynecologic surgery. The ureters can be easily visualized along the pelvic sidewall in most abdominal operations. If visualization is difficult, an incision can be made in the peritoneum lateral to the infundibulopelvic ligament. If necessary, the round ligament may be clamped, cut, and ligated. As the peritoneum is dissected medially away from the lateral pelvic sidewall, the ureter comes away with it and can be traced fairly easily from the pelvic brim above down to its disappearance beneath the uterine vessels where it enters its tunnel in the cardinal ligament. It most cases, the ureter can be palpated in normal cardinal ligament tissue and should be felt in every case when clamps are placed adjacent to the cervix in total abdominal hysterectomy. Dissection of the lowest 3 cm of ureter may be done but is more difficult than dissection of the upper ureter and could itself result in injury to the ureter if not done carefully. Dissection, palpation, and/or visualization of the ureter has been recommended as a routine in every abdominal gynecologic operation as the best way to prevent ureteral injury.

When intraoperative bleeding occurs, there is a tendency to place clamps blindly deep in the pelvis in a pool of blood attempting to clamp bleeding vessels. Ureters may be clamped and ligated by such desperate maneuvers. It is far better to control the hemorrhage with temporary measures using the pressure of the finger, a stick sponge, or a pack and then to suction away the blood, replace the blood lost if necessary, request appropriate instruments and sutures, and arrange for proper exposure. Then the bleeding vessel can be definitively ligated or clipped hopefully without injuring adjacent structures such as the ureters.

Where the Ureter Is at Greatest Risk of Injury

Of course, the ureter may be injured at any point along its course in the pelvis. When the infundibulopelvic ligament is clamped, cut, and ligated, the ureter that has a normal relationship lies only 1 cm away. Distortion of anatomy by tubo-ovarian abscess, endometriosis, paraovarian cysts, or ovarian tumor may result in a shortened infundibulopelvic ligament that may be even closer to the ureter. The location of this segment of the ureter should be verified by visualization, palpation, and/or dissection before the lowest clamp is placed across the ovarian vessels. After the lowest clamp has been safely placed, the other clamps can be placed above it.

Along the lateral pelvic sidewall, the ureter is at risk of injury in removing adherent residual adnexa or ovarian remnants, freeing adnexal structures adherent to the posterior broad ligament, suspending the posterior vaginal fornix to the uterosacral ligaments, closing the cul-de-sac with a Moschcowitz operation, and reperitonizing the pelvis. In all of these procedures, the ureter must be identified before clamps and sutures are placed.

The ureters are in even greater danger of injury when the uterine vessels are clamped and ligated. Injury is avoided by first skeletonizing the vessels and then clamping them with three clamps after palpating the ureter in the cardinal ligament. The lowest clamp is placed first, at a right angle to the uterus, at the level of the internal cervical os. The other two clamps are placed above the lowest clamp. The uterine vessels are cut between the upper and middle clamps. The two lower clamps are replaced by suture ligatures that should contain only the uterine vessels. This technique is designed to ligate the uterine vessels securely while at the same time avoiding ureteral injury.

In my experience, the most common site of ureteral injury is in the lowest 3 to 4 cm, between the level of the uterine vessels and the entrance of the ureter into the bladder. This is the part of the dissection involved with removing the cervix. It is the removal of the cervix in performing a total abdominal hysterectomy that causes the largest number of ureteral injuries. As mentioned earlier, the ureters are only about 2 cm away from the cervix, but this distance is not always constant, as described by Sampson. Several maneuvers will help to avoid ureteral injury here. The bladder must be well mobilized inferiorly and laterally. The ureter should be palpated in the cardinal ligament and even pushed laterally if possible before clamps and sutures are placed in the cardinal ligament. When induration and fibrosis of paracervical tissue occur, the ureters may be drawn abnormally close to the cervix, may be difficult to palpate, and will not fall away from the cervix and vagina as the dissection proceeds. In these cases and in every total abdominal hysterectomy for benign disease, development of the pubovesicocervical fascia will be helpful. If clamps are placed beneath this fascia, as in the Richardson intrafascial technique, ureteral injury should not occur. Finally, if necessary, the ureter may be identified by dissecting it free and retracting it out of harm's way.

If one is uncertain of the location of the ureters when doing a suprapubic urethropexy, it may be helpful to open the lower anterior bladder wall and pass ureteral catheters up through the ureteral orifices. This is not often necessary as long as the urethropexy sutures are placed in anterior paravaginal fascia adjacent to the urethra and not higher up.

When one is operating vaginally, the ureter may be at risk of injury at several points. When anterior colporrhaphy is performed, the ureters may be only 0.9 cm away from sutures, as measured by Hofmeister using a special intraoperative cineradiographic fluoroscopic technique. It is difficult to explain why the ureters are not injured more frequently with this operation. When downward traction is made on the cervix during vaginal hysterectomy, ureters are drawn further down into the operative field by exaggerating the knee of the ureter (Fig 13–4). Complete development of the vesicocervical space with retractor elevation of the bladder will help to lift the ureters away from clamps and sutures. This may be further facilitated by clamping the bladder pillars adjacent to the cervix on each side of the vesicocervical space. Locating the ureter by palpation in the cardinal ligament may also be helpful in avoiding ureteral injury (Fig 13–5). Care must be exercised in the placement of clamps and sutures on the cardinal ligaments and uterine vessels. A single rather than double clamp technique should be used, taking only small bites of tissue. And again, when the posterior cul-de-plasty technique is used to support the posterior vaginal fornix after the uterus is removed vaginally, the sutures must be placed

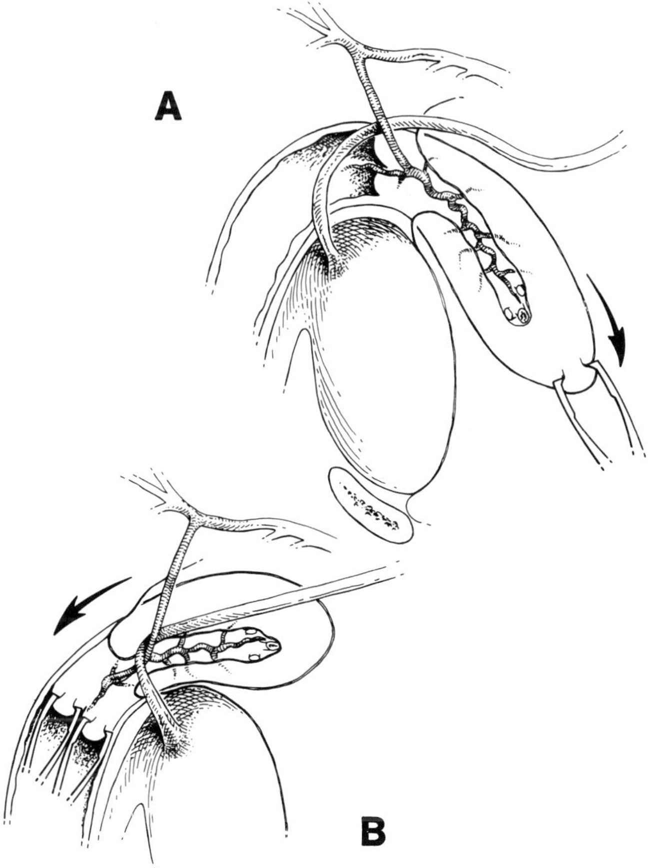

FIG 13–4.
A, in abdominal operation, upward traction on the uterine fundus pulls the uterine vessels away from the ureters. **B,** in vaginal operation, downward traction on the cervix exaggerates the knee of the ureter and draws it into the operative field. (From Mattingly RF, Thompson JD: *TeLinde's Operative Gynecology,* ed 6. Philadelphia, JB Lippincott Co, 1985. Used by permission.)

carefully and only in the uterosacral ligaments. If sutures are placed higher on the pelvic wall, the ureters may be incorporated. Clamping the infundibulopelvic ligament vaginally to remove the tubes and ovaries is hazardous since the ureter is only 1 cm away.

Ureteral Integrity

In our series of ureteral injuries, when the injury was recognized and repaired at the operation of injury, no kidneys were lost, and only one reoperation was required. Immediate recognition and repair of injury to the ureter are extremely important in prevention of secondary serious postoperative morbidity and loss of kidney function. It is important to keep in mind the wise statement of many pelvic surgeons, to wit "the venial sin is injury to the ureter; the mortal sin is failure of recognition." Emphasis is generally placed on prevention of ureteral injuries during difficult and complicated operations for extensive pelvic disease. However, ureteral injury may also occur during a standard uncomplicated operation. Symmonds believes that "the easy hysterectomy (or other straightforward gynecologic operation),

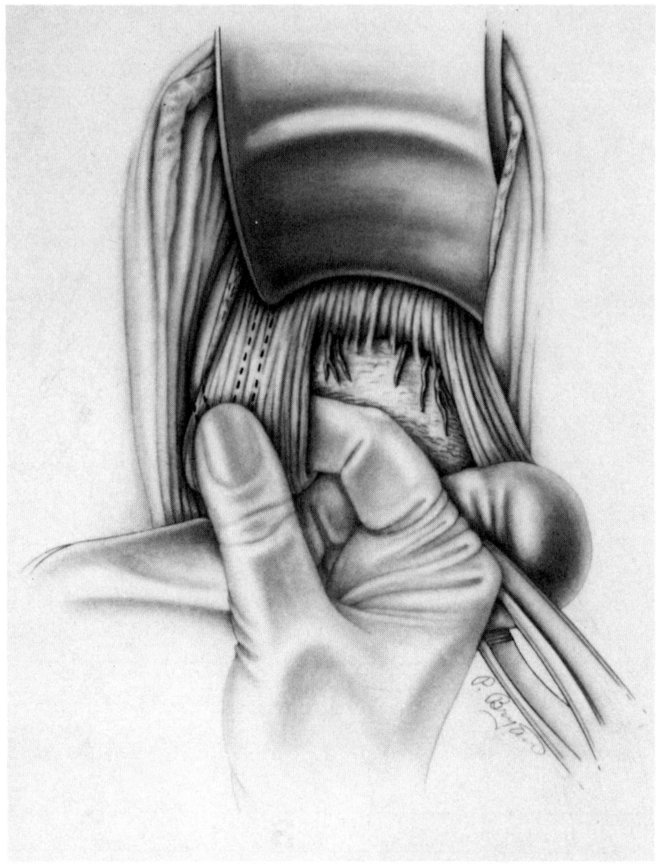

FIG 13–5.
The ureter may be palpated in the bladder pillar during vaginal hysterectomy, thus allowing placement of clamps to avoid injury. (From Mattingly RF, Thompson JD: *TeLinde's Operative Gynecology,* ed 6. Philadelphia, JB Lippincott Co, 1985. Used by permission.)

not the hazardous or difficult dissection, is responsible for most of the genitourinary tract injuries (and fistulas) in this country."

Because of the importance of detecting ureteral injuries at the operation of injury, I recommend that gynecologic surgeons adopt a routine and effective method of accurately determining ureteral integrity before the operation is ended, whether this be by palpation, mobilization and inspection, ureteral catheterization, or some other means. I have adopted an intravenous dye test that I use routinely at the end of each major gynecologic operation, both abdominal and vaginal. Before the incision is closed in abdominal operations, ureteral integrity may be quickly ascertained by injecting 5 mL of indigo carmine intravenously, placing a cystoscope in the bladder, and observing efflux of the dye from each ureteral orifice in 3 to 5 minutes. This single procedure is facilitated by having placed the patient in Allen Universal stirrups for the laparotomy. Of course, for vaginal operations, this simple procedure is even easier to perform since the external urethral meatus is a part of the operative field. Should the dye not spurt from a ureteral orifice (even after adequate hydration), the corresponding ureter should be explored along its course and the problem identified and corrected. It is my contention that adoption of this simple procedure as a routine measure would result in discovery of all ureteral injuries at the operation of injury.

Ureteral Consciousness

The level of consciousness about the ureter in the mind of the gynecologic surgeon has much to do with primary prevention of ureteral injury. It begins preoperatively with a careful assessment of the extent of pelvic disease, preoperative cystoscopy and excretory urography when indicated, and preoperative ureteral catheterization in a few selected patients. It must continue with an appropriate level of consciousness throughout the entire pelvic dissection and especially at certain key points in the operation. A heightened level of ureteral consciousness is required to prove ureteral integrity at the end of each major gynecologic procedure, and it must continue in the postoperative period. Patients with persistent postoperative fever, persistent abdominal distention, costovertebral angle tenderness, hematuria, and, of course, urinary drainage from the vagina should be investigated with postoperative excretory urography and other appropriate studies to determine the presence of ureteral injury as early as possible in the postoperative period in case it was not recognized at operation. "Out of sight, out of mind" is unfortunately responsible for many ureteral injuries and the damage they can cause to the kidneys. "Taking a chance," either consciously or subconsciously, that the ureter is in its normal position anatomically, is uninvolved with the disease process, and will not or has not been injured at operation is not a wise course.

Types and Sequelae of Ureteral Surgical Injury

A ureter may be injured during the course of an easy, difficult, or careless pelvic dissection. It may be kinked or partially or completely ligated with a suture. It may be crushed with one or more clamps. It may be cut or partially or completely resected either unintentionally or sometimes intentionally usually during the course of operations for gynecologic malignancy. Or it may undergo ischemic necrosis of the ureteral wall usually from stripping the blood supply from around the ureter for several centimeters, especially in the presence of infection and irradiation. The injuries may be single or multiple, unilateral or bilateral.

Depending on many different circumstances, a variety of sequelae to ureteral injury may occur. When injury has been minor, spontaneous resolution and healing may occur with only temporary and minimal interference with function. A minor degree of kinking or obstruction may eventually disappear. Spontaneous healing of more serious injuries, such as ureterovaginal fistula, is possible but should not be expected and is unlikely to occur without impaired kidney function.

When it is not recognized that the ureter has been ligated completely, it is inevitable that the kidney function will gradually disappear. Silent atrophy of the kidney as a result of unrecognized ureteral ligation at gynecologic operations is very uncommon, although undoubted cases have been reported. More commonly, infection supervenes, and the patient may be seriously ill before the ureteral ligation is recognized. A silent renal atrophy is possible only in the absence of infection. There have been reports of ureteral obstruction lasting more than 100 days in which relatively normal kidney function returned after relief of the obstruction.

When the ureter is ligated, the pressure within the lumen of the ureter rapidly rises from a mean of approximately 6.5 mm Hg to 50 to 75 mm Hg within 1 hour. Patients experience flank pain at the higher pressures. The pressure gradually decreases over time. Atrophy in the distal renal nephron begins in the first week and extends to the cortical region in the second week. Protein casts are deposited in Bowman's space of glomeruli. Urine escapes by pyelocanalicular and pyelosinus backflow and by the lymphatic and venous systems. The afferent arterioles are constricted, and the glomerular filtration rates and total renal blood flow are reduced. Even incomplete obstruction can destroy kidney function given sufficient time. The recovery potential following release of obstruction is dependent on many factors, including the length of time the kidney has been obstructed, the completeness of the obstruction, the presence or absence of infection, the degree of backflow, and the degree of functional impairment of the opposite kidney. After the obstruction is relieved, most kidneys will continue to show some impairment of function. The longer the obstruction is allowed to exist, the more likely the kidney function will be severely or permanently impaired.

A ligated ureter will usually not stay ligated. As pressure distends the lumen and pushes the thinned ureteral wall more and more tightly against the suture, an ischemic area will rupture, allowing escape of urine. A urinoma will form that is sometimes palpable on pelvic or abdominal examination. If a fresh incision exists in the vaginal apex, urine will dissect there and escape, thus creating a ureterovaginal fistula. Sometimes an overzealous stripping of the blood vessels of the periureteral arterial plexus occurs during extensive hysterectomy for invasive cervical cancer. Necrosis of the ureteral wall with extravasation of urine can result.

Eventually, at the site of injury, a stenosis of the ureteral lumen will develop and will progressively cause more and more hydroureter and hydronephrosis above. When the stenosis is complete, the kidney function is in danger of being lost if the stenosis is not relieved.

Bilateral ureteral injury with obstruction will quickly result in uremia if not relieved. Ligation of the ureter of a solitary kidney will also result in uremia.

Surgical Repair of Ureteral Injuries

The ureter should be handled gently, preferably with the operator's fingers or with noncrushing clamps or forceps. The ureter should not be freed from its bed except as necessary for repair of the injury. However, mobilization of the ureter must always be sufficient to allow repair without tension on the suture line. Reanastomosis or reimplantation must always be done without tension.

The ureter is capable of regenerating uroepithelium and smooth muscle, thus bridging the site of repair. This will be facilitated by carefully approximating the ureteral mucosa, by taking measures to avoid tension on the suture line, and by minimizing urinary leakage through the repair site. The success of repair will also depend on the health of the tissues that surround the ureters. If the periureteral tissue is rigid and fibrotic, there will be interference with healing of the repair site, but this can be enhanced by wrapping the ureter in omental fat.

The controversy regarding use of ureteral stints in repairing ureteral injuries has not been resolved. I prefer to use stents across the repair site to stabilize and immobilize the ureter and to prevent angulation during healing, to encourage an orderly regeneration of uroepithelium and smooth muscle, to reduce urinary extravasation at the repair site, and to prevent stenosis of the lumen. The stent must fit the lumen size comfortably without distending the ureter. Single or double-ended pigtail or J catheters are popular since they are not likely to be pushed into the bladder after placement. A Silastic tubing is well tolerated without causing inflammation but becomes soft and pliable at body temperature with a tendency to be expelled unless reinforced with stainless steel wire. A plastic pediatric feeding tube of proper caliber may also be used as a stent.

The decision regarding urinary diversion above the repair site is critical to the success of the repair. Unless the repair is a simple one with no technical difficulty and minimal urinary extravasation, diversion of the urinary stream with percutaneous nephrostomy is required. A Jackson-Pratt drain should be used to remove extravasated urine from the repair site.

The repair should be made with a minimal number of fine delayed absorbable no. 4-0 sutures, either polyglycolic acid or polyglactin. Permanent nonabsorbable sutures should not be used. The lumen at the repair site should be enlarged by angulated incisions. The edges should be carefully approximated without strangulation. Magnification with surgical loupes may be helpful.

As emphasized earlier, the best time to diagnose and repair ureteral injury is at the operation of injury. Should the diagnosis not be made until later, there is controversy regarding the correct timing of surgical repair. A number of different circumstances must be considered, including the patient's condition; the extent, location, and duration of the injury; and the condition of periureteral tissues. In general, it is now regarded as acceptable to attempt early repair of simple injuries in the immediate postoperative period should circumstances be ideal. Otherwise, percutaneous nephrostomy is the treatment of choice with definitive repair delayed until the induration of periureteral tissues has resolved. This may require a delay of 6 to 8 weeks, during which time a percutaneous nephrostomy may be required. Those situations in which extensive devascularization of the ureter has occurred, as with extensive hysterectomy, should not be repaired immediately. Definitive repair should be delayed in the presence of significant pelvic infection, cellulitis, or postoperative abscess formation or in any patient with a chronic, debilitating disease in whom primary healing of the repaired ureter may be impaired.

Finally, one additional principle must be emphasized. If a suture is found tied around a ureter, it should, of course, be removed. Inspection may then reveal a fairly normal appearing ureter. However, if the suture has been in place for any length of time (sometimes even less than 30 minutes), a defect will usually develop in the wall of the ureter after the suture has been removed. The defect may not be apparent at the time of disligation but may develop later. Simple disligation of a ureter is not usually sufficient for a ureter that has been ligated more than a few minutes. Ureteroneocystostomy or ureteroureterostomy will also be necessary in most cases. The same principle applies to a crushing injury to the ureter.

Ureterovaginal Fistula

Although mentioned earlier as a sequela of ureteral injury, ureterovaginal fistula deserves additional comment. Urine may drain from the vagina in the immediate postoperative period if the ureter has been cut and not ligated. This is unusual since the ureter is ordinarily included in a ligated pedicle. Usually after a febrile postoperative course that may also be complicated by persistent abdominal distention and costovertebral angle tenderness, urine may begin leaking from the vagina in 10 to 14 days as the suture loosens or the ureteral wall undergoes necrosis. When ureteral damage results from stripping the ureter of its blood supply as in extensive hysterectomy for cervical cancer, a longer period of time may elapse before ischemia has progressed to the point of necrosis of the ureteral wall and fistula formation. When urine begins draining through the vagina, the patient's clinical condition may improve temporarily and the fever may subside.

Excretory urography is one of the first studies indicated after appearance of urine from the vagina. Hydroureteronephrosis will usually be present on the same side of the injured ureter. A concomitant vesicovaginal fistula can be ruled out by instilling methylene blue dye into the bladder through a transurethral catheter. If a tampon placed in the vagina is wet but unstained with methylene blue, a ureterovaginal fistula is suspected. The location of the fistula can be identified more precisely by cystoscopy, with inspection of ureteral orifices for efflux of indigo carmine dye injected intravenously, and by attempting passage of a ureteral catheter on the side suspected of injury by these previous tests. As a rule, the ureteral catheter will not pass above the point of injury. A retrograde pyelogram will confirm the point of obstruction. It may also demonstrate periureteral extravasation of dye and a fistula tract. If by chance a catheter can be passed beyond the point of obstruction, it should be left in place for 14 to 21 days during which time the ureteral wall will hopefully heal. Before the catheter is removed, a retrograde pyelogram should be done to demonstrate healing of the fistula.

Usually, a ureteral catheter cannot be passed beyond the obstruction. In these patients, there is a tendency for progressive stenosis of the ureter to occur at the site of injury with the passage of time. If a repair operation is to be delayed, such patients must be followed by excretory urography every 2 to 3 weeks to be certain that the kidney is still functioning well. A reasonable period of expectant management may be permissible without establishing kidney drainage with percutaneous nephrostomy. However, cessation of urinary leakage through the vagina usually associated with recurrent pyelitis is an ominous sign and an indication that the obstruction is complete. Urinary drainage by either percutaneous nephrostomy or ureteral reimplantation will be required to salvage kidney function. Cessation of urine flow through a ureterovaginal fistula is almost never a good sign that the ureter has healed without stenosis. Only when excretory urography is normal, demonstrating an intact ureter, can it be considered a good sign.

Whether done immediately or delayed, the operation to correct a ureterovaginal fistula associated with injury to the lowest 3 to 4 cm of ureter is reimplantation of the ureter into the bladder. Fashioning a bladder flap may be necessary to bridge the gap if a direct ureteroneocystostomy cannot be done without tension.

Bilateral Ureteral Ligation

Bilateral ureteral ligation is a rare complication of gynecologic surgery but must be suspected when a patient is anuric in the first 24 to 48 hours following surgery. Soon thereafter the blood urea nitrogen and creatinine levels begin to rise and the patient may experience back pain and bilateral costovertebral angle tenderness. Failure to relieve the obstruction will result in progressive uremia and renal failure. Ureteral obstruction is easily demonstrated by excretory urogram that will show evidence of bilateral faintly visible nephrograms and hydroureteronephrosis on delayed films. Before emergency surgery is undertaken, cystoscopy with attempt to pass catheters beyond the point of obstruction should be done, but will usually be unsuccessful. When the diagnosis of bilateral ureteral ligation is certain, a decision must be made regarding the most appropriate management. If the diagnosis is made within the first 48 to 72 hours before the patient is profoundly ill from uremia and other circumstances are absolutely ideal, immediate operation to perform disligation and establish ureteral patency is the treatment of choice. Bilateral percutaneous nephrostomies are preferable to attempting disligation or anastomosis in a seriously ill patient who is not a candidate for surgery. After nephrostomy drainage is established, ureteral repair may be deferred for several weeks until the patient is a good surgical candidate. But before a definitive operation is done, another attempt at passing ureteral catheters beyond the point of obstruction should be made upward through the cystoscope or downward through the nephrostomy tube. Whether the problem is solved by operative or nonoperative means, the patient must have frequent excretory urograms to assess ureteral patency and kidney function.

Ureteroureterostomy

Ureteroureteral anastomosis may be done at the time of injury (always preferable) or at the time of subsequent delayed repair. The procedure is performed for injuries just above or below the pelvic brim. Ureteroureterostomy is technically difficult to do on the lowest 3 to 4 cm of ureter, and the results are not satisfactory. A transperitoneal approach is preferred. The site of injury is usually in the vicinity of the common iliac artery and vein and the hypogastric artery and vein, so dissection of the ureter must be done carefully. Locating the site of injury is facilitated by cystoscopic passage of a ureteral catheter as high up as possible. The peritoneum is incised and reflected along the lateral border of the ureter. The point of injury is identified, and the traumatized ureteral tissue is excised to the point of viability along with edematous, indurated, and/or infected periureteral tissue and suture fragments. The freshened ends of the ureter must have an adequate blood supply. If there is doubt about this, fluorescein dye and Wood's lamp may be used for confirmation. The ureter above and below the site of injury must be mobilized sufficiently to allow anastomosis without tension (Fig 13–6). The free ends of the ureter are cut obliquely and spatulated for 5 mm to ensure a wide lumen at the anastomotic site. A double J or pigtail ureteral stent is passed upward to the renal pelvis and downward into the bladder. With the ureter splinted by a splint of proper caliber, the two ends of the ureter are brought together snugly by four to six interrupted no. 4-0 delayed absorbable sutures placed through the ureteral wall above and below. The sutures are tied securely but without strangulating the tissue. Before the abdomen is closed, extraperitoneal drainage of the operative site is established by placing a Jackson-Pratt drain through a small stab wound. The drain should not touch the site of anastomosis.

Silastic tubing may be used as an alternate method of splinting the ureter. It may be passed to the renal pelvis. A suture should be placed to identify the end that is passed into the bladder. If there is any question regarding whether or not the stent is patent and draining, the end in the bladder can be easily identified and withdrawn through the urethra with a cystoscope. It can then be irrigated whenever urinary drainage seems inadequate.

If the anastomosis is entirely satisfactory, I tend to use only the indwelling stent left in place for 14 to 21 days, depending on a variety of circumstances. However, in difficult cases where the outcome is not as certain, one may also consider

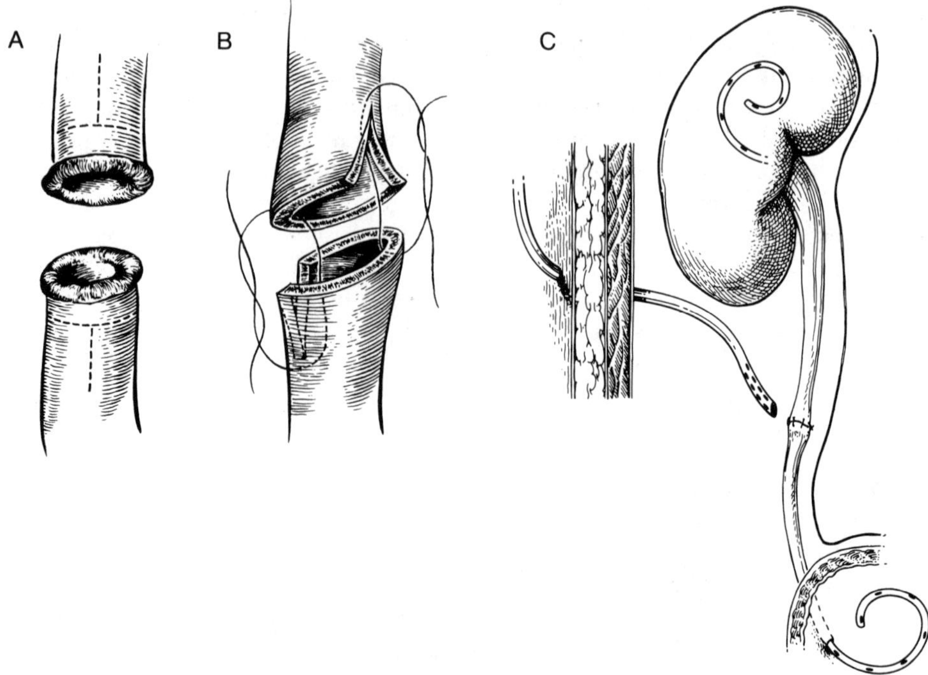

FIG 13–6.
A, the ends of the ureters are trimmed and spatulated. **B,** fine delayed absorbable sutures are used to approximate the ends of the ureter. **C,** the anastomosis is done over a double J or pigtail stent. A suction catheter is placed retroperitoneally to the side of the anastomosis. (From Mattingly RF, Thompson JD: *TeLinde's Operative Gynecology,* ed 6. Philadelphia, JB Lippincott Co, 1985. Used by permission.)

placing a percutaneous nephrostomy drainage tube for decompression of the anastomotic site until healing is secure. In addition, in cases where the anastomosis lies in a bed of indurated, infected, and unhealthy tissue, an omental pedicle should be mobilized and sutured beneath the ureter.

Ureteroneocystostomy

When injury has occurred in the lowest 4 to 5 cm of the ureter, implantation into the bladder gives better results than attempts to do a ureteroureterostomy. Again, a transperitoneal approach is usually preferred. The ureter may be directly implanted into the bladder through a small incision in the bladder wall. This operation is referred to as the "fish-mouth" procedure since the ends of the ureter are incised on each side for approximately 5 mm to produce ureteral flaps that are sutured to the bladder wall from inside out. The no. 4-0 delayed absorbable sutures are placed on each side of the incision in the bladder wall in such a way that the split ends of the ureter are held open. Any remaining defect in the bladder is closed with no. 3-0 delayed absorbable sutures. Adjacent peritoneum may be used to reinforce the anastomosis and to prevent tension on the suture line. A ureteral stent is usually employed (Fig 13–7).

Because of the high incidence and associated risk of vesicoureteral reflux, this simple direct implantation of the ureter into the bladder is not used often, although it has served gynecologic surgeons well on emergency occasions when more com-

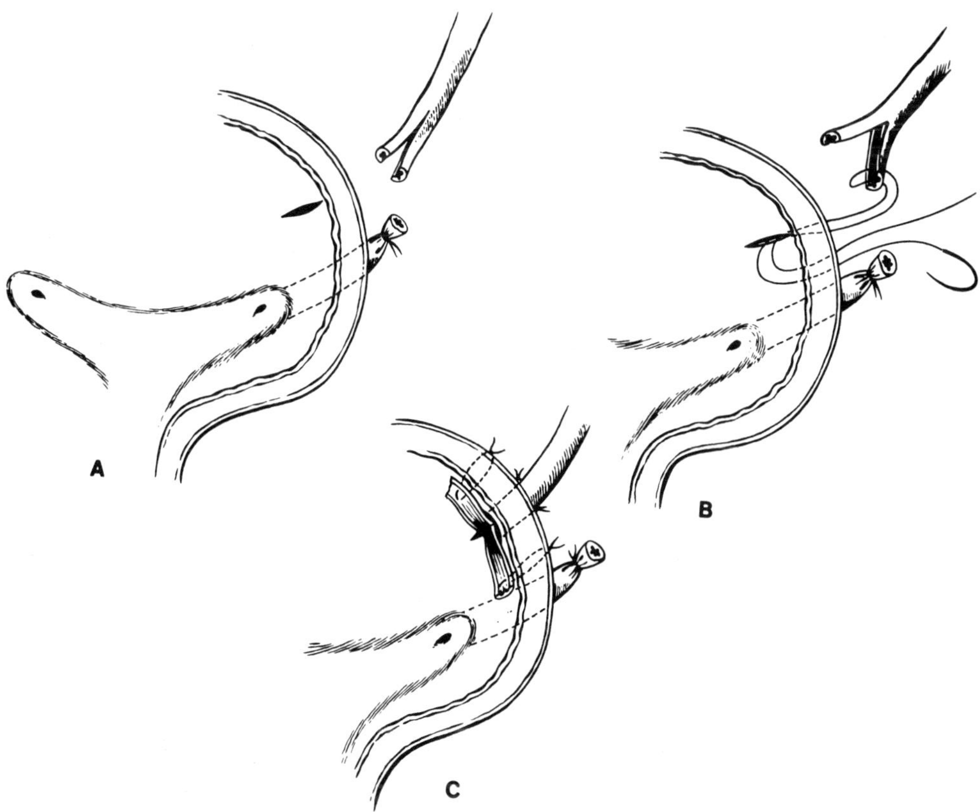

FIG 13–7.
Ureterovesical implantation, fish-mouth technique. **A,** excised free end of ureter is spatulated for 1 to 2 cm. New ureteral orifice has been made by scalpel above the trigone in position to reach excised ureter. **B,** each end of ureteral flap is anchored with a mattress suture of no. 4-0 delayed absorbable suture and passed through new ureteral orifice and full thickness of bladder wall. **C,** bladder flaps are tied on external surface of the bladder and reinforced with seromuscular sutures in bladder wall and ureter at site of implantation. (From Mattingly RF, Thompson JD: *TeLinde's Operative Gynecology,* ed 7. Philadelphia, JB Lippincott Co, 1990. Used by permission.)

plicated operations are not appropriate. In the absence of urinary tract infection or chronic renal disease, ureteral reflux, if it occurs, has not usually produced serious problems such as chronic recurrent ascending infection with loss of renal function.

The preferred method of ureteral implantation is the submucosal tunnel technique since it more nearly establishes the normal intramural anatomy of the ureter and avoids reflux. The distal ureter is carefully dissected from the site of traumatic injury. All devitalized tissue is debrided. Unhealthy tissue at the distal end of the ureter must be excised. Mobilization of the ureter and bladder base should help ensure that the anastomosis can be made without tension. The bladder dome is opened transversely. The most dependent portion of the posterior bladder wall that will allow a tension-free anastomosis is selected, and a submucosal tunnel 1 to 1.5 cm long is fashioned. The incision is extended through the entire thickness of the bladder wall at the superior margin of the tunnel. The ureter is drawn through and sutured to its new orifice at the lower end of the tunnel. Size 4-0 delayed absorbable sutures and an indwelling splinting catheter are used. The transverse incision in the anterior bladder wall is closed longitudinally in two layers. A Jackson-Pratt drain is placed extraperitoneally, and the operative site is peritonized. The splinting catheter is left in place for 14 to 21 days before removal (Fig 13–8).

An alternate method of using a submucosal tunnel for ureteroneocystostomy is shown in Figure 13–9.

When extensive trauma to the lower ureter results, after debridement, in a ureter that is too short for ureteroneocystostomy without tension, some special techniques of bridging the gap must be employed. The bladder base can be mobilized by incising the lateral peritoneal attachments of the bladder. The bladder base can be sharply dissected and mobilized from its fascial attachments to the vagina. The ureter can be mobilized for a greater distance above. If anastomosis without

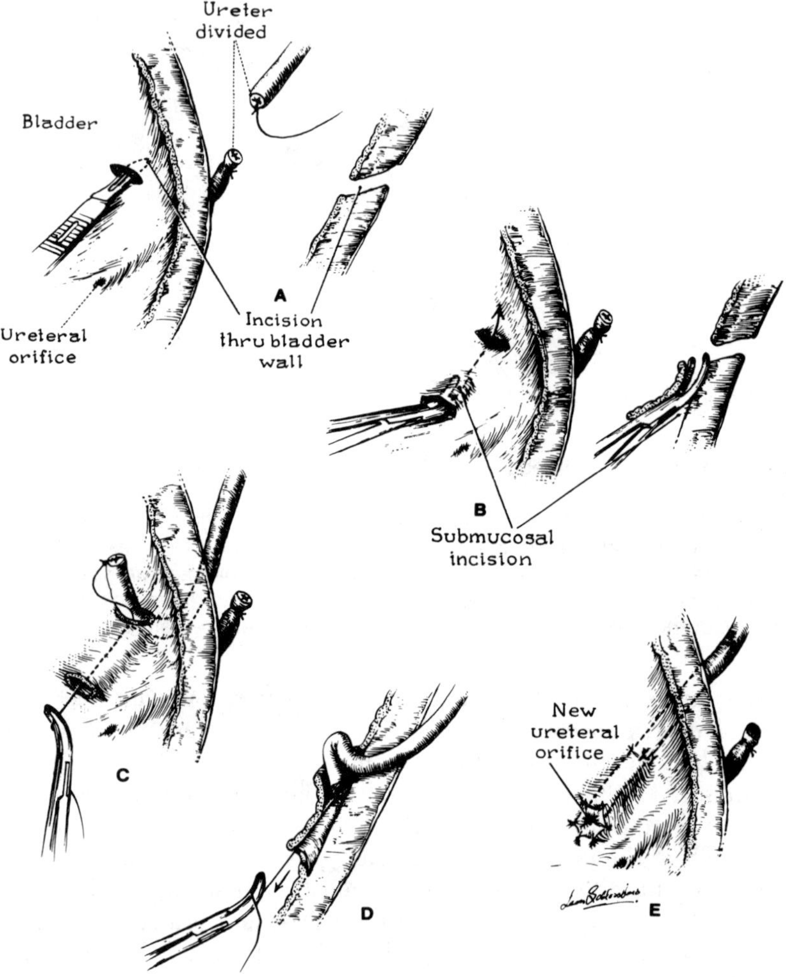

FIG 13–8.
Submucosal tunnel technique of ureterovesical implantation. **A,** bladder mucosa is incised above trigone at planned site of implantation; oblique incision through bladder wall is made from exterior. **B,** Adson clamp is inserted through new orifice and tunneled beneath mucosa for 1.5 cm to upper mucosal incision. **C,** ureter is guided through bladder wall and upper mucosal orifice and gently guided through submucosal tunnel. **D,** by traction suture. **E,** mucosa-to-mucosa anastomosis of ureter to bladder; upper incision is closed with fine suture. (From Mattingly RF, Thompson JD: *TeLinde's Operative Gynecology,* ed 7. Philadelphia, JB Lippincott Co, 1990. Used by permission.)

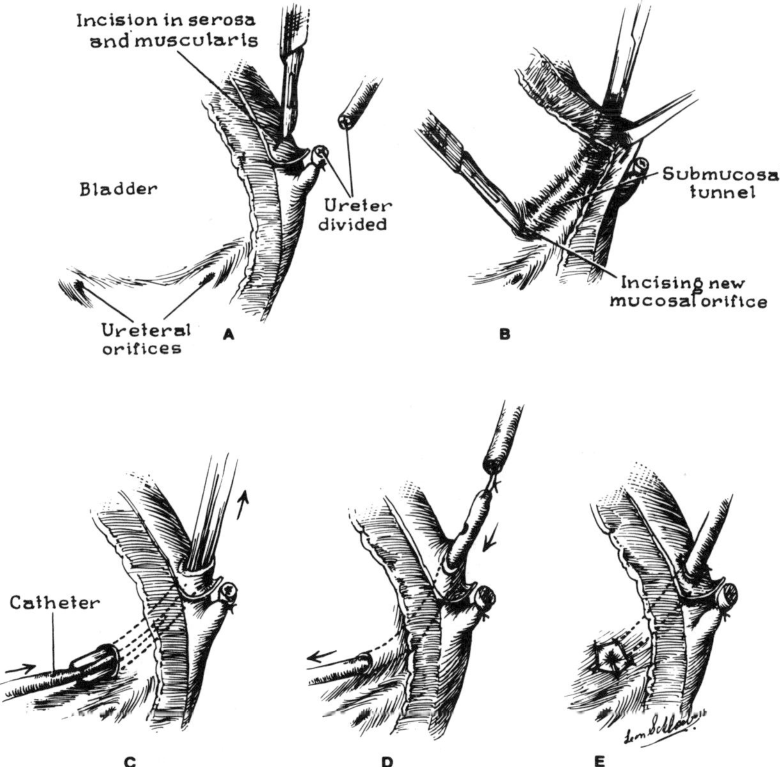

FIG 13–9.
Submucosal tunnel procedure for ureterovesical anastomosis, external technique. **A,** oblique incision through bladder wall initiated on external surface. **B,** Adson clamp passed through muscular wall and beneath mucosa for 1.5 cm (tunnel formation); bladder mucosa incised over tip of clamp at site of new ureteral orifice. **C,** small, straight rubber catheter drawn through tunnel and bladder wall. **D,** catheter sutured to excised ureter; ureter guided through bladder wall and tunnel by traction on catheter. **E,** mucosa-to-mucosa anastomosis of ureter to bladder. (From Mattingly RF, Thompson JD: *TeLinde's Operative Gynecology,* ed 7. Philadelphia, JB Lippincott Co, 1990. Used by permission.)

tension is still not possible, a transverse incision should be made in the anterior bladder wall. A finger is placed inside, and the cornu of the bladder is elevated and sutured to the psoas muscle tendon as high as possible. The transverse bladder incision then should be closed longitudinally. Following mobilization and elevation of the bladder to the psoas muscle, a ureteroneocystostomy can usually be done without tension according to the most appropriate technique (Fig 13–10).

This psoas muscle hitch method of bridging the gap between the bladder and a short ureter is superior to developing a Boari flap of bladder muscle. The flap procedure is frequently associated with reflux and may also become ischemic and stenotic. Ingenious techniques of developing bladder flaps should be used as a last resort to bridge the gap to a short ureter, especially if the pelvis has been irradiated.

Vaginal Repair of Ureteral Injuries

In special circumstances, transvaginal repair of simple injuries to the lower ureter may be possible and entirely satisfactory, especially if the injury was the result of a vaginal operation in which only the lowest 3 cm of ureter might be involved.

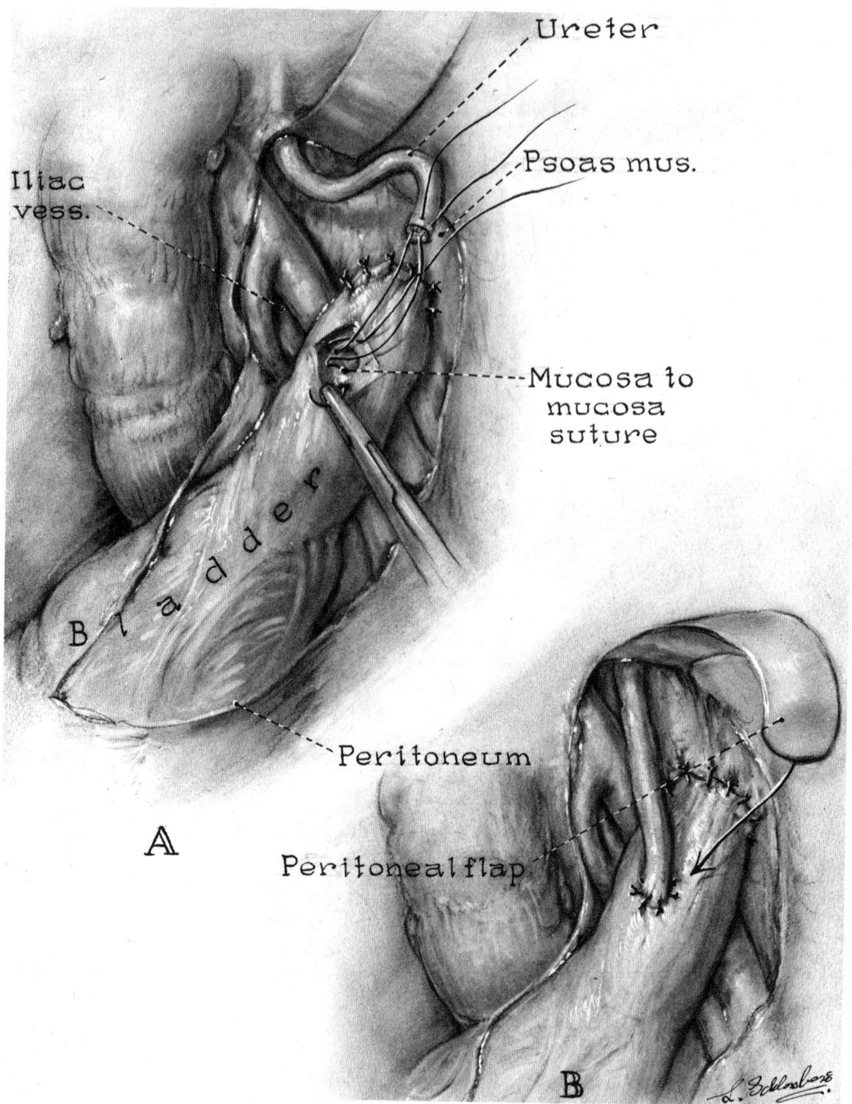

FIG 13–10.
Ureterovesical anastomosis of the short ureter–psoas muscle hitch procedure. **A,** bladder peritoneum is incised from lateral pelvic wall, and bladder is mobilized and anchored to psoas muscle at pelvic brim (psoas muscle hitch) near site of planned ureterovesical anastomosis. Mucosa-to-mucosa anastomosis of ureter to bladder is performed. **B,** ureterovesical anastomosis is reinforced with fine serosal sutures and peritoneum is advanced over anastomotic site. (From Mattingly RF, Thompson JD: *TeLinde's Operative Gynecology,* ed 7. Philadelphia, JB Lippincott Co, 1990. Used by permission.)

The surgeon must be familiar with the anatomy of the lower ureter as seen through the vagina. Developing the paravesical space will facilitate the dissection and make it possible to locate the dilated ureter above the site of injury. Identification is also facilitated by passage of a catheter up as far as possible on the side of the injury. After the site of injury is located and examined, a decision regarding the proper operative procedure for repair is made. Depending on the extent and location, the injury may be repaired with simple disligation or with ureteroneocystostomy. A

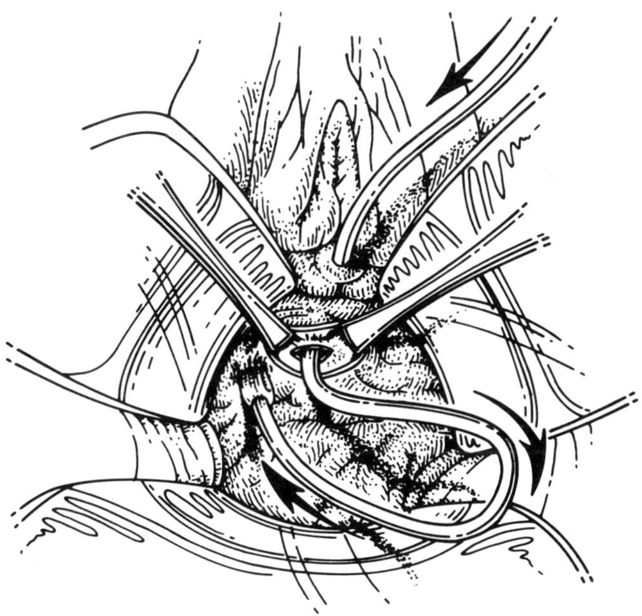

FIG 13–11.
After the ureter is identified, debrided, mobilized, spatulated, and catheterized, the catheter is brought into the bladder and out through the urethra through a cystostomy incision. A ureteroneocystostomy is then performed. (From Mattingly RF, Thompson JD: *TeLinde's Operative Gynecology,* ed 6. Philadelphia, JB Lippincott Co, 1985. Used by permission.)

simple technique of implanting the ureter into the bladder is used. Both are usually done using a splinting catheter that is left indwelling for 14 to 21 days (Fig 13–11). On occasion it may be advisable to reinforce the repair site with a bulbocavernosus fat flap developed from the labia. This fat flap will serve as a protective shield between the repair site and the vaginal vault, which should be left open for drainage.

Other Procedures

Other more complicated procedures usually beyond the scope of most gynecologic surgeons have been used in the management of patients with extensive ureteral injuries. Transureteroureterostomy (i.e., anastomosis of the upper ureter on one side to the intact ureter on the opposite side through a subperitoneal tunnel) can be successful in selected cases. There is the potential for compromising the function of the kidney on the normal side.

Many ingenious techniques have been devised for substituting a segment of ileum for a ureter that has been damaged too extensively to be repaired or implanted into the bladder. In fact, the ileum may be substituted for the entire course of the ureter on one or both sides. Of course, both ureters may be anastomosed to the ileum, which may then be anastomosed to the skin (Bricker's pouch) if the bladder is not present or is not suitable for implantation.

Autotransplantation of the kidney to the pelvis may be considered in a patient who has no possibility of repair of the injured ureter and poor function of the opposite kidney. It has the potential for excellent results when done by an experienced renal transplant surgeon.

OPERATIVE INJURIES TO THE BLADDER

Currently throughout the world, injury to the bladder resulting from prolonged obstructed labor and producing vesicovaginal fistula causes tragic social and medical problems for many young women, especially in developing countries. Tahzib studied 1,443 patients with vesicovaginal fistulas between 1969 and 1980 in Northern Nigeria, the largest series of vesicovaginal fistulas ever reported. Eighty-three percent were caused by prolonged obstructed labor. Thirteen percent resulted from gishiri cut, a traditional tribal practice of cutting the anterior vaginal wall with a razor blade to treat a variety of conditions including backache, dyspareunia, goiter, infertility, and obstructed labor. In this series, only 1% of vesicovaginal fistulas resulted from operative injuries to the bladder. This major health problem for women in the world deserves greater attention. Measures for prevention must include not only improved and accessible medical services (including contraceptive services) but also universal education and improved status for women. For example, in Ethiopia, young girls are frequently married by age 10 years. There are only 87 hospitals and 800 physicians for 45 million people. Under these circumstances, it is difficult to conceive of doing cesarean sections for all patients with obstructed labor and providing contraceptive services to teenagers.

In many countries in the world, including the United States, vesicovaginal fistulas of obstetric etiology are rare. In the last 30 years at Grady Memorial Hospital in Atlanta, no vesicovaginal fistulas have occurred during the course of 180,000 obstetric deliveries in a predominantly black and indigent population. Major contributors to prevention have been improved management of obstetric problems and techniques of delivery, especially the more liberal use of cesarean section with a concomitant decrease in the number of difficult forceps operations, and improvements in the management of labor. Because of this, few American gynecologists have or need experience in the repair of vesicovaginal fistulas of obstetric origin.

In the United States today, the most important measures for reducing the incidence and morbidity of vesicovaginal fistulas must be directed to proper techniques of gynecologic surgery. Although a rare vesicovaginal fistula results from other causes (e.g., radiation therapy for cervical cancer), gynecologic surgery is the most common etiology in the United States and in many other developed countries in the world. The principles of repair of vesicovaginal fistula of obstetric etiology established in the 19th century, although still applicable today for obstetric fistulas, must be modified for management of the postsurgical fistulas of the 20th century. The modifications are necessary to recognize that the subject of vesicovaginal fistula is not a single subject but many different subjects depending on etiology, location, size, and so forth. This discussion will emphasize that part of the subject of trauma to the bladder that results from the operative management of gynecologic disease and conditions.

Prevention

When gynecologic surgery is done properly, postoperative vesicovaginal fistula may be a very rare occurrence. Between 1970 and 1985, 24,883 patients underwent major gynecologic surgery at the Mayo Clinic. Only one patient developed a postoperative vesicovaginal fistula (after primary radical hysterectomy). In spite of this commendable record, the bladder is the most common site of injury to the urinary tract and occurs in approximately 1% of patients undergoing gynecologic surgery.

Bladder injury occurs most commonly during hysterectomy. Among 75 posthysterectomy vesicovaginal fistulas reported by Miller and George, 54 followed total abdominal hysterectomy, 18 followed total vaginal hysterectomy, and 3 followed radical hysterectomy. None followed subtotal abdominal hysterectomy. In the past several decades, total rather than subtotal abdominal hysterectomy has become the routine procedure. Thus, injury to the base of the bladder occurs more frequently now than before and is reported in 0.5% to 1% of patients undergoing a total abdominal hysterectomy. To reduce the risk of vesicovaginal fistulas, Baker has suggested that the gynecologic surgeon consider leaving the cervix in place by doing a subtotal hysterectomy when the cervix is benign, when removing the uterine corpus will remove the patient's pathology, and when there are conditions such as endometriosis or tubo-ovarian abscess that may increase the risk of bladder injury when the cervix is removed. I subscribe to this principle of using good surgical judgment. No operation should be routine for every patient. However, it should be possible for the experienced gynecologic surgeon to remove the cervix without injury to the bladder in almost every patient. This is especially important in younger women who may be exposed to cervical carcinogens for many years to come. Certainly if in the judgment of the gynecologic surgeon the danger of removing the cervix is greater than the danger of leaving it in, a subtotal hysterectomy should be done. In addition, the danger of removing the cervix includes the possibility of injury not only to the bladder but also to the ureters and rectum as well.

The gynecologic surgeon must be thoroughly familiar with the anatomy of the bladder and especially its boundaries in relation to the lower uterine isthmus, the cervix, the anterior vaginal wall, and the anterior abdominal wall. The base of the bladder above the interureteric ridge rests on and is draped across the anterior lower uterine isthmus, the cervix, and the upper anterior vaginal wall. The bladder trigone is at a lower level below the cervix and rests on the middle third of the anterior vaginal wall. It is, therefore, less susceptible to injury when a total hysterectomy is done. If the bladder is injured during its dissection away from the cervix and vagina, the injury will fortunately be located above the interureteric ridge and trigone in almost all cases. This anatomic relationship is extremely important to keep in mind (Fig 13–12). If one places a cystoscope in the bladder and watches as an index finger pushes up along the anterior vaginal wall, one can easily confirm this relationship.

Injury to the bladder base is more common with total abdominal hysterectomy than with vaginal hysterectomy. This is probably because patients with more extensive disease (e.g., endometriosis, large leiomyomas, tubo-ovarian abscess, and gynecologic malignancy) are usually operated on abdominally. Some injuries to the bladder base from total abdominal hysterectomy are caused by vigorous or blunt dissection in the wrong plane between the bladder base and the pubovesicocervical fascia covering the cervix. This dissection should be done precisely and sharply with scissors. Pushing down vigorously against the vesicovaginal attachments with a sponge will weaken the bladder wall and should be discouraged. Injury may also result from inadequate mobilization of the bladder inferiorly and laterally so that clamps and sutures placed in the cardinal ligament and anterior vaginal cuff may "pinch" the bladder base (Fig 13–13). The vesicocervicovaginal space should be developed completely and the bladder thoroughly mobilized both inferiorly and laterally. Pulling the uterine corpus superiorly while retracting the bladder base anteri-

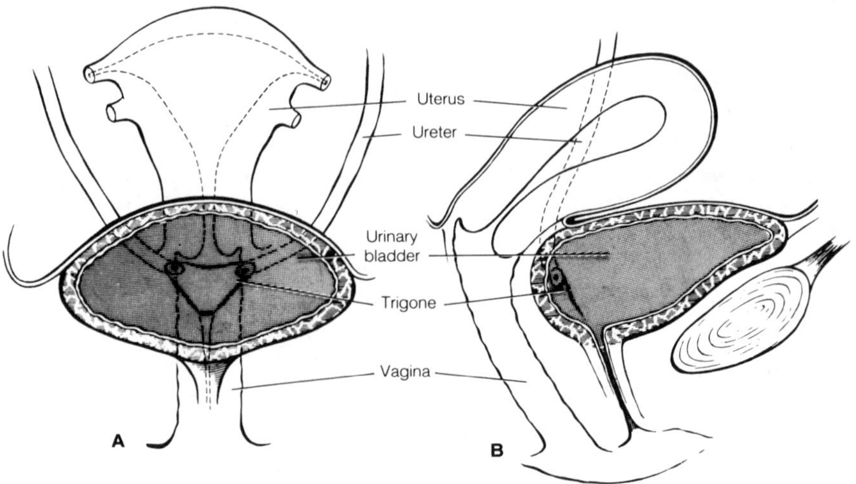

FIG 13–12.
A, anterior view of the normal anatomy of ureter and bladder. The terminal end of the ureter passes medially from the lateral pelvic wall and crosses over the anterior fornix, where it enters the trigone of the bladder, which rests on the upper one third of the anterior vaginal wall. **B,** Sagittal view of anatomic relationship of ureter and bladder base. Note that the ureter enters the trigone in the area of the upper one third of the vagina. (From Mattingly RF, Thompson JD: *TeLinde's Operative Gynecology,* ed 7. Philadelphia, JB Lippincott Co, 1990. Used by permission.)

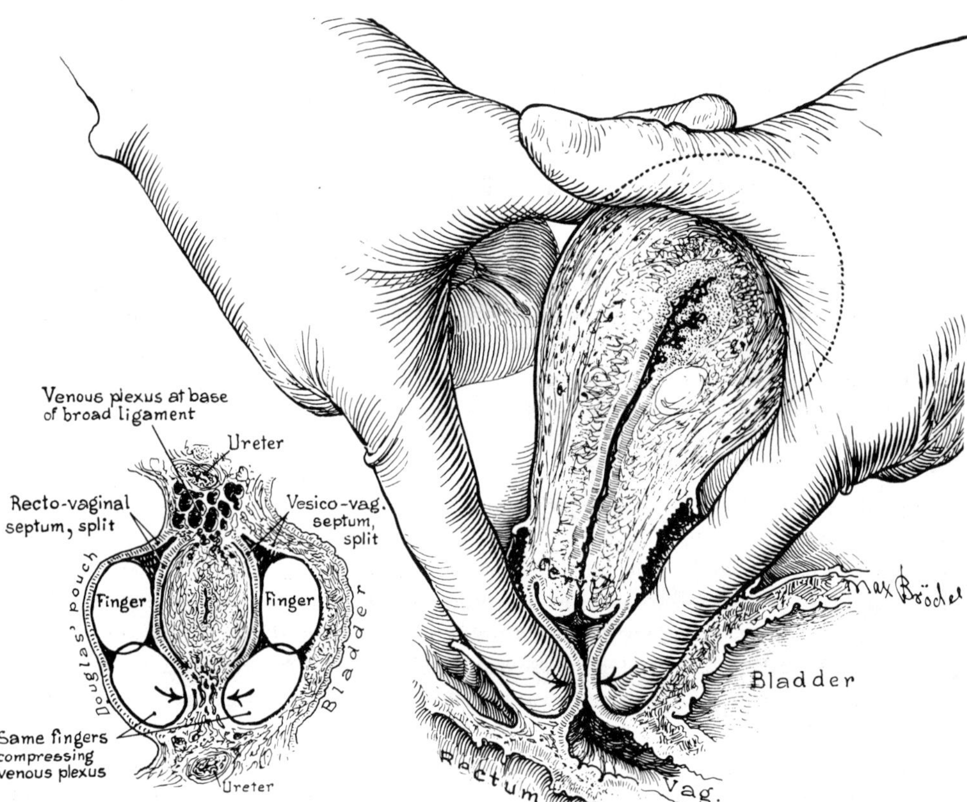

FIG 13–13.
Total abdominal hysterectomy. Testing the depth of the anterior and posterior dissections. The *inset* shows the method of segregating the vascular plexus on each side into a narrow zone adjacent to the basal segment of the broad ligament. (From Richardson EH: *Surg Gynecol Obstet* 1929; 48:248.)

orly will facilitate the full development of the vesicocervicovaginal space and help prevent bladder injury. Also helpful is the utilization of the intrafascial technique of removing the cervix, described by Richardson of the Johns Hopkins Hospital in 1927. This technique employs an inverted V or T incision in the pubovesicocervical fascia covering the cervix. When the cervix is removed, the anterior arm of the cardinal ligament clamp is placed beneath the pubovesicocervical fascia and actually peels the fascia off the cervix as the clamp is closed. Clamps placed beneath the pubovesicocervical fascia will not include the bladder wall. But before clamps are placed across the cardinal ligaments and before an incision is made in the anterior vaginal wall, the vesicocervicovaginal space must be developed completely and the bladder thoroughly mobilized inferiorly and laterally. Some vesicovaginal fistulas are caused by placing sutures through the bladder base when the cuff is sutured. Again, this results from inadequate mobilization and retraction and inadequate exposure, possibly because of a limited incision in the abdominal wall. When a suture catches the bladder base, gradual necrosis of the bladder wall will lead to vesicovaginal fistula formation about 7 to 10 days after surgery.

As with total abdominal hysterectomy, the bladder is most frequently injured during total vaginal hysterectomy when the bladder is dissected away from the cervix and the lower anterior uterine isthmus. The location of the injury is the same as in total abdominal hysterectomy. Ordinarily the plane of dissection between the cervix and bladder is easy to identify and relatively avascular. The dissection may be facilitated by injecting sterile saline beneath the vaginal mucosa. I prefer not to use a vasopressor in the injecting solution because of experimental and clinical evidence that vasopressors interfere with the local tissue resistance to infection, and vasopressors are not necessary to control bleeding. An incision is made through the vaginal mucosa at its point of attachment to the cervix just above the anterior lip. It is extended to the 3 and 9 o'clock positions laterally. The blade of the electrosurgical Bovie unit, slightly bent at the tip, can be used for this dissection. Strong traction is made downward with a tenaculum placed on the anterior cervical lip. Countertraction beneath the bladder above will expose the tissues that need to be cut. With the tip pointed downward toward the cervix, the operator uses the Bovie as an artist might use a brush on a canvas, taking brief short strokes and cutting tissue that is under stretch. Small bleeding vessels may be coagulated along the way. Scissor dissection with the handles elevated and the points against the uterus can also be used. However, dissection with a gauze-covered finger is too blunt and may injure the bladder wall. When the dense attachment of the bladder has been dissected through, the loose space above covered only with the vesicouterine peritoneal reflection can be felt with the finger. It should not be pushed away. With proper retraction and lighting, the peritoneum can be identified and incised. When one is able to see contents of the peritoneal cavity through this small incision, confirming that the peritoneal cavity and not the bladder has been entered, the incision in the peritoneum may be extended. After this, the bladder is held up and out of the way with a retractor.

Unfortunately, development of the vesicocervical space is not always easy. When the dissection is misdirected and difficult, or there is abnormal adherence between the bladder and cervix, troublesome bleeding may obscure the operative field. The dissection may be too deep in the muscle of the anterior lower uterine isthmus, the most frequent and understandable error since the operator may be trying to avoid bladder injury. Or the dissection may be too anterior and the bladder wall may be weakened or the bladder actually entered. Hopefully, the operator will not extend the dissection into the bladder before recognizing the error. If there is a possibility that the dissection has been directed too far anteriorly, two helpful suggestions may prevent final entry into the bladder. First, one should place an instrument (a Kelly clamp or uterine sound will do nicely) into the bladder through the urethra. The tip of the clamp can be felt and will identify the location of the bladder wall in relation to the plane of dissection. Second, 5 mL of methylene blue or indigo carmine can be instilled into the bladder through the urethra. The dye will stain the bladder mucosa, making it more visible to avoid an entry into the bladder. This simple measure can be adopted as a routine before every vaginal hysterectomy since it is not possible to predict when the dissection will be difficult. It might be especially useful in patients who have had a previous cesarean section and who can be expected to have an abnormal adherence between the bladder and the lower anterior uterine isthmus. Previous cesarean section or sections can cause this difficulty when total vaginal or total abdominal hysterectomy are done. As the number of cesarean sections in the United States increases, the frequency with which the gynecologic surgeon encounters this problem will also increase. In my experience, the dissection is less difficult with vaginal hysterectomy because one is able to pass an instrument transurethrally to help identify a proper plane for dissection. Of course, transurethral passage of an instrument is also possible when one is operating abdominally if the patient has been positioned in Allen Universal stirrups for the operation.

Jaszczak and Evans have proposed an intrafascial technique for vaginal hysterectomy designed to avoid injury to the bladder. Although the idea may be sound, it has not been evaluated extensively. Bladder injury and vesicovaginal fistula resulting from vaginal hysterectomy are best prevented by finding the proper plane of dissection between the bladder base above and the cervix and anterior lower uterine isthmus below, by opening the vesicouterine fold of peritoneum carefully, by mobilizing the bladder laterally by clamping and cutting the bladder pillars on each side, by placing a retractor beneath the bladder for its protection, and by properly placing clamps and ligatures on small bites of paracervical and parametrial tissue as close to the uterus as possible.

Although much less common, there are several other situations in which bladder injury may occur. Finding a proper plane for dissection for repeat anterior colporrhaphy may be difficult. The operator will be well advised to inject sterile saline just beneath the vaginal mucosa and dissect carefully between the mucosa and the fascia beneath rather than trying to find a deeper plane for dissection. If a patient has had a previous suprapubic urethropexy, the space of Retzius may be difficult to develop in any subsequent operation because of adherence between the anterior bladder wall, the symphysis, and the pubic rami. Bleeding from large veins may obscure dissection in the proper plane. Sharp dissection will usually be required to release the dense fibrous adhesions. Blunt dissection is risky and may tear into the bladder. Repeat suprapubic urethropexy and Goebel-Stoeckel suburethral sling operations must be done with care to avoid injury to the anterior bladder wall.

When the bladder is mobilized away from the uterus to perform a cesarean section (especially a repeat cesarean section), abnormal adherence and dissection in the wrong plane may result in accidental bladder entry. This may be even more likely when the cesarean section is done for emergency indications.

Distortion of the lower anterior uterine isthmus by leiomyomas can cause diffi-

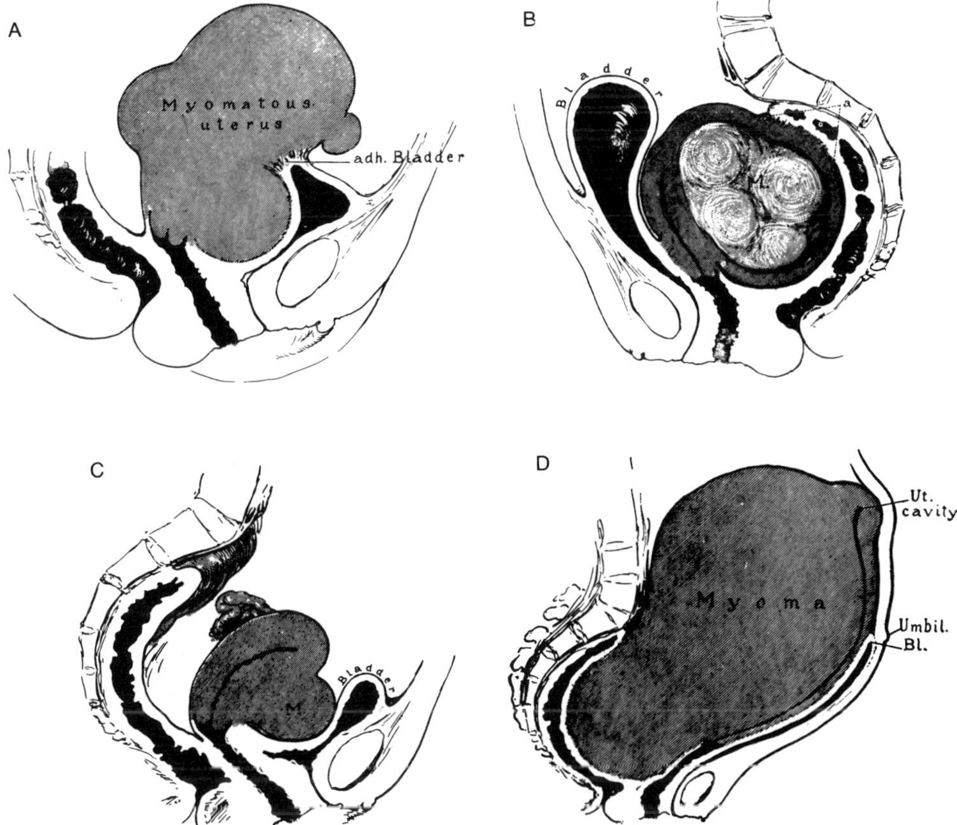

FIG 13–14.
Abnormal relationships of the uterus and bladder caused by uterine leiomyomas. **A,** the uterus is abnormally adherent to the bladder. **B,** a large posterior myoma pushes the bladder against the symphysis. **C,** an anterior myoma pushes the bladder against the symphysis. **D,** a large myoma causes obstruction of the vesical neck with bladder hypertrophy extending to the umbilicus. (From: Kelly HA, Cullen TS: *Myomata of the Uterus.* Philadelphia, WB Saunders Co, 1909. Used by permission.)

culty in finding the proper plane of dissection beneath the bladder (Fig 13–14,A–C). If uterine leiomyomas obstruct the vesical neck, considerable hypertrophy of the bladder muscle will result over time much the same as in men with benign prostatic hypertrophy. The bladder can become so large as to reach to the umbilicus and will definitely be encountered when an incision is made in the lower abdomen (Fig 13–14,D). In extreme cases, it may be necessary to begin a midline incision above the umbilicus, identify the top of the bladder, dissect it free laterally, and fold it down over the patient's thighs to gain access to the pelvis to remove the leiomyomas. Fortunately, such extreme cases are not as commonly seen in the United States today as in previous decades. Before a transverse Maylard or Cherney incision is made across the lower abdomen, the bladder must be completely empty. Otherwise, the incision may go through the dome of the bladder.

It is common practice in reperitonizing the pelvis following subtotal abdominal hysterectomy to pull the edge of the bladder peritoneum over the top of the cervix and suture it posteriorly. If removal of the cervix either vaginally or abdominally is indicated later, the operator will do well to recognize this abnormal position of the bladder. The exact boundaries of the bladder will be obscured by its abnormal adherence to the top and back of the cervix.

In patients with the Mayer-Rokitansky-Küster-Hauser syndrome (congenital absence of the uterus and vagina), the Abbe-Wharton-McIndoe operation attempts to develop a space for sexual intercourse between the urethra and bladder anteriorly and the rectum posteriorly. Definition of the correct plane for dissection can be easy or difficult. A difficult dissection can be facilitated by placing an instrument in the urethra and a double-gloved finger in the rectum to avoid injury to the bladder and rectum.

One percent to 3% of patients will develop vesicovaginal fistulas following extensive hysterectomy as primary treatment for invasive cancer of the cervix. If such an extensive operation is done after previous pelvic irradiation, the incidence is higher. Boronow and Rutledge found a fourfold increase in vesicovaginal fistula formation even when simple hysterectomy was performed on patients who had been previously irradiated. Hysterectomy, especially extensive hysterectomy, further compromises the blood supply to the base of the bladder already compromised by the obliterative endarteritis caused by radiation treatment. Since postirradiation fistulas are the most difficult to close, every precaution should be taken to prevent their formation. For example, Petty and associates reported five patients who developed new cervical or uterine neoplasms 1 to 27 years after initial radiation therapy for cervical cancer. All underwent abdominal hysterectomy without postoperative vesicovaginal fistula formation. Success was attributed to cautious surgical technique and the use of an omental pedicle graft to bring new vascularity to the bladder base. Such a preventive measure makes good sense.

Operative Repair of Bladder Injury

If an injury to the bladder can be discovered at the operation of injury and properly repaired, a vesicovaginal fistula is not likely to occur. Indeed, the gynecologic surgeon can even be encouraged to intentionally enter the bladder when it is necessary to define the anatomic limits of pathology or a proper plane for dissection. In an analysis of 77 cases of recognized bladder entry, Everett and Mattingly found no case that failed to heal when repaired at the time of initial entry. The unirradiated bladder is rich in collateral blood supply. Defects will heal when closed correctly. Healing is not dependent on the placement of large numbers of sutures. Accurate placement of a correct number of sutures is more important. Injury to the bladder should not be considered a dreaded and serious complication when recognized and closed correctly.

One of the most frequent sites of injury is the dome of the bladder, especially in when an incision is made in a patient who has had a previous incision or in a patient in advanced pregnancy. Fortunately, entry into the bladder dome is easy to recognize and repair. A double-layered closure should be used. An initial continuous no. 3-0 delayed absorbable suture in the bladder mucosa is reinforced by another layer of continuous suture in the bladder muscle. In closing the abdominal incision later after the operation is completed, the site of repair of the bladder should be extraperitonized if possible. An indwelling transurethral catheter should be left indwelling for 7 to 10 days postoperatively depending on the extent of injury, security of repair, and whether the repair site in the dome is intraperitoneal or extraperitoneal.

Injuries to the base of the bladder are more likely to result in fistula formation if they are not recognized and repaired correctly, probably because the bladder base is the most dependent portion. Injury in this site is usually the result of removal of the cervix in total hysterectomy, either abdominal or vaginal. Once the bladder has been entered, the dissection can be redirected into the proper plane and the operation completed before the defect is repaired. Then the extent of the injury should be carefully determined, especially its proximity to the ureteral orifices inside the bladder. Ordinarily, the defect will be above the interureteric ridges. If one cannot be certain of the location of the ureteral orifices, injection of 5 mL of indigo carmine dye intravenously will cause blue urine to spurt from the orifices in 3 to 5 minutes. Ureteral catheters can be passed, but this is not often necessary. After careful assessment of the limits of the defect in all directions, the first layer of closure is usually a continuous no. 3-0 delayed absorbable suture that care-

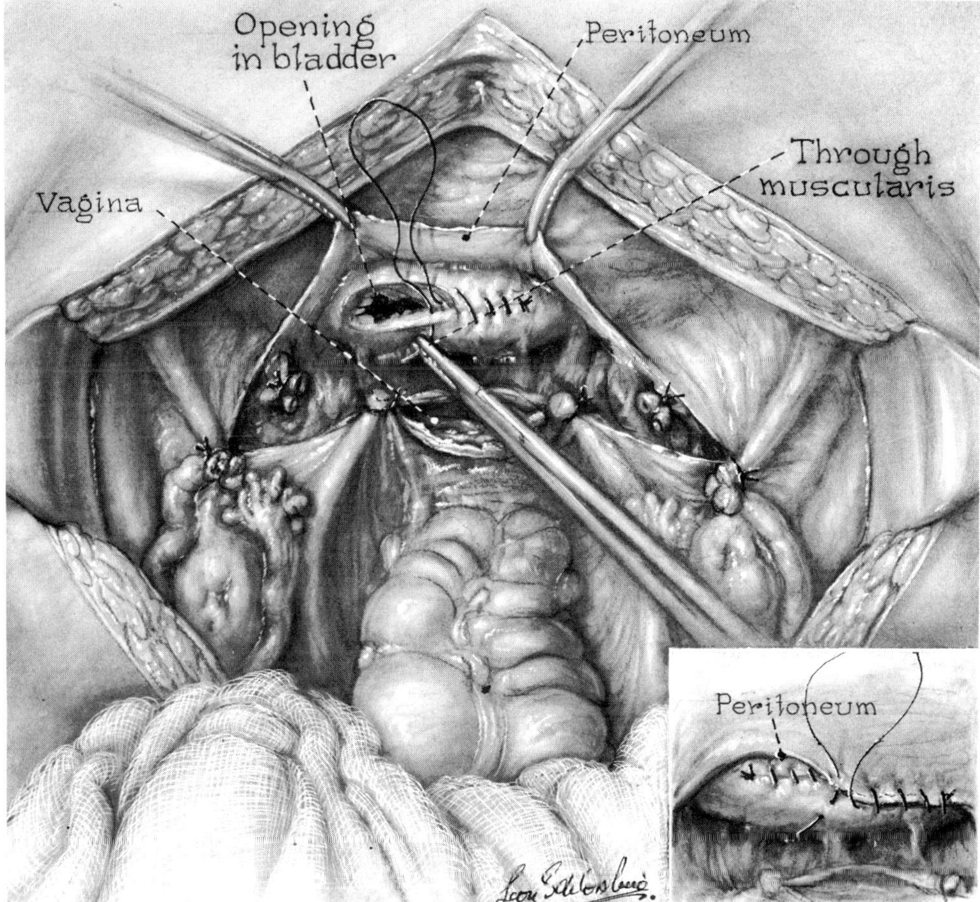

FIG 13–15.
Closure of accidental opening of bladder during total abdominal hysterectomy. The bladder is closed with a continuous no. 3-0 delayed absorbable suture, inverting mucosa into the bladder. A second muscular layer of interrupted sutures should support the initial layer. The suture line is then reinforced by bringing the peritoneum over the operative defect and suturing it in place. Advancement of the bladder peritoneum over the suture line will protect it from postoperative pelvic cellulitis and make certain that no leakage occurs into the vagina. (From Mattingly RF, Thompson JD: *TeLinde's Operative Gynecology*, ed 7. Philadelphia, JB Lippincott Co, 1990. Used by permission.)

fully approximates and inverts the bladder mucosa, making certain that the closure goes beyond the limits of the defect (Fig 13–15). The security of this first layer of closure should be tested by instilling 200 mL of sterile milk or dilute methylene blue into the bladder. Any point of leakage should be reinforced with additional sutures. The closure must be without tension. There will usually have been sufficient mobilization of the bladder base to accomplish closure without tension, especially if the suture line is horizontal. A second and possibly third layer of sutures is placed in the bladder muscle. These may be interrupted vertical mattress sutures or continuous sutures.

The next step is most important. The edge of the vesical peritoneum is sutured to the anterior vaginal cuff. This superimposes another layer between the bladder mucosa and the vaginal vault and also helps to relieve tension on the suture line. This is a very useful maneuver and should be used to reinforce any suspected area of weakness in the bladder wall, even if the bladder has not actually been entered. The peritoneum is interposed between the vaginal apex and the bladder defect.

Finally, at the end of the operation, cystoscopy should be performed. Indigo carmine is injected intravenously. Dye spurting from each ureteral orifice assures ureteral integrity. The bladder side of the repair should be inspected for bleeding. The bladder should be kept as empty as possible with an indwelling suprapubic or transurethral catheter. A suprapubic catheter is preferred if the repair of the defect involves the bladder trigone. The catheter may be removed in 7 to 14 days depending on the extent of the defect, the security of the closure, the condition of the tissues, and the condition of the patient.

This technique of repairing a defect in the bladder base may be used whether the defect results from abdominal or vaginal hysterectomy.

Whenever there is a suspicion of bladder weakness or injury but the problem is not clearly determined by examination, 200 to 300 mL of sterile saline should be instilled to distend the bladder wall. A careful inspection for leakage of fluid or weakness in the muscle should be carried out. If there is any concern that the bladder wall is too thin at a particular point, several sutures should be placed for reinforcement.

Vesicovaginal Fistula

Diagnosis

When a patient develops a vesicovaginal fistula, review of the operative and postoperative record may show nothing to suspect that such a complication would occur. On the other had, such a review will often show that the patient had serious and extensive pelvic disease (e.g., adhesions, pelvic infection, malignancy, or endometriosis) at operation or a history of previous irradiation or gynecologic surgery. In addition, the operation may have been difficult because of obesity, difficulty with anesthesia, or poor exposure. The postoperative recovery may have been complicated by persistent fever, unusual discomfort, prolonged ileus, or hematuria. When the index of suspicion that a vesicovaginal fistula is developing is high, sterile saline stained with methylene blue may be instilled into the bladder through a urethral catheter for confirmation.

When definite leakage of urine from the vagina does begin sometime during the first 3 weeks of the postoperative period, successful treatment depends on an exact diagnosis. Leakage may come through the urethra, through a vesicovaginal fistula, through a ureterovaginal fistula on one or both sides, or through various combinations of any and all of these. A fistula opening may or may not be found by speculum examination of the vaginal apex. Regardless, a dilute solution of methylene blue should be instilled in the bladder. If the fistula is small and cannot be demonstrated with the patient in the dorsal lithotomy or knee chest positions, the three-tampon test of Moir should be used. In this test, three dry cotton tampons are placed in the vagina in tandem. Dilute methylene blue (200 mL) is instilled into the bladder. The patient is asked to walk about for 10 to 15 minutes, and the tampons are then removed and inspected. If the lowest tampon is wet and stained blue, the patient is presumed to have transurethral incontinence. If the upper tampon in the vaginal apex is wet and blue, a vesicovaginal fistula is indicated. If the upper tampon is wet but not stained blue, a ureterovaginal fistula is indicated. The vaginal orifice of the fistula may be located by noting the position of the staining or wetness on the tampon in relation to its position in the vaginal apex.

These simple tests require confirmation by excretory urography and cystoscopy. If the vesicovaginal fistula is so large that the bladder cannot be distended with running sterile water, air cystoscopy may be done using a regular cystoscope with the patient in the knee chest position. The bladder orifice of a small fistula can be demonstrated more easily if a probe is passed into the bladder through the vaginal orifice of the fistula. Cystoscopy is necessary to confirm the diagnosis of vesicovaginal fistula, to look for other fistula sites, and to determine the size of the fistula and its proximity to the ureteral orifices and the internal urethral meatus. Intravenous indigo carmine spurting from the ureteral orifices will rule out ureterovaginal fistula or fistulas.

There may be very little incontinence of urine when the vesicovaginal fistula is very small, and the amount may depend on the position of the patient. Voiding in large quantities may still be possible. More often with larger fistulas, the incontinence is total and voiding is absent. With such marked incontinence, the patient will become depressed and reclusive. Some patients will become frankly psychotic with despair if the incontinence remains for an extended period. The vulva becomes excoriated, reddened, and tender from the constant wetness of urine and the irritation of perineal pads, diapers, and rubber pants. The odor of urea is offensive and embarrassing to the point of precluding social interaction.

Except for vulvar irritation, most traumatic fistulas are painless. However, fistulas caused by radiation may be painful and surrounded by encrustations and necrotic tissue.

Management and Repair

For this discussion of management, vesicovaginal fistulas will be divided into two categories: simple and complicated. Simple vesicovaginal fistulas are small fistulas that develop as a result of relatively minor trauma to an otherwise healthy bladder during the course of total hysterectomy, abdominal or vaginal. Complicated fistulas are those that are large, develop in irradiated tissue, involve a ureteral orifice, follow extensive hysterectomy, are associated with other fistulas (rectovaginal, ureterovaginal, urethrovaginal, etc.), or have had previous unsuccessful attempts at repair. The major emphasis in this discussion will be given to the management of patients with simple vesicovaginal fistula, by far the largest group.

Simple Fistulas. ***Preoperative Management.***—There is very little that can be done to help patients stay comfortable before the fistula repair is done. A vulvar cream containing lanolin may relieve some discomfort. Some patients prefer to spend long periods of time in the water (tub, swimming, pool, etc.). A variety of collecting devices have been tried, but none is satisfactory because of the difficulty in maintaining a tight seal. Some patients prefer to wear a transurethral catheter in the bladder with a leg bag and some do not. Some patients require tranquilizers and some do not. Antibiotics are not required since cystitis and pyelitis are uncommon in patients with vesicovaginal fistulas. Patients who are postmenopausal or young patients who have had both ovaries removed should be placed on oral estrogen therapy. The patient will always need the encouragement and support of her family and friends and her physician during this trying time.

In my experience, spontaneous healing of a simple vesicovaginal fistula is a rare occurrence. However, it has been reported to occur in 15% to 20% of patients. The fistula must be very small, and there must be no extenuating circumstances. Spontaneous healing may be facilitated by inserting a large-caliber indwelling transurethral catheter. If the transvaginal urinary leakage stops, there is a better chance of spontaneous healing. In 3 weeks, the catheter is removed and the outcome determined. Fistulas that heal spontaneously have been known to break apart at some later time. Superficial bladder fulguration has been successful in closing some minute vesicovaginal fistulas according to some reports. Most experts do not recommend fulguration since it may increase rather than decrease the caliber of the opening. Prolonged catheter drainage with or without fulguration is only occasionally successful and is usually just another disappointment for a patient who desperately wants the urine leakage to stop now!

Timing of Repair.—Simple vesicovaginal fistulas, that is, those small fistulas that develop from relatively minor trauma to an otherwise healthy bladder during the course of total hysterectomy (abdominal or vaginal), can usually be repaired soon after the diagnosis is made. The concept of early repair began with the report of Collins and Prent in 1960. In 15 cases, all were operated on within 8 weeks and most within 4 weeks of the diagnosis; successful closure was achieved in 13 cases on the first attempt. The fistulas resulted from operations for benign disease. All repairs were done transvaginally. In another report in 1971, Collins and associates achieved a 72.4% success rate on the first attempt in 29 patients without malignancy when the operation was done in the first 2 weeks after fistula discovery. The most recent Tulane University experience with early repair was reported by O'Quinn in 1984. Fifty-four patients with acute fistulas were operated on within 8 weeks of the discovery of the fistula. Forty-three of the 54 patients were operated on within 4 weeks. Forty-eight of the 54 patients had successful first-attempt closures. Four patients were reoperated on 12 days later with successful closure on the second attempt. The remaining two patients had a successful second attempt at closure 5 and 6 weeks later. All patients had a simple transvaginal operation for repair of the fistula.

Cruikshank reported his experience with early repair of posthysterectomy vesicovaginal fistulas. A simple transvaginal repair was used in nine patients who had a simple, small, noncomplicated fistula. All of the repairs were done between 13 and 19 days following diagnosis which was made between six and fifteen days following hysterectomy. The repair was successful in all nine patients on the first attempt.

Our experience at Emory University in a small series of patients has been similar.

The Tulane University group has always advised preoperative administration of cortisone to bring about "resolution of inflammatory reaction" around the fistula. However, our experience and that of others suggest that success can be regularly achieved without using steroids. We no longer recommend their use. Also, based on our experience and that of others we have no hesitation in recommending repair of simple posthysterectomy vesicovaginal fistula shortly after the diagnosis is made. A simple transvaginal Latzko partial colpocleisis will be successful in more than 80% of cases.

Some experienced gynecologists prefer to wait 3 to 4 months to repair a vesicovaginal fistula, believing that the tissue should be completely normal and without edema, infection, or induration so that dissection, suturing, and healing will result in the best possibility of successful closure. Of course, in the meantime the patient is terribly uncomfortable, irritated, embarrassed, depressed, and restricted in social and marital activities. During this long period of delay, not having been completely convinced that she should be required to remain in this unpleasant state for months, she is likely to seek other advice. Much unpleasantness can be avoided by offering an early repair with a reasonable chance of success.

Consider the following description of two hypothetical groups of patients. In the first group, 100 patients with simple posthysterectomy vesicovaginal fistulas have a repair after 3 months with a 95% success. The remaining 5 patients are repaired successfully with a second attempt 3 months later. The calculated total number of "wet days" in this group is 9,450. Contrast this with 100 patients in the second group who have a repair within 1 month with an 80% success. The remaining 20 patients have a successful attempt at repair 3 months later. The calculated total number of wet days in this group is 4,800. In other words, in this hypothetical comparison, the total number of wet days is reduced by almost 50% by early repair. Certainly it is always important to think in terms of a successful repair. However, it is also important to do everything possible to relieve the patient's misery. If given the facts and an opportunity to choose, most patients will opt for early repair.

The Operation.—All simple posthysterectomy vesicovaginal fistulas should be closed with a transvaginal Latzko partial colpocleisis. The operation is simple and rapid, and recovery is prompt with few postoperative problems. Extensive transperitoneal-transvesical operations are not needed for these simple fistulas. Many complicated vesicovaginal fistulas can also be closed with a transvaginal operation.

My preference is to place all patients in the dorsal lithotomy position for transvaginal vesicovaginal fistula repair. I rarely use the Sims lateral or knee-chest positions.

A cystoscope should be available to examine the bladder orifice of the fistula just before the repair is done and to also perform cystoscopy at the end of the operation. If necessary, ureteral catheters may be inserted.

Most fistulas can be repaired with a basic instrument set with a few additions such a long-handled, fine-pointed scissors; long delicate needle holders; an assortment of long scalpel handles and blades; the extender for the needle point Bovie; and an assortment of vaginal retractors.

Some of the technical difficulties in performing transvaginal fistula repair may be solved by innovations in the use of special instruments. However, it is more

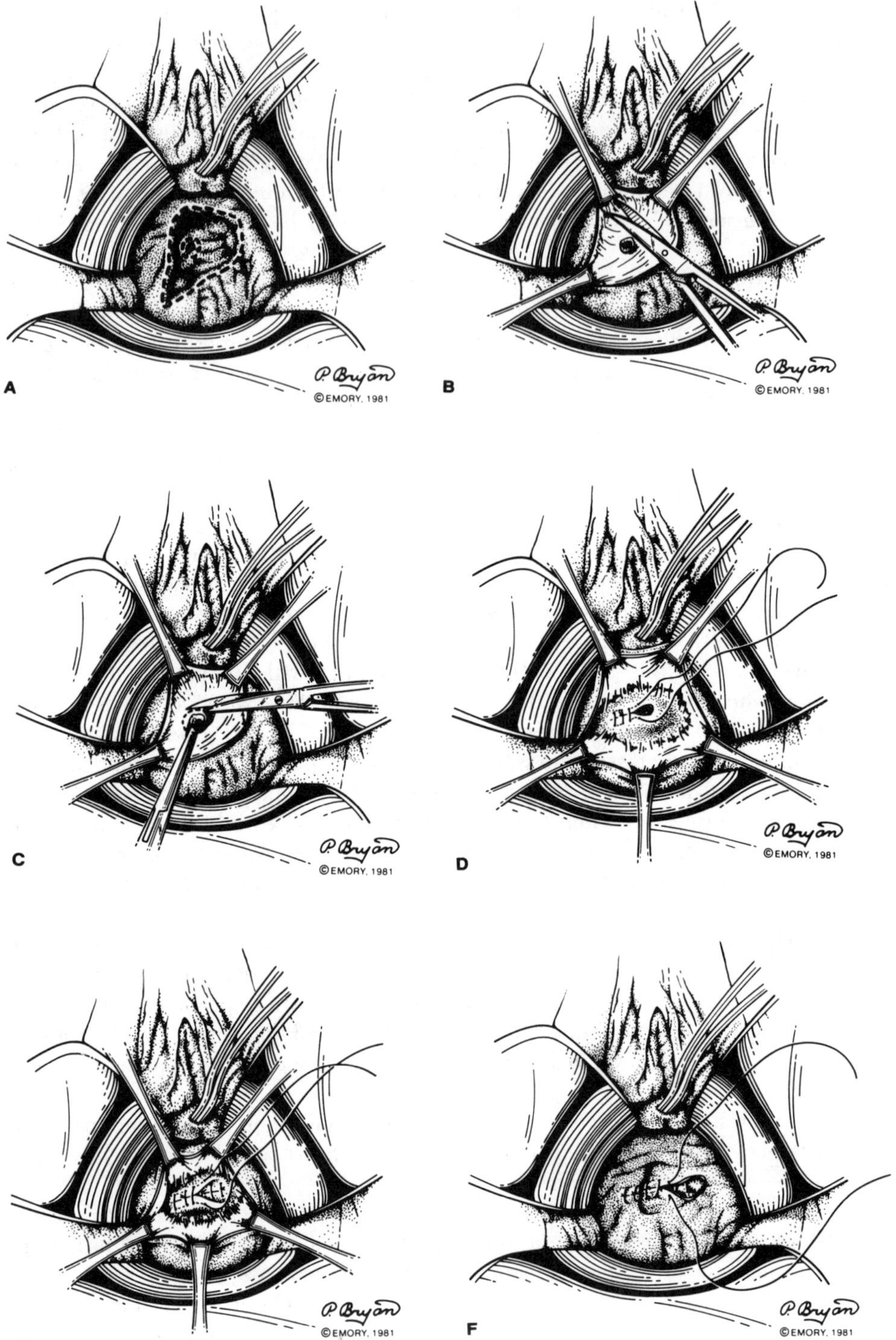

FIG 13–16.
Operation for a closure of a simple posthysterectomy vesicovaginal fistula by the Latzko technique. **A,** ureters have been catheterized to prevent encirclement of a ureter by a suture. Incisions about the fistula opening and about the indurated vaginal mucosa margin are marked by the *dotted*

likely that the technical difficulties will be solved by improved exposure and accessibility of the fistula itself. In the ordinary case, sufficient exposure is achieved simply by retracting the vaginal walls. On the other hand, if there is a narrow subpubic arch, a rigid vagina scarred from recent operations, a tight vaginal outlet, or a well-supported deep vaginal vault, an episiotomy or Schuchardt's incision may be needed and should be made without hesitation. Such a simple maneuver can convert a technically difficult and possibly unsuccessful operation into an easy operation with a successful result. Sometimes exposure can be improved by placing traction sutures in the vaginal wall at several points around the fistula or by placing a pediatric Foley catheter into the bladder through the fistula. When the bulb is distended in the bladder and downward traction is made on the catheter, the fistula is more accessible to repair.

If the fistula is fresh and the tissue is still indurated, the entire tract, including the vaginal and bladder orifices, should be excised (Fig 13–16,A). Excision of the tract will inevitably result in a larger hole in the bladder, and this is as it should be. For the repair of a fresh fistula to be successful, all of the indurated tissue surrounding the tract must be removed so that normal tissue can be approximated for better healing (Fig 13–16,B and C).

If the fistula is mature and the tissue is no longer indurated but completely epithelialized with fibrotic scar tissue, the tract may not need to be excised. Instead, when sufficient mobilization has been achieved, the tract may simply be entropionized by the first layer of sutures.

The vaginal mucosa must be widely mobilized for several centimeters around the fistula in all directions. If the fistula is fresh, wide mobilization will also include an extensive debridement of all infected and indurated tissue back to healthy bleeding tissue. Success in closing a fresh fistula depends on the willingness of the operator to remove all the unhealthy tissue.

The correct plane of dissection is just beneath the vaginal mucosa. All fascia and muscle should be left intact on the bladder side. Dissection in the proper plane is facilitated by injecting sterile saline just beneath the vaginal mucosa. The vaginal mucosa must be excised for several centimeters around the fistula, leaving the vaginal vault denuded. Care should be taken not to enter the peritoneal cavity. Any entry should be closed.

The vaginal orifice of the fistula will always sit on the transverse scar across the top of the vagina where the anterior and posterior vaginal cuff were approximated at the time of hysterectomy or were allowed to heal together in case the vagina was left open.

My suture preference for closure of vesicovaginal fistula is no. 3-0 delayed absorbable polyglactin or polyglycolic acid suture. This suture retains its tensile strength longer and causes less tissue reaction than catgut and may be partly re-

---

lines. **B,** the vaginal mucosa is dissected back from the fistula opening for a sufficient distance to mobilize the bladder wall about the fistula. **C,** the fistula tract is sharply and completely excised. **D,** no. 3-0 delayed absorbable interrupted mattress sutures taken parallel to the edge of the fistula tract are used as the initial suture line, inverting tissue into the bladder. The security of the closure should be tested by instillation of 100 to 200 mL of dilute methylene blue or sterile milk into the bladder. **E,** two or three additional layers should approximate the bladder muscularis broad surface to broad surface without tension. Size 3-0 delayed absorbable interrupted mattress sutures should be used. **F,** the vaginal mucosa is closed transversely with interrupted no. 3-0 delayed absorbable sutures. (Copyright © 1981, Emory University.)

sponsible for better results with early repair. The suture is swaged onto a fine, semimalleable, round needle of small caliber. This suture can be used for all layers and does not need to be removed. Permanent sutures should not be used.

The bladder orifice of the fistula is carefully closed by approximating the bladder mucosa with a horizontal line of no. 3-0 delayed absorbable interrupted mattress sutures (Fig 13–16,D). This first row of sutures is most important to the success of the closure. Good bites should be taken in healthy tissue to close the hole securely. This first layer of closure should be tested by instillation of 200 mL of dilute methylene blue or sterile milk into the bladder. Any point of leakage is noted and reinforced with additional sutures. If the first layer of closure is water tight, the chance of success is good. A vesicovaginal fistula repair is not likely to be successful unless the bladder orifice of the fistula is closed securely.

After the bladder orifice of the fistula is closed securely, the closure is reinforced by two or three additional lines of no. 3-0 delayed absorbable horizontal mattress sutures to approximate the anterior and posterior vaginal walls (Fig 13–16,E). This approximation of broad surface to broad surface without tension is another important axiom in fistula repair. If the layers do not come together without tension, a wider dissection of the bladder base is required. The excess vaginal mucosa is trimmed, but generous flaps are left for approximation without tension. All suture lines should be transverse to the longitudinal axis of the vagina (Fig 13–16,F).

At the end of the operation, cystoscopy is performed to confirm hemostasis in the bladder and to test for ureteral integrity. Five milliliters of indigo carmine dye are injected intravenously. In 3 to 5 minutes, the dye will spurt from each ureteral orifice, proving that the intramural portion of the ureter has not been incorporated in the repair.

There is no hard and fast rule about postoperative bladder drainage after initial repair of simple vesicovaginal fistulas. The determination regarding the type and duration of bladder drainage should be made at the end of the operation and will depend on a number of factors, including the operator's impression of the security of the closure and the location of the repair site inside the bladder. When the operation has gone extremely well and there is every reason to expect a successful result, I have left an indwelling transurethral catheter in overnight and removed it the next morning. The patient is discharged after demonstrating a satisfactory voiding pattern with instructions to void frequently and not allow the bladder to become distended. On other occasions, the catheter has been left in for 7 to 14 days. Suprapubic catheters are very seldom used after initial repair of a simple posthysterectomy vesicovaginal fistula.

Care must be taken to make certain that the catheter does not become obstructed. Many good vesicovaginal fistula repairs have been ruined by an obstructed catheter and an overdistended bladder. Patients who are discharged with a catheter should be instructed to cut the catheter with scissors and remove it immediately if there is any sign of inadequate drainage and bladder distention and then to report for assessment of the situation. The best way to keep the catheter open and to avoid urinary tract infection is to ensure an adequate intake of fluids sufficient to produce output of a large quantity of dilute urine, preferably at least 100 mL/hour.

Complicated Fistulas.—Again, complicated vesicovaginal fistulas are those that are large; those that have had previous unsuccessful attempts at repair; those that involve the one or both ureters, vesical neck, or urethra; those that are associated with intestinal fistulas; and those that result from extensive surgery or radiation therapy (or both) for gynecologic malignancy. Many complicated fistulas can still be closed using a transvaginal Latzko partial colpocleisis. The basic principles of fistula repair just described for simple fistulas still apply when complicated fistulas are repaired and perhaps should be applied even more strictly. For very difficult fistulas, the repair may need to be done in stages. For example, if a patient has a radiation-induced vesicovaginal and rectovaginal fistula associated with bilateral ureteral stenosis and hydroureter, such a complicated problem may require three operations for solution. The first operation would include bilateral ureteroileocutaneous anastomosis and colostomy; the second operation would be closure of the fistulas; and the third operation would be closure of the colostomy and anastomosis of the ileal conduit to the bladder if the second operation is successful.

Special techniques and management principles may be needed to achieve continence in a patient with a complicated vesicovaginal fistula. Although early repair of simple posthysterectomy vesicovaginal fistula is appropriate, the repair of a complicated fistula should be delayed until the tissue around the fistula is healed and healthy. This may take 3 to 6 months. In the case of a radiation-induced fistula, it may take much longer, and one must wait until the effects of the acute irradiation injury have subsided and the fistula has finally achieved its ultimate size. This may take many months.

Very complicated vesicovaginal fistulas may require a combined transvaginal-transvesical-transperitoneal approach for final closure. A dissection from below might mobilize the vaginal mucosa and possibly bring in a bulbocavernosus fat flap. The vaginal mucosa is closed before making an abdominal incision to open the bladder. Ureteral catheters can be passed and the bladder mucosa mobilized and closed. Then a peritoneal flap and/or omental flap can also be mobilized to be interposed between the bladder and vagina. A technique of abdominal closure of vesicovaginal fistula using bisection of the bladder and wide mobilization of the bladder from the vagina, allowing for closure of the vagina and bladder in separate layers, described by O'Connor, is illustrated in Figure 13–17.

When local tissue healing is impaired by radiation, diabetes, chronic infection, or other factors, hard sclerotic and fibrotic tissue with occluded arterioles may extend a considerable distance beyond the fistula margins. Neovascularization from fresh, well-vascularized tissue pedicles brought to the fistula site will support the repair and promote healing. Small arterioles migrate from the normal tissue pedicles into the ischemic tissues at the repair site.

Various techniques of autografting have been described by Zacharin. The most common techniques are the bulbocavernosus labial fat pad, the omental pedicle grafts, and the gracilis muscle graft. These techniques may be extremely useful in surgical closure of complicated vesicovaginal fistulas since the key to successful closure of these fistulas is to bring in a new blood supply to devitalized vaginal and bladder tissues.

After repair of a complicated vesicovaginal fistula, prolonged drainage of the bladder is usually required. Depending on a variety of circumstances, suprapubic or transurethral drainage (or both) is used. On rare occasions, for very complicated fistulas, patients are asked to lie on their abdomen with a suprapubic catheter draining directly into a bottle on the floor through the mattress.

Only when the closure of a vesicovaginal fistula is considered technically impossible to close should urinary diversion above the bladder be advised. This is most often necessary for painful postirradiation fistulas. Ureteral anastomosis to the intact functioning sigmoid colon is not an appropriate operation because of the attendant metabolic and electrolyte problem of hyperchloremic acidosis, because of chronic hydroureteronephrosis with pyelonephritis, and because of the development of colon malignancies at the anastomotic site. Anastomosis of the ureters to an ileal conduit is my preferred procedure. Newer procedures using intestinal segments in ingenious but complicated ways to provide urinary continence on the abdominal wall are available.

Unusual Fistulas.—In the United States, serious urethral damage causing fistula is uncommon from any cause. Urethral damage from prolonged obstructed labor or difficult forceps operations caused urethral injuries many years ago. A urethrovaginal fistula may be seen after suburethral diverticulectomy or anterior colporrhaphy or radiation therapy for carcinoma involving the anterior vaginal wall or urethra. The urethra may be damaged if the bulb of an indwelling catheter is accidentally inflated in the urethral lumen, but this does not ordinarily result in fistula formation. Lymphogranuloma may destroy the urethra. Operations to repair urethral injuries are technically tedious and difficult. An operation to repair urethral damage, first described by Symmonds, is shown in Figure 13–18.

Vesicouterine and vesicocervical fistulas are uncommon and today will usually result from injury and necrosis of the bladder wall directly over the dehiscence of a lower uterine segment cesarean section incision. The patient may complain of some

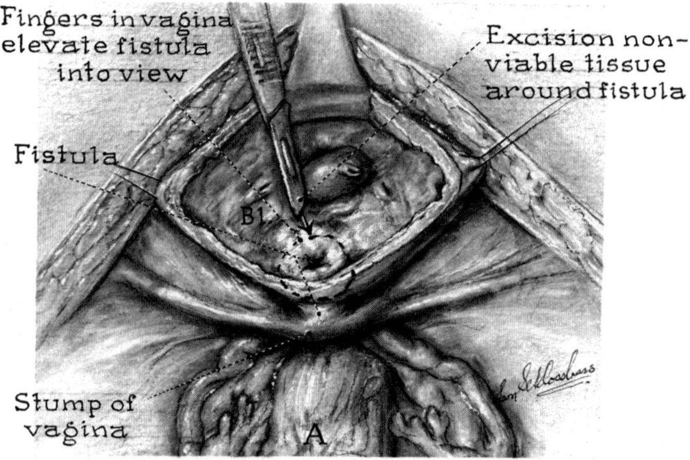

FIG 13–17.
Transabdominal, transvesical closure of vesicovaginal fistula. **A,** a longitudinal incision in the bladder dome illustrates the vesical opening of the fistula and its relationship to the vagina and the ureteral orifices. **B,** the incision in the bladder wall is extended around the orifice of the fistula. The fistulous tract and its vaginal orifice are completely excised. **C,** interrupted no. 3-0 delayed absorbable sutures are used to close the vaginal opening in one or two layers. **D,** a continuous no. 3-0 delayed absorbable suture closes the bladder mucosa longitudinally. **E,** a suprapubic catheter is placed through the bladder dome in an extra-peritoneal location. The bladder is distended to check for security of closure. **F,** the bladder muscularis is closed with no. 3-0 delayed absorbable continuous or interrupted sutures. **G,** in complicated fistulas, an omental flap may be developed and sutured between the bladder closure and the vaginal closure. (From Mattingly RF, Thompson JD: *TeLinde's Operative Gynecology,* ed 7. Philadelphia, JB Lippincott Co, 1990. Used by permission.)

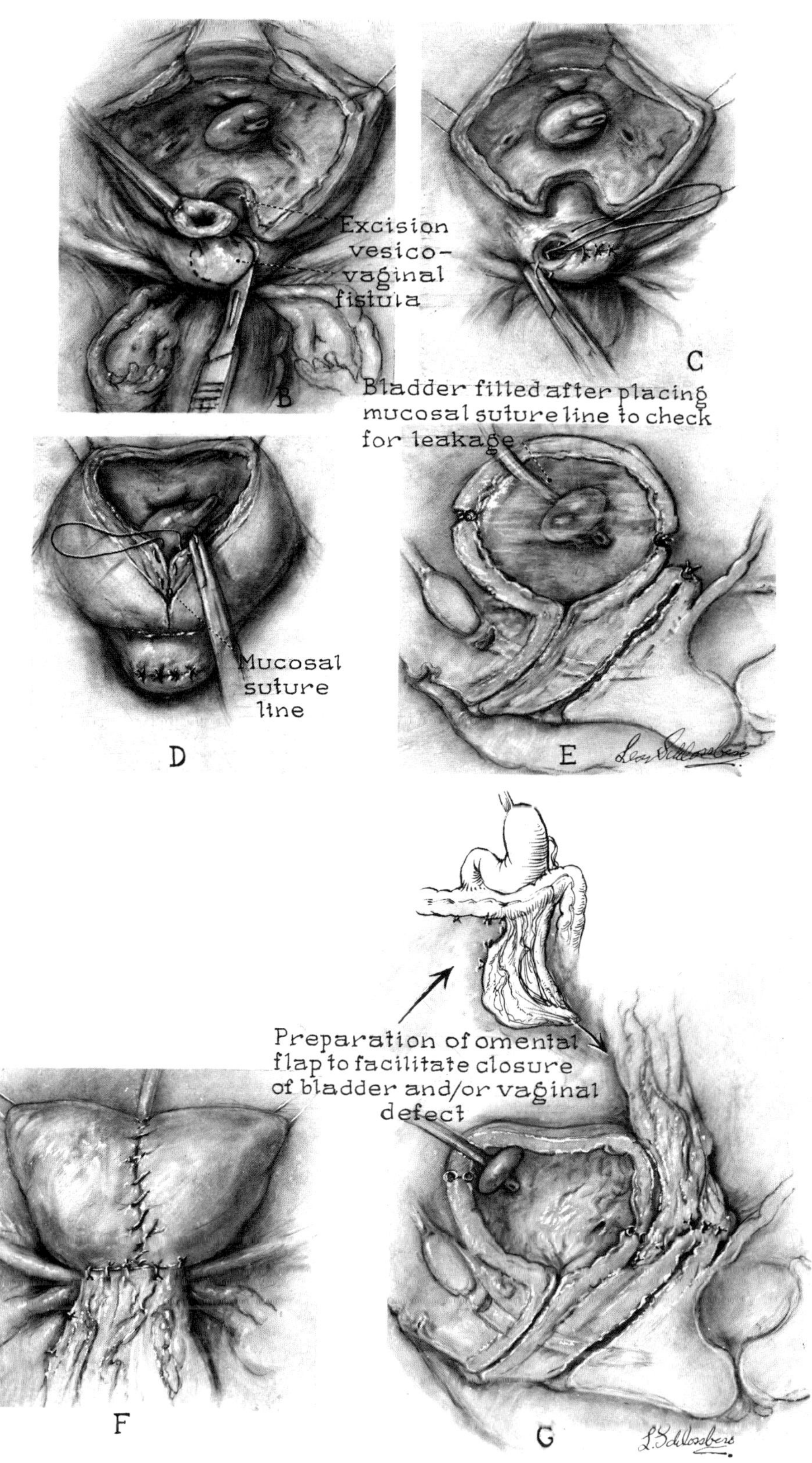

FIG 13–17 (cont.).

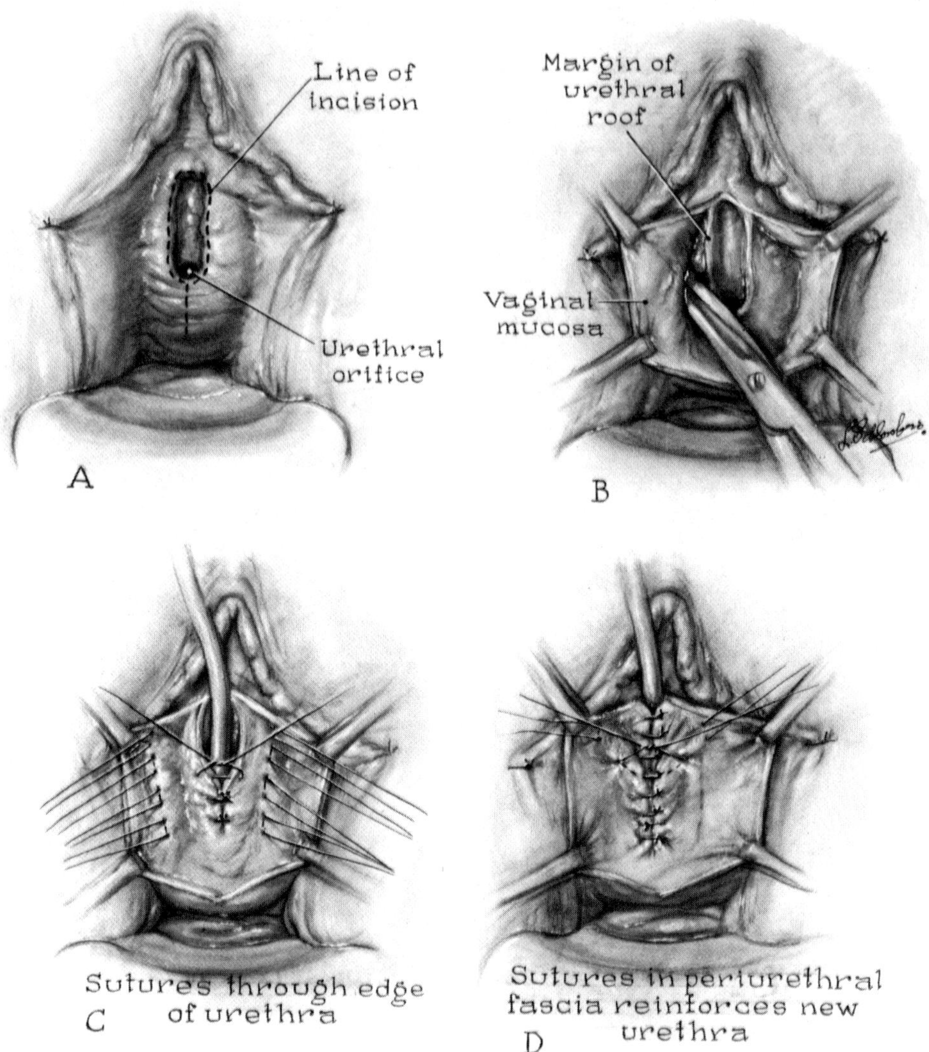

FIG 13–18.
Reconstruction of total or partial loss of urethral floor. **A,** line of incision along lateral margin of roof of urethra and beneath bladder base. **B,** enough of the urethral margins and fascia are freed from the vagina to permit approximation of the urethral mucosa in the midline. **C,** urethral edges are approximated in the midline over a no. 12 French catheter with interrupted no. 3-0 delayed absorbable sutures. Mobilized urethral fascia is sutured on each side of the total length of the urethra. The lower strand of each suture is tied beneath the urethral floor, **D,** and the upper strands of the two sutures are used to pull the fascia beneath the urethra, where they are tied.

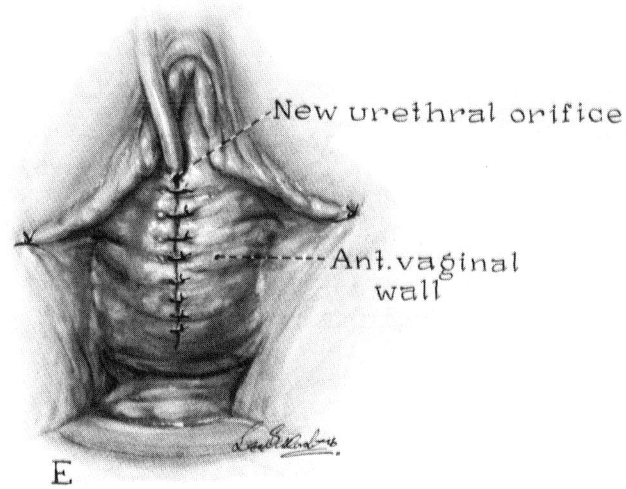

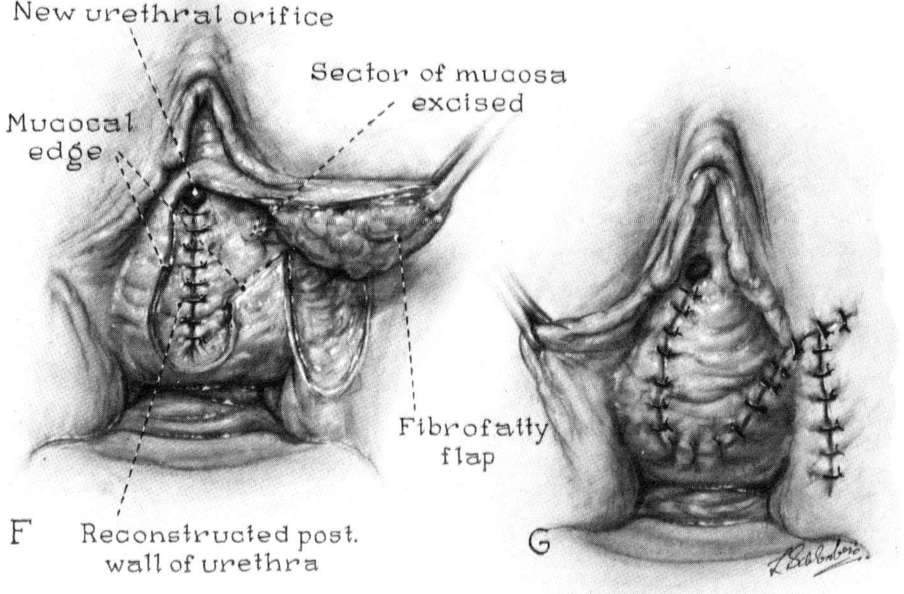

FIG 13–18 (cont.).
E, the vaginal mucosa is closed without tension. The bladder is filled with sterile water before the catheter is removed, and a suprapubic tube is inserted. **F,** alternatively for additional reinforcement, a labial fat pad is developed by a U-shaped incision along the lateral and medial aspects of the labia, leaving a broad pedicle superiorly. The lateral vaginal mucosa is resected between the urethral operative site and the labial graft, **G.** The skin margins of the labial graft are sutured to the vaginal margins with no. 3-0 interrupted delayed absorbable suture. The labial skin margins are closed so as to produce a flat vulvar surface. (From Mattingly RF, Thompson JD: *TeLinde's Operative Gynecology*, ed 7. Philadelphia, JB Lippincott Co, 1990. Used by permission.)

involuntary loss of urine through the vagina or she may remain continent of urine. Instead, she may experience cyclic hematuria (menouria) and amenorrhea. Cystoscopy, cystogram, and hysterogram are useful diagnostic procedures. The fistula will always be supratrigonal. The operation to repair the fistula can be done abdominally or vaginally depending on a variety of circumstances. The bladder is dissected free from the lower anterior uterine isthmus. Following identification of the fistula tract, the bladder and uterine orifices are closed separately. A layer of peritoneum should be mobilized and sutured between the repair sites. A hysterectomy is not required for successful repair. If a hysterectomy is done, it should be indicated from some other reason, including the presence of a large defect in the uterine wall, repair of which appears to be technically unsatisfactory.

Complications of Fistula Repair

Except for breakdown of the repair, there are few complications of fistula repair. Injury to the intramural portion of the ureter can be diagnosed and corrected if cystoscopy with the indigo carmine dye test is performed at the end of the repair. Cystoscopy will also diagnose intravesical bleeding, providing an opportunity for control before clot formation inside the bladder with bladder distention and obstruction of catheter drainage damaging the repair site.

The most dreaded complication of all is, of course, failure of the fistula repair to heal. This is usually evident 7 to 10 days after the operation. If the repair breaks down, a large-bore catheter should be placed in the bladder and allowed to remain for several weeks. This will provide an opportunity for the fistula to heal spontaneously or, if not, to heal with the smallest defect possible so that the next attempt at repair will have the best chance of success. During this time, the gynecologic surgeon will need to make the best possible effort to provide emotional support to the patient. Fortunately, almost all fistulas can be closed eventually, even complicated ones.

REFERENCES

Baker HW: Selective indications for subtotal hysterectomy. *J Ky Med Assoc* 1985; 83:355.

Beland G: Early treatment of ureteral injuries found after gynecological surgery. *J Urol* 1977; 118:25.

Bergman H (ed): *The Ureter.* New York, Springer-Verlag New York, 1981.

Betson JR: Bulbocavernosus fat pad transplant. *Obstet Gynecol* 1980; 9:303.

Boyce WH: Use of the internal ureteral stent in surgery of the kidney and ureter, in Boyarksy S, Gottschalk EA, Tanagho EA, et al (eds): *Urodynamics: Hydrodynamics of the Ureter and Renal Pelvis.* New York, Academic Press, 1971.

Boronow RC: Repair of radiation-induced vaginal fistula utilizing the Martius technique. *World J Surg* 1986; 10:237.

Boronow RC, Rutledge F: Vesicovaginal fistula, radiation, and gynecologic cancer. *Am J Obstet Gynecol* 1971; 111:85.

Clarke DH, Holland JB: Repair of vesicovaginal fistulas: Simultaneous transvaginal-transvesical approach. *South Med J* 1975; 68:1410.

Collins CG, Collins JH, Harrison BR, et al: Early repair of vesicovaginal fistula. *Am J Obstet Gynecol* 1971; 111:524.

Collins CG, Prent D: Results of early repair of vesicovaginal fistula with preliminary cortisone treatment. *Am J Obstet Gynecol* 1960; 80:1005.

Cruikshank SH: Early closure of post-hysterectomy vesicovaginal fistulas. *South Med J* 1988; 81:1525.

Cruikshank SH: Surgical method of identifying the ureters during total vaginal hysterectomy. *Obstet Gynecol* 1986; 67:277.

Ehrlich RM, Melman A, Skinner DG: The use of vesicopsoas hitch in urologic surgery. *J Urol* 1978; 119:322.

Elkins TE, Drescher C, Martey JO, et al: Vesicovaginal fistula revisited. *Obstet Gynecol* 1988; 72:307.

Everett HS, Mattingly RF: Urinary tract injuries resulting from pelvic surgery. *Am J Obstet Gynecol* 1956; 71:502.

Falk HC, Orkin LA: Nonsurgical closure of vesicovaginal fistulas. *Obstet Gynecol* 1957; 9:538.

Fearl CL, Keizur LW: Optimum time interval from occurrence to repair of vesicovaginal fistula. *Am J Obstet Gynecol* 1968; 104:205.

Flynn JT, Tiptaft RC, Woodhourse CR, et al: The early and aggressive repair of iatrogenic ureteric injuries. *Br J Urol* 1979; 51:454.

Fry DE, Milholen L, Harbrecht PJ: Iatrogenic ureteral injury: Options in management. *Arch Surg* 1983; 118:454.

Garlock JH: The cure of an intractable vesicovaginal fistula by the use of a pedicled muscle flap. *Surg Gynecol Obstet* 1928; 47:225.

Gillenwater JY: The pathology of urinary obstruction, in Walsh PC, Gittes RF, Perlmutter AL, et al (eds): *Campbell's Urology*, ed. 5. Philadelphia, WB Saunders Co, 1986, pp 542–578.

Graham JB: Painful syndrome of postradiation urinary vaginal fistula. *Surg Gynecol Obstet* 1964; 121:1260.

Hache L, Pratt JH, Cook EN: Vesicouterine fistula. *Mayo Clin Proc* 1966; 41:150.

Harrow BR: A neglected maneuver for ureterovesical implantation following injury at gynecologic operation. *J Urol* 1968; 100:280.

Hatch KD, Parham G, Shingleton HM, et al: Ureteral strictures and fistulae following radical hysterectomy. *Gynecol Oncol* 1984; 19:17.

Hedgegaard CK, Wallace D: Percutaneous nephrostomy: Current indications and potential uses in obstetrics and gynecology. Literature review and report of a case. *Obstet Gynecol Surv* 1987; 42:671.

Hofmeister FJ: Pelvic anatomy of the ureter in relation to surgery performed through the vagina. *Clin Obstet Gynecol* 1982; 25:821.

Hyman RM: Coagulation therapy for small vesicovaginal fistulas. *Clin Obstet Gynecol* 1968; 8:465.

Iloabachie GC, Njoku O: Vesicouterine fistula. *Br J Urol* 1985; 57:438.

Jaszczak SE, Evans TN: Intrafascial abdominal and vaginal hysterectomy: A reappraisal. *Obstet Gynecol* 1982; 59:435.

Kaplan Jo, Winslow OP, Sneider SE, et al: Dilatation of a surgically ligated ureter through percutaneous nephrostomy. *AJR* 1982; 39:188.

Kiricuta I, Goldstein AMB: The repair of extensive vesicovaginal fistulas with pedicled omentum: A review of 27 cases. *J Urol* 1972; 108:724.

Krupp P, Hoffman M, Roeling W: Terminal ileum as ureteral substitute. *Obstet Gynecol* 1970; 35:416.

Kursh EC, Morse RM, Resnick MI, et al: Prevention of the development of a vesicovaginal fistula. *Surg Gynecol Obstet* 1988; 166:490.

Larson DM, Malone JM Jr, Copeland LJ, et al: Ureteral assessment after radical hysterectomy. *Obstet Gynecol* 1987; 69:612.

Latzko W: Postoperative vesicovaginal fistulas. *Am J Surg* 1942; 58:211–228.

Lee RA, Symmonds RE: Ureterovaginal fistula. *Am J Obstet Gynecol* 1971; 109:1032.

Lee RA, Symmonds RE, Williams TJ: Current status of genitourinary fistula. *Obstet Gynecol* 1988; 72:313.

Mann WJ, Arato M, Patsner B, et al: Ureteral injuries in an obstetrics and gynecology training program: Etiology and management. *Obstet Gynecol* 1988; 72:82.

Martius H: Vesicovaginal Therapy especially by plastic transplantation of flaps. *Z Geburtshilfe Gynakol* 1932; 103:22.

Mattingly RF, Thompson JD: *TeLinde's Operative Gynecology*, ed 6. Philadelphia, JB Lippincott Co, 1985, Chapters 14 and 27.

Miller NF, George H: Lower urinary tract fistulas in women. A study based on 292 cases. *Am J Obstet Gynecol* 1954; 68:436.

Moir JC: Vesicovaginal fistula. *Proc R Soc Med* 1966; 59:1019.

Murphy M: Social consequences of vesicovaginal fistula in Northern Nigeria. *J Biosoc Sci* 1981; 13:139.

O'Connor VJ, Jr: Repair of vesicovaginal fistula with associated urethral loss. *Surg Gynecol Obstet* 1978; 146:251.

O'Quinn AG, Degefu S, Batson HK, et al: Early repair of vesicovaginal fistula following preliminary corticosteroid treatment. Paper presented at the Society of Pelvic Surgeons, New Orleans, November 1984.

Patil V, Waterhourse K, Laungani G: Management of 18 difficult vesicovaginal and urethrovaginal fistulas with modified Ingelman-Sundberg and Martius operations. *J Urol* 1980; 123:653.

Pettit PD, Lee RA: Ovarian remnant syndrome: Diagnostic dilemma and surgical challenge. *Obstet Gynecol* 1988; 71:580.

Persky L, Herman G, Geurrier K: Non-delay in vesicovaginal fistula repair. *Urology* 1979; 13:273.

Petty WM, Lowy RO, Oyama AA: Total abdominal hysterectomy after radiation therapy for cervical cancer: Use of omental graft for fistula prevention. *Am J Obstet Gynecol* 1986; 154:1222.

Piscitelli JT, Simel DL, Addison WA: Who should have intravenous pyelograms before hysterectomy for benign disease? *Obstet Gynecol* 1987; 69:541.

Podratz K, Symmonds RE, Hagen JV: Vesicovaginal fistulae. *Baillieres Clin Obstet Gynaecol* 1987; 1:4124.

Ponig BF Jr: Microsurgical ureteroureterostomy in ureteral injuries. *J Urol* 1982; 128:594.

Richardson EH: A simplified technic for abdominal panhysterectomy. *Surg Gynecol Obstet* 1929; 48:248.

Ridley JH: Indirect air cystoscopy. *South Med J* 1951; 44:114.

Sampson JA: Ligation and clamping of the ureter as complications of surgical operations. *Am Med* 1902; 4:693.

Sampson JA: The relation between carcinoma cervicis uteri and the ureters and its significance in the more radical operations for that disease. *Johns Hopkins Med Bull* 1904; 156:72.

Sampson JA: Ureteral fistulae as sequelae of pelvic operations. *Surg Gynecol Obstet* 1909; 8:170.

Shapiro SR, Bennett AH: Recovery of renal function after prolonged unilateral ureteral obstruction. *J Urol* 1976; 115:136.

Shoenwald MB, Orkin LA: Bilateral intravesical ureteral ligation. Complication of Cooper's ligament suspension. *J Urol* 1974; 3:787.

Symmonds RE: Incontinence: Vesical and urethral fistulas. *Clin Obstet Gynecol* 1984; 27:499.

Symmonds RE: Ureteral injuries associated with gynecologic surgery: Prevention and management. *Clin Obstet Gynecol* 1976; 19:623.

Symmonds RE, Hill M: Loss of the urethra: A report on 50 patients. *Am J Obstet Gynecol* 1978; 130:130.

Tahzib F: Epidemiological determinants of vesicovaginal fistulas. *Br J Obstet Gynecol* 1983; 90:387.

Tancer ML: The post total hysterectomy (vault) vesicovaginal fistula. *J Urol* 1980; 123:839.

Taylor JS, Hewson AD, Rachow P: Synchronous combined transvaginal transvesical repair of vesicovaginal fistulas. *Aust NZ J Surg* 1980; 50:23.

Thompson IM: Bladder flap repair of ureteral injuries. *Urol Clin North Am* 1977; 4:51.

Thompson JD, Benigno BB: Vaginal repair of ureteral injuries. *Am J Obstet Gynecol* 1971; 3:601.

Turner-Warwick R: The use of the omental pedicle graft in urinary tract reconstruction. *J Urol* 1976; 116:341.

Turner-Warwick R: The use of pedicle grafts in the repair of urinary tract fistulae. *Br J Urol* 1972; 44:644.

Turner-Warwick R, Worth PH: The psoas bladder hitch procedure for the replacement of the lower third of the ureter. *Br J Urol* 1969; 41:701.

Youssef AF: "Menouria" following lower segment cesarean section: A syndrome. *Am J Obstet Gynecol* 1957; 73:759.

Witters S, Cornelissen J, Vereecken R: Iatrogenic ureteral injury: Aggressive or conservative treatment. *Am J Obstet Gynecol* 1986; 155:582.

Zacharin RF: Grafting as a principle in the surgical management of vesicovaginal and rectovaginal fistulae. *Aust NZ J Obstet Gynaecol* 1980; 20:10.

Zacharin RF: *Obstetric Fistula.* New York, Springer-Verlag New York, 1988.

Chapter 14

Recurrent Rectal Fistula

David H. Nichols, M.D.

In the evaluation of a patient with recurrent rectal fistula, the surgeon must first rule out active inflammatory bowel disease, such as Crohn's disease, tuberculosis, or lymphopathia venerum, which may be suspected by a patient history of frequent bowel movements, weight loss, passage of mucus, and on physical examination of the fistula, finding pain to touch, induration and edema, and granulations. The surgeon must further exclude by history and biopsy the presence of invasive neoplastic disease at the site of fistula formation. (Biopsies should be performed on areas suspected of neoplasia, including ulceration with palpably hard margins that often are whitish and occasionally are bloody.)

Intestinal diverticulosis may be recognized from the patient's history, and perforation through the internal genitalia may lead to fistula formation at the vault of the vagina; however, this is usually colovaginal and not rectovaginal, because diverticulosis does not involve the rectum. The diagnosis is confirmed by barium enema and sigmoidoscopy or colonoscopy.

When the patient's history includes previous pelvic radiation, often in the distant past, the presence of a degree of endarteritis obliterans can be assumed or suspected. In the previously irradiated patient, a history of prior vaginal or rectal biopsy of some reddish or granular area on the surface of the posterior vaginal wall of the vagina may be the cause of the fistula. Although such an area is usually not malignant, the biopsy site may not heal well, and due to the local devascularization, a rectovaginal fistula may develop. A better primary approach to the evaluation of such a postradiation redness would be the use of cytology from a surface smear and colposcopy, with careful biopsy only of a site found likely to be malignant. Repair of such a postradiation rectovaginal fistula from which malignancy has been excluded should not be attempted until the patient has experienced at least 1 year of intravaginal estrogen supplementation, and the technique of repair must include meticulous dissection with a layered closure and interposition between the rectum and vagina of a Martius bulbocavernosus graft between the two layers. If the tissues and layers can be closed without tension, hemostasis is adequate, and the surgery is carried out precisely and with the most gentle handling of tissue, a complimentary diverting colostomy may not be necessary.

Most recurrent lower intestinal fistulas in women are either anoperineal or rectovaginal. There is as large a world of pathologic and surgical difference between a recurrent anal fistula and rectovaginal fistula as there is between their previously unrepaired counterparts. In most instances, both etiology and treatment of the two conditions are quite distinctively different.

ANAL FISTULA

Anal fistula is frequently associated with anal abscess but may follow trauma to anal tissue and may be associated with inflammatory bowel disease such as Crohn's. Parks has demonstrated that anal glands may penetrate the internal anal sphincter at the base of the anal crypt and theorizes that infection of such a glandular duct can result in an abscess that can spread in various directions, not infrequently leading to subsequent development of anal fistula. Some of these sites of abscess formation with fistula are shown in Figure 14–1. Although incision and drainage are critical to resolution of the abscess, it is essential to determine by gentle probing the relationship between the abscess, a fistula, and the internal or external anal sphincter and whether or not the abscess is above or below the patient's levator ani. It must be remembered that supralevator abscess may be associated with inflammatory bowel disease. Ischiorectal abscess should be drained through an incision close to the anal canal and usually under hospital operating room anesthesia. If by examination an opening into an anal crypt is identified, often by noting the escape of pus from the abscess into the crypt, this should be noted in the operative report for a reference during subsequent search and surgery. Culture of a perianal abscess should be taken. If it shows predominantly *Escherichia coli*, recurrence is more likely than if it shows *Staphylococcus aureus*, because the former suggests fistulous communication with the rectum. Search for a probable fistula should be undertaken anoscopically about 2 weeks after evacuation of the abscess cavity.

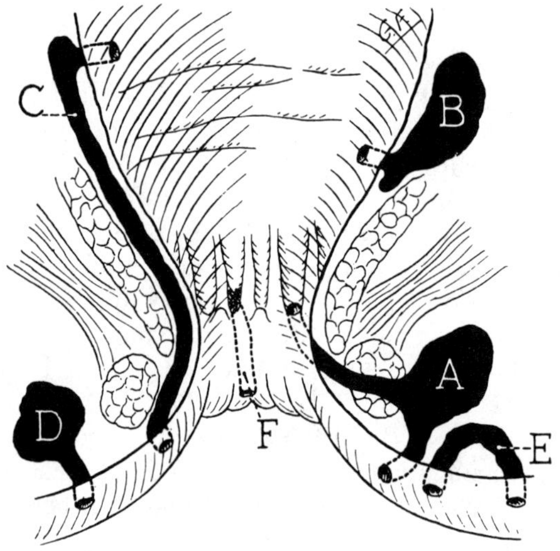

FIG 14–1.
Various locations of anorectal fistulas and sinuses. **A,** complete fistula between an internal opening in an anal crypt, tunneling through the external sphincter and external opening on the perineum. **B,** internal rectal sinus. **C,** complete rectal fistula. **D,** perianal sinus. **E,** complete external perianal fistula. **F,** complete submucocutaneous fistula. (From Hirschman LJ: *Synopsis of Ano-Rectal Diseases,* ed 2. St Louis, CV Mosby Co, 1942, p 169. Used by permission.)

Abscess between the internal and external anal sphincters (in contrast to a submucosal abscess between the internal sphincter and the rectal mucosa) should be excised transrectally, including the crypt-bearing area, leaving the wound open for subsequent healing by granulation.

Most anal fistulas are preceded by a history of an abscess that either ruptured spontaneously or was drained. The surgery to correct anal fistula may be far more difficult than that for a rectovaginal fistula, because severe anal incontinence may develop postoperatively consequent to disruption in fibrosis of the anal sphincter mechanism. Goodsall's rule describes the relationship between the fistulous tract and the two ends of the fistula, which is important because the lining of the tract should be exposed and curetted or excised due to its probable glandular content. The rule states that when the external fistulous opening lies anterior to a horizontal plane drawn through the center of the anal canal, the internal opening tends to be located radially at the end of a straight line from the external opening. When the external opening lies posterior to this plane, the tract is usually curved, and the internal opening is located in the posterior midline. Application of this rule is a great help in locating and probing a fistulous tract. Fistulas of the intersphincteric plane most commonly have a single external opening, but transsphincteric fistulas may have multiple openings arising from the ischiorectal fossa and postanal space, producing the horseshoe-type fistula, each tract of which must be separately exposed and curetted. Failure to expose all of this gland-bearing tissue in the tract will cause a recurrence first of an abscess, then of a fistula. Injections of milk, which are nonstaining, or of a solution of indigo-carmine, which stains the tissues very deeply, using a short blunt or Marx needle may help demonstrate the tract. Probing of the tract should precede excision of each of its segments. This will cure most intrasphincteric and transsphincteric fistulas, but the supralevator extension should not be drained into the rectum. Probably the advice of a surgeon with special experience in this area should be obtained, because there is a great chance of fecal incontinence developing from division of the puborectalis sling.

When a lower fistula transgresses the external sphincter, the surgeon during excision of the tract may incise a part of the sphincter, anticipating its reunion by scar tissue during the healing phase. If this appears to risk sphincter integrity, a seton of no. 2 polyglycolic acid (Dexon) or silk may be used (Fig 14–2). Its use, as

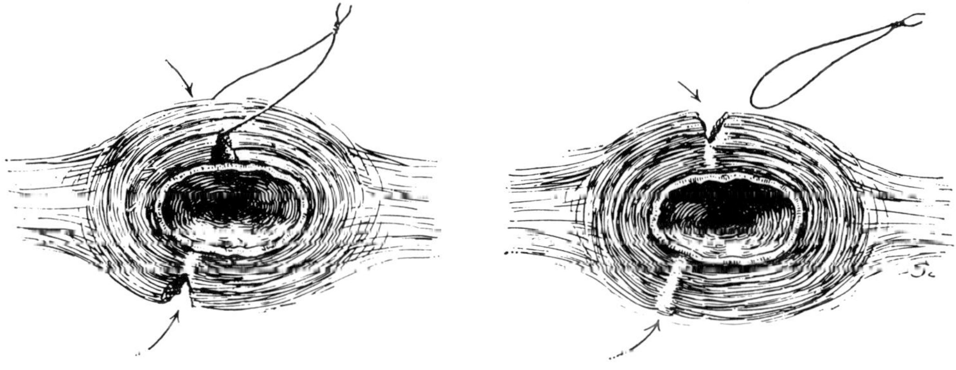

FIG 14–2.
Details of division of sphincter by seton *(arrows)*. (From Hirschman LJ: *Synopsis of Ano-Rectal Diseases*, ed 2. St Louis, CV Mosby Co, 1942, p 185. Used by permission.)

Corman suggests, is similar to the principle of a wire cutting through a block of ice, which, if in continuous contact, will readhere after division by the wire. After the skin between the anal canal and the perineum is excised, the seton of doubled no. 2 Dexon or silk is placed around the sphincter and tied very tightly, and the ends are cut long. It is retightened in about 2 weeks, by which time the muscle and tract will have been cut through and the latter reunited by scar tissue. One week later, the retightened seton will have cut through the remainder of the muscle, the suture removed, and the wound permitted to heal. This can be used through the puborectalis sling during treatment of the extrasphincteric fistula, particularly when the internal opening of the fistula is above the levator ani. Complete excision of an extrasphincteric fistula risks postoperative wound breakdown of any sphincter repair with subsequent incontinence, which may be difficult to repair.

RECTOVAGINAL FISTULA

A genital fistula has a high-pressure side and a low-pressure side, and material flows from the high-pressure side to and through the low-pressure side and not the other way around. With rectovaginal fistula, the high-pressure side is the rectum, and the low-pressure side is the vagina. For this reason, symptomatic material does not flow from the vagina into the rectum but flows from the rectum into the vagina; therefore, the effective closure or removal of the *rectal* opening (the high pressure side of the equation) is the primary goal. If the rectal opening of the fistula is removed and the opening closed, the vaginal opening generally requires little or no attention, because it will granulate in and become reepithelialized. This may occur a little faster if the epithelialized edges have been trimmed, but the vaginal opening need be closed only by one or two loosely placed sutures.

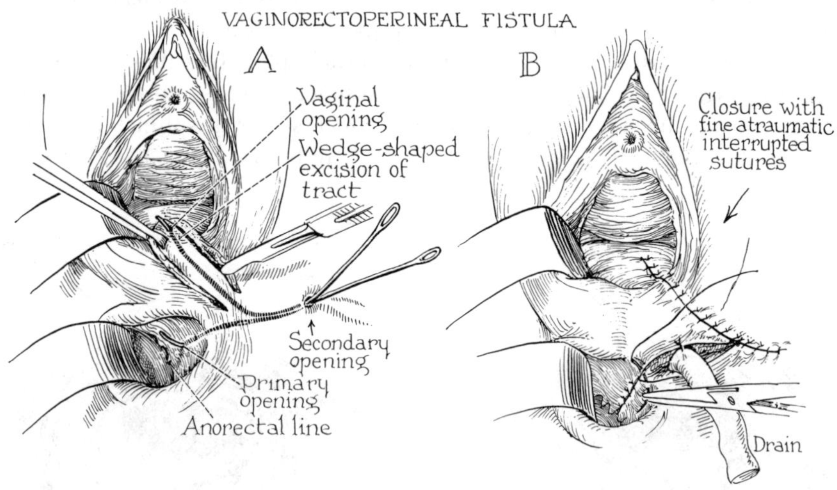

FIG 14–3.
Extrasphincteric vaginorectoperineal fistula excision. Malleable probes have been inserted into the fistulous tracts and an incision made through the skin and subcutaneous tissue **(A)**, excising each tract. A small Penrose drain may be inserted subcutaneously and the incision closed with interrupted sutures **(B)**. Alternately, the incisions may be left open for healing by granulation and secondary intention (From Ball TL: *Gynecologic Surgery and Urology*, ed 2. St Louis, CV Mosby Co, 1963. Used by permission.)

One must determine that a suspected recurrence of fistula is not, in fact, a previously undiagnosed second rectovaginal fistula, because the surgical prognosis is considerably more favorable for the latter.

When recurrent rectovaginal fistula follows previous surgical repair, one must consider that the initial repair may have been surgically satisfactory from a mechanical and technical standpoint and therefore consider and exclude or treat any previously undiagnosed inflammatory bowel disease that may be a significant etiologic factor. Characteristically, such recurrent and usually larger fistulas will be unexpectedly evident several weeks or months following the initial repair. When a patient with Crohn's disease requests surgical repair, she should be made fully aware of the risks and prognosis. The repair should be performed during the period of remission of the disease and following 1 month's preparation using 1,000 mg of metronidazole daily and 20 mg of prednisone daily in divided doses. The transperineal rectal flap operation, shown in (Fig 14–4) is most useful for such fistulas in the lower third of the vagina. It exteriorizes the rectal fistula, which will be removed with the resection of the anterior rectal wall.

Recurrent rectovaginal fistula in the midvagina may be repaired by a layered technique in which the rectal wall containing the fistula is carefully mobilized about 2 cm in each direction lateral to the fistula's opening, which is then excised. The rectal muscularis is approximated by transversely applied interrupted mattress sutures of fine polyglycolic acid or chromic suture material, inverting the cut mucosal edge into the rectal lumen. A second layer of mattress stitches inverts and reinforces the first layer from which it removes much of the tension, which otherwise might tend to draw the suture layer apart. A layer of intervening tissue must be inserted between the rectum and vagina if the blood supply here is poor, often by a bulbocavernosus fat pad transplant, and the full thickness of the vagina approximated in a direction at right angles to the suture line in the rectal wall. If the external anal sphincter is not intact, it should be repaired by appropriate transvaginal sphincterplasty and perineorrhaphy. Occasionally so little tissue will be present that the technique is much like that of freshening the edges and repairing a fourth-degree perineal laceration.

Because the external anal sphincter is usually competent with recurrent rectovaginal fistula, easily assessed by asking the patient to contract her perineal muscles during preoperative examination, one will find it often to be functional and intact. It is not necessary or even desirable to cut it to facilitate repair of a fistula cranial to this site.

For recurrent rectovaginal fistulas in the lower third of the vagina, the most common site, a transperineal rectal flap sliding operation is most satisfactory. For all operations involving the voluntary muscle sphincter repair, a light general anesthetic without muscle relaxants is preferable so that skeletal muscle remnants can be easily recognized for incorporation in the repair.

Transperineal Flap Sliding Operation

I usually perform this operation by a semicircular incision through the rectal wall beneath the external anal sphincter (Fig 14–4). If scarring is extensive, one may choose an alternate dissection directly beneath the vaginal wall, over the perineal body, and into the rectovaginal space. The latter is opened widely, and the fistula's tract is transected. The epithelialized portions are excised, and the rectal muscularis is closed transversely with two layers of interrupted mattress stitches, inverting the wound into the rectum. An intervening layer of soft tissue (i.e., levator fascia) may be brought in to insulate the area, and the vagina is loosely approximated with a single interrupted full-thickness suture so placed that the axis of the vaginal approximation is at right angles to that of the rectum.

In rare instances, as with a very large recurrent fistula in a patient with previous massive pelvic radiation, the fistula may be closed by a modified colpocleisis, in which the anterior vaginal wall and bladder are sewn to the defect in the anterior rectal wall.

PRINCIPLES OF REPAIR

1. A time for fistula repair should be chosen when granulation tissue, infection, edema, and pain are minimal.
2. The repair must interrupt the continuity of the fistula.
3. The epithelialized fistulous tract should be excised.
4. Unless the anterior rectal flap sliding operation has been performed and the exteriorized rectal wall, including the fistula, excised, the rectal side of the fistula should be closed with a layer of interrupted mattress stitches placed in the muscularis in such a fashion that the cut edge of rectal mucosa will be everted into the rectal lumen. A second layer of sutures should be placed, inverting the first layer.

Preoperative Preparation

A clear liquid diet is begun 2 days before admission to the hospital, and one-half bottle of citrate of magnesia or two bisacodyl (Dulcolax) tablets are given the afternoon before admission.

Although mechanical cleansing of the bowel lumen reduces the total fecal mass, it does not significantly reduce the number of bacteria present on the intestinal epithelium. The patient is given a whole-gut lavage with GoLytely by mouth, as much of the solution as can rapidly be swallowed, beginning at 7:30 pm the evening before surgery.

One-half hour before surgery, 2 gm of a broad-spectrum antibiotic such as cefoxitin (Mefoxin) is administered intravenously. This may be repeated 2 hours later.

If whole-gut lavage is not used, the patient may be given two Fleet enemas 1 hour apart the evening before admission and plain water or saline enemas the morning of surgery until the return is clear.

Postoperative Care

A clear liquid diet is advised for the first 3 postoperative days, followed by a low-residue diet for the next 3 weeks.

A stool softener, such as docusate sodium (Colace) should be given for 5 weeks to keep the stool on the soft side. If intestinal cramps are troublesome, the patient may be given 10 drops of tincture of opium in water three times daily for 5 days.

There should be a bowel movement between the fifth and seventh day postop-

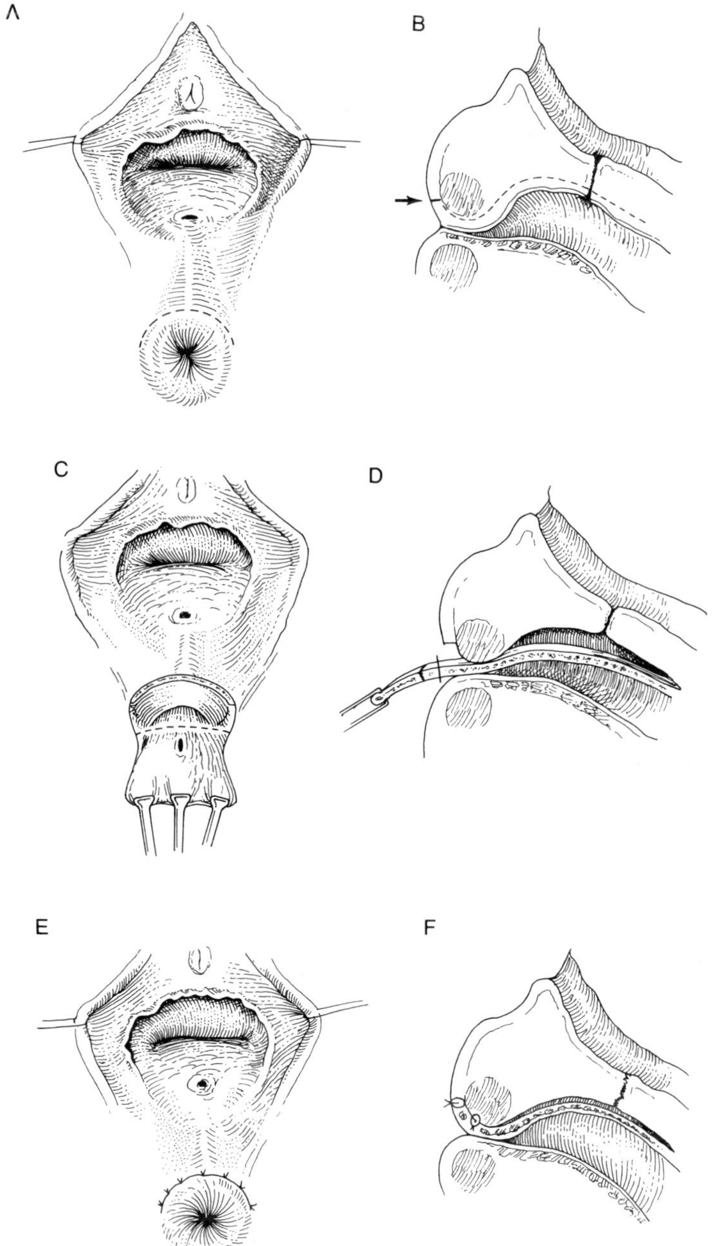

FIG 14–4.
Transperineal rectal flap operation. There is a rectovaginal fistula proximal to an intact external anal sphincter. All tissue to be dissected has been infiltrated with 0.5% lidocaine in 1:200,000 epinephrine. The site for the initial incision is identified by the *dashed line* **(A).** This is shown in sagittal section **(B),** where *V* indicates the vagina and *R* the rectum. The dissection continues beneath the perineal body to the rectovaginal space. Traction to the anterior rectal wall stretches it until the fistulous opening in the rectum has been exteriorized **(C),** shown in sagittal section in **D,** where the fistula *(a)* has been exteriorized. The rectal flap is excised along the *dashed line* that corresponds to *b* in the sagittal view. The remaining anterior rectal wall is tacked to the capsule of the external anal sphincter and the edge sewn to the perineal skin **(E),** completing the operation. The sagittal view **(F)** shows the interruption in the continuity of the fistula. The vaginal side of the tract will granulate in and quickly disappear. It, too, may be excised during the operation and edges loosely approximated by one or two stitches postoperatively (Redrawn from Nichols DH, Randall CL: *Vaginal Surgery,* ed 3. Baltimore, Williams & Wilkins Co, 1989.)

eratively. If none has occurred spontaneously, a small oral dose of GoLytely is preferable to an enema.

No coitus is permitted for 3 months postoperatively.

BIBLIOGRAPHY

Ball TL: *Gynecologic Surgery and Urology,* ed 2. St Louis CV Mosby Co, 1963.

Beecham CT: Recurring rectovaginal fistulas. *Obstet Gynecol* 1972; 40:323–326.

Boronow RC: Management of radiation induced vaginal fistulas. *Am J Obstet Gynecol* 1971; 110:1–8.

Corman ML: *Colon and Rectal Surgery.* Philadelphia, JB Lippincott Co, 1984, pp 108–112.

Goligher JC: *Surgery of the Anus, Rectum, and Colon,* ed 3. Springfield, Ill, Charles C Thomas, Publisher, 1975.

Goodsall DH: Anorectal fistula, in Goodsall DH, Miles WE (eds): *Diseases of the Anus and Rectum: Part I.* London, Longmans, Green and Co, 1900, pp 92–173.

Hirschman LJ: *Synopsis of Ano-Rectal Diseases,* ed 2. St Louis, CV Mosby Co, 1942, pp 168–193.

Nichols DH, Randall CL: *Vaginal Surgery,* ed 3. Baltimore, Williams & Wilkins Co, 1989, pp 388–402.

Nichols RL: Bowel preparation: Perioperative care, in Wilmore DW, Brennan MF, Harken AH, et al (eds): *Care of the Surgical Patient.* New York, Scientific American, 1989, vol 1, chapter 4.

Parks AG: Fistula-in-ano, in Morson BC (ed): *Diseases of the Colon, Rectum, and Anus.* New York, Appleton-Century-Croft, 1969, p 277.

Rosenshein NB, Genadry RR, Woodruff JD: An anatomic classification of rectovaginal septal defect. *Am J Obstet Gynecol* 1980; 137:439–442.

Solla JA, Rothenberger DA: Preoperative bowel preparation. *Dis Colon Rectum* 1990; 33:154–159.

Thompson JD: Transperineal repair of a rectovaginal fistula, in *OB-GYN Illustrated.* New Scotland, NY, Learning Technology, 1985.

Chapter 15

Recurrent Anal Incontinence

David H. Nichols, M.D.

Anal incontinence is socially devastating to the afflicted patient, because it includes the inability to control and retain rectal gas as well as stool, both of which may be lost involuntarily under most inappropriate circumstances. The patient probably will have already undergone one or more external anal sphincter plication procedures with or without a coincident perineorrhaphy, which did not restore continence. In such patients, the surgeon must make a distinction between frequent bowel movements, as might be seen with an irritable colon or diverticulosis, and anorectal incontinence, the latter characterized by the addition of involuntary rectal soiling. Presumably, rectovaginal fistula, ulcerative colitis, and Crohn's disease of the colon have been excluded by suitable examinations.

Recurrent anal incontinence may be seen with disruption of the external anal sphincter, usually of traumatic obstetric origin, often unrecognized or imprecisely repaired. Such a patient may secondarily develop a state of continence consequent to hypertrophy of the pelvic diaphragm through long-standing exercise of habitual voluntary isometric pubococcygeal contractions (e.g., 15 3-second contractions six times daily over several years). A generation ago, Kelly described such acquired continence among Pennsylvania farm women whom he had seen with unrepaired fourth-degree lacerations sustained many years previously. If the levator ani is intact, voluntary overdevelopment may produce an almost sphincter-like action that can be most effective.

Recurrent or persistent rectal incontinence may also be demonstrated in a patient in whom the external anal sphincter is intact but suffers a faulty innervation. The pelvic diaphragm and levator ani are supplied primarily by the paired pudendal and accessory pudendal nerves, which also supply the muscular fibers of the external anal sphincter. These muscles function in concert with one another. It is important to review briefly the normal mechanism for rectal continence so that we can pinpoint its possible disorders.

RECTAL CONTINENCE

There is a network of neuromuscular receptors within the levator ani that not only can detect rectal fullness but also can discriminate between gas, liquid, and solid content of the bowel. Stimulation of these receptors by increasing rectal content is followed by an increase in the tone of these muscles, which are never entirely at rest. The levator ani muscles are innervated by branches of the pudendal nerve, which similarly innervate the external anal sphincter. These muscles contract simultaneously and synergistically. They differ from the other voluntary muscles of the body in that they maintain, via this network of neuromuscular receptors, a constant state of tone proportional to the quantity of the rectal contents. Their unique capacity for discrimination can permit the slow escape of rectal gas even during sleep while retaining solid content. Because intestinal peristalsis continues even during sleep, it is this reflex contraction of these voluntary muscles that maintains continence. The ability of these muscles to contract effectively depends, therefore, on both their intrinsic integrity and that of their nerve supply, primarily the pudendal or the accessory pudendal nerves. Disruption of either nerve through congenital weakness, as might be noted with spina bifida or from acquired trauma as from a pathologic degree of stretching during childbirth or chronic straining at stool, may result in a loss of this major component of rectal continence.

Ordinarily, the gastrocolic reflex regularly assists defecation by promoting large intestinal peristalsis, which becomes part of the habit pattern of regular defecation. If, however, this reflex is consistently inhibited by voluntary postponement of this cleansing process, constipation may occur.

A backup system of continence occurs through the internal anal sphincter, which is an involuntary smooth muscle continuation of the wall of the large intestine. By a complex interaction, the internal sphincter reflexively relaxes preceding and during the act of defecation to permit the unimpeded transit of stool. When the levator ani or external anal sphincter or its nerve supply have been effectively compromised, the internal anal sphincter may remain as the sole barrier to rectal incontinence.

In addition to the previous mechanism, reflex contraction of the intact pubococcygei creates an anorectal valve that can be identified by the angulation of the anorectal junction, the anterior wall of the rectum covering the central lumen when the pubococcygei are contracted. Relaxation of this angulated valve promotes transit of stool.

There is an indirect role of the levator ani in providing a similar mechanism assisting urinary continence. When this mechanism has been disrupted, there may be associated stress incontinence of urine as well as anorectal incontinence. A sudden onset of both urinary and anal incontinence following a fall leads one to consider the possibility of acute herniation of an intervertebral disc, which may interfere with the pudendal nerves at their origin between S3 and S4. Careful neurologic examination is important in establishing this diagnosis, since disc herniation into the cauda equina may be present, though not demonstrated by myelography.

PERINEAL DESCENT SYNDROME

The pelvic diaphragm and its innervation by the pudendal may be damaged to varying degrees by pathologic stretching, either as might result from bearing down during childbirth or, more commonly, chronic straining at stool. These stresses appear mechanically to stretch the pudendal nerve at its angulation around the ischial spine. The resulting progressive damage to the pudendal nerve over a period of time may compound the inability of the pelvic diaphragm and external anal sphincter to function at maximum efficiency. Pathologic funneling of the pelvic diaphragm is produced and is manifested by a visible descent of the perineum and anus (Fig 15–1). The patient then actually sits on her anus, which becomes the most dependent portion of the perineum. With straining, the perineum and anus may descend further as the pelvic diaphragm becomes more and more funneled.

Initially this excessive funneling reduces the width of the hiatus between the levatores ani. In some patients, obstipation, an inability to empty the rectum no matter how hard the patient strains, may develop. Difficulty evacuating may become progressively worse, along with a noticeable decrease in the diameter of the stool to an almost ribbon-like extrusion.

An important anatomic deformity in perineal descent syndrome is loss of the anorectal angle, consequent to pathologic stretching of the pelvic diaphragm. It often coexists with cystocele, rectocele, uterine prolapse, and enterocele. When symptomatic, all of these elements should be effectively treated. Strong consideration should be given to correcting the symptomatic perineal descent by a coincident retrorectal levatorplasty. In this operation, an incision is made between the anus and the tip of the coccyx, the anococcygeal ligament is divided, and the dissection is carried directly into the retrorectal space (Fig 15–2). A series of plication stitches are placed in the posterior wall of the rectum, tied, but not cut. When all of these have been placed, they are sewn to the periosteum of the undersurface of the sacrum with care taken to avoid the middle sacral artery. When tied, the sutures will bring the rectum back into the hollow of the sacrum. The bellies of the pubococcygei are brought together behind the rectum with a series of interrupted stitches, tied only tightly enough to hold them together but not to strangulate the tissue. This surgery reestablishes and lengthens the levator plate (which is the fusion of the pubococcygei posterior to the rectum).

Each elongated pubococcygeus may be shortened by a Z stitch or two as necessary to reestablish the horizontal orientation of the levator plate. An effective anorectal angle is thus reestablished but in a fashion by which it can be temporarily and voluntarily straightened out during the normal evacuation process, unlocking

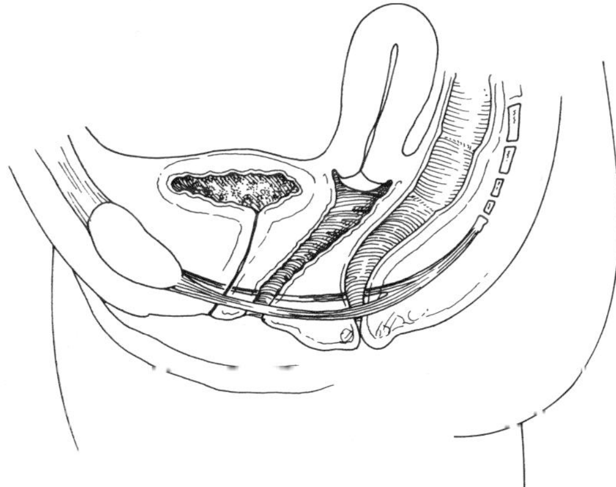

FIG 15–1.
A sagittal section of the pelvis shows elongation and sagging of the levator plate. The usual angle between the anal canal and the rectum as well as the horizontal axis of the rectum and the upper portion of the vagina have been lost. (Redrawn from Nichols DH, Randall CL: *Vaginal Surgery,* ed 3. Baltimore, Williams & Wilkins Co, 1989.)

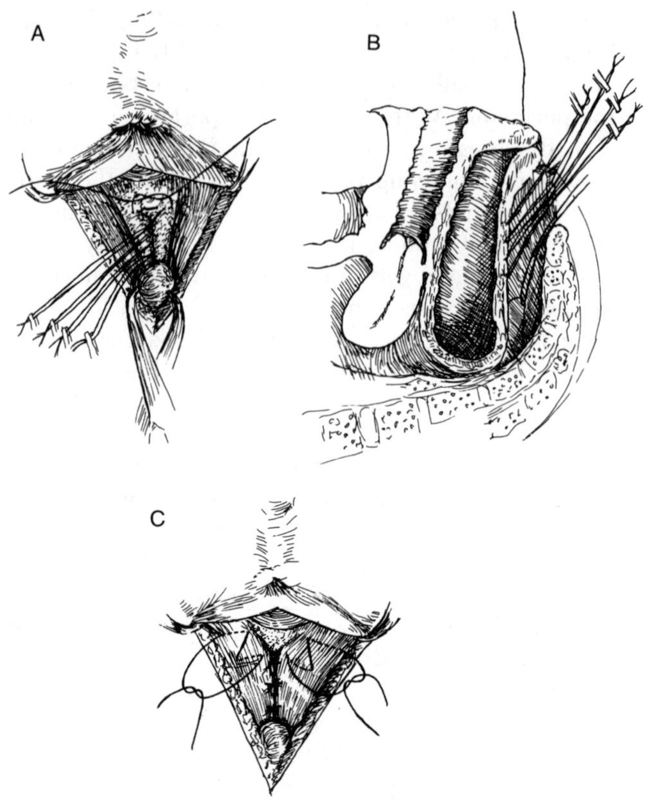

FIG 15–2.
The essential steps of retrorectal levatorplasty include an incision through the skin beneath the anus and the coccyx, transection of any anococcygeal ligament that may be present, and an opening established into the retrorectal space. A series of plication stitches are placed in the posterior wall of the rectum and tied **(A).** These are then sewn to the periosteum of the hollow of the sacrum and tied **(B).** A number of interrupted stitches are placed reuniting the right to the left pubococcygeus **(C)** and reestablishing the levator plate and helping to form a new anorectal angle. These are tied loosely so as to avoid strangulation. A markedly elongated pubococcygeus may be further shortened by a Z stitch on each side, which, when tied, will shorten the pubococcygeus. (Redrawn from Nichols DH, Randall CL: *Vaginal Surgery,* ed 3. Baltimore, Williams & Wilkins Co, 1989.)

its protective valvelike function. Repair of coincident cystocele, rectocele, enterocele, and uterine prolapse follows immediately. If a reconstruction of this sort is not performed in a symptomatic patient, the perineal descent and pudendal nerve damage will progress.

Function of the levator ani can be measured by electromyography, but it can also be evaluated more conveniently by asking the patient to contract her pelvic diaphragm voluntarily during pelvic examination. Failure in the ability to voluntarily contract her pubococcygei suggests the presence of a pudendal neuropathy. Such damage may be permanent. For such a patient, the sole means for rectal continence may lie with the already described involuntary mechanism within her internal anal sphincter. Continence and evacuation will depend on her ability to program the necessary relaxation of her internal anal sphincter. If this last mechanism is lost, there may be total sphincter deficiency, and the patient may become rectally incontinent, an unwelcome event for which effective treatment is almost impossible. The patient may present anywhere along the spectrum of symptoms from evacuation difficulty to complete incontinence. Early diagnosis is essential to encourage reeducation about bowel habit to eliminate straining and prevent incremental pudendal nerve damage.

Both perineal descent syndrome and genital prolapse may be associated with coincident rectal prolapse, an actual intussusception of the bowel on itself. When present, rectal prolapse should be treated by a separate surgical procedure, usually transabdominal, and the intussusception reduced either by large bowel resection or by suspension as in a Ripstein-like procedure.

PHYSICAL EXAMINATION

Pelvic examination should establish the depth and axis of the vagina and rectum. Normally the upper part of the vagina rests on the rectum, which rests on an intact levator plate. The anorectal angle is established as the rectum bends over the edge of this intact levator plate. When the vaginal or rectal axis is vertical in the resting position, there is damage to the levator plate, either structural or neurologic.

When the patient is asked to contract voluntarily her pubococcygei, her ability to perform this action is noted carefully. When the patient cannot demonstrate effective contraction of these muscles, a neuropathy may be present. One should similarly test the integrity of the external anal sphincter by asking the patient to voluntarily contract it. Its reflex contraction may be noted by the insertion of a finger into the rectum. When the reflex is found wanting, one must seek to determine whether the failure is the consequence of disruption of the external anal sphincter from unrepaired trauma, the consequence of a neuropathy, or both. An intact, but patulous external anal sphincter suggests the latter, although that condition may be temporarily induced by a coincident rectal prolapse. In the latter, intussusception of the rectum causes the rectal mucosa to protrude through the external anal sphincter and acts as a dilating wedge, disturbing the reflex contraction of the muscle.

If both pubococcygeus and external anal sphincter appear to be nonfunctional, a primary pudendal neuropathy is likely. If only one component is nonfunctional, usually the external anal sphincter, traumatic disruption of the sphincter is likely.

Brief neurologic examination may identify changes in sensitivity of the pelvic skin, with or without demonstrable leg pain. When these are present, further examination of that portion of the nervous system is indicated, as by selective electromyography of the pelvic diaphragm or external anal sphincter, and evaluation of function, as by defecogram and barium enema. Fasting blood glucose levels can be examined to determine more effectively the possibility of a neuropathy secondary to an abnormality in carbohydrate metabolism.

The pelvic examination of the integrity of the pelvic floor should be repeated when the patient is standing, with one foot resting on a shelf or stool at the end of the examining table. In this position, the patient first holds by voluntarily contracting her pelvic muscles to the best of her ability and then pushes using a Valsalva maneuver.

Physical examination at times may identify a perineal prolapse that is synonymous with the descending perineum syndrome. In this situation, there is pathologic stretching and funneling of the levator ani, usually as the result of obstetric damage or straining at stool. The defect may result from abnormality in the integrity of the pubococcygei themselves or in their nerve supply. The ability or inability of the patient to contract these muscles voluntarily suggests which of the two abnormalities is present.

Descending perineum syndrome is suggested by the finding that the anus is the most dependent portion of the patient's perineum, a situation made worse by voluntary straining, as the funneling of the muscles pathologically increases. During the development of this syndrome, there may at first be no symptoms, but later there will be progressive obstipation and narrowing of stool. These symptoms are made worse the harder the patient strains. If the condition at this state remains undiagnosed and untreated, further progression is a distinct possibility, with development of a progressive pudendal neuropathy. If the condition becomes permanent, the mechanism of anal continence will be severely disturbed.

Coincident rectal prolapse suggests pathologic elongation of the large intestine and its mesentery, allowing an actual intussusception of the bowel. As mentioned before, the leading edge of the intussusception may constitute a dilating wedge of tissue pushing through the anorectal valve and external anal sphincter. Coincident progressive anal incontinence often results. Henry suggested this relationship as follows:

> I think the primary pathology is one of neuropathy affecting the pelvic floor—in many patients a consequence of damage to the pudendal nerve inflicted by traumatic childbirth. Incontinence may not develop initially if the internal anal sphincter is functioning normally. Pelvic floor denervation initiates rectal prolapse because of disruption of the anorectal flap valve. The prolapse starts with descent of the anterior rectal wall and at a later stage a circumferential complete prolapse intussuscepts through the anus. The dilatation of the internal anal sphincter caused by the prolapsing rectum then destroys the only mechanism protecting anorectal continence and a major functional problem results. Because the internal sphincter recovers, many patients recover a reasonable degree of control after successful repair of the prolapse. If continence is not recovered within 6 months, we will offer the patient a transperineal post-anal repair [of the puborectalis and the pelvic diaphragm].

TREATMENT OF RECTAL PROLAPSE

The treatment of rectal prolapse is primarily surgical, involving usually a transabdominal rectopexy using the Ripstein-type pinup operation, and when there is an unusually long segment of bowel, treatment is an appropriate transabdominal resection of this extra intestine with reanastomosis and sacral fixation of the colon. The transperineal bowel resection of Dunphy may be considered as a second choice, though it is technically more difficult to judge the amount of intestine to be removed and proximal sacral fixation cannot be done. For the elderly or infirm, the insertion of a Thiersh wire reinforcement of the external anal sphincter may be performed. This latter must be very delicately gauged, however, so as not to create a mechanical obstruction that would precipitate increased straining at stool.

The retrorectal levatorplasty or the Parks post–anal repair may correct the descending perineal syndrome before a total neuropathy has developed. There should be a meticulous attempt to correct abnormal bowel habits to lessen the need for straining at stool. If such reeducation is neglected, increased damage to the pudendal nerve is likely to result.

The patient might be placed on dietary fiber supplement such as bran used daily at breakfast. Redevelopment of good bowel habits should include heeding the morning gastrocolic reflex with adequate time for effective evacuation at the same time every day. Estrogenic hormone supplementation for the postmenopausal woman may increase the pelvic blood supply and muscular nutrition. When the pubococcygei can be contracted, even though weakly and ineffectively at first, an intense program of Kegel perineal resistive exercises will be useful. A series of 15 voluntary firm contractions of this muscle for 3 seconds each six times daily should be employed. Increased muscular strength will often be reflected in an improvement in rectal continence. The exercise should be continued indefinitely. In some resistive cases, some improvement may be obtained from courses of galvanic stimulation of the anal sphincter and pelvic diaphragm.

When mechanical disruption of the levator ani or the external anal sphincter has been demonstrated, the treatment is surgical. Though unusually patulous, a sphincterplasty either anterior or posterior may be performed with or without coincident perineorrhaphy. Correction of any defect of the supports of the posterior vaginal wall, including treatment of such rectocele as may be present, may thus be done at the same procedure. For the perineal descent syndrome, a retrorectal levatorplasty with colporrhaphy will usually be indicated if the patient is symptomatic. For genuine rectal prolapse, a transabdominal rectopexy with coincident excision of any pathologically long dilated loops of large bowel would be indicated.

Some patients may require a combination of these procedures. The surgeon should be mindful of the coincident or future development of urinary stress incontinence in such patients, as well as the possibility of progression of bowel symptoms. Patients should be encouraged to participate in a long-term follow-up program that includes attention to improving bowel habits and elimination of straining at stool so that the natural progression of this most troublesome disorder can be arrested.

BIBLIOGRAPHY

Corman ML: *Colon and Rectal Surgery.* Philadelphia, JB Lippincott Co, 1984, pp 115–138.

Goligher JC: *Surgery of the Anus, Rectum and Colon,* ed 3. Springfield, Ill, Charles C Thomas, Publisher, 1975, pp 409–419.

Henry MM, Swash M: *Colpoproctology and the Pelvic Floor.* Stoneham, Mass, Butterworth, 1985, pp 217–281.

Henry MM, Porter NH: *A Colour Atlas of Faecal Incontinence and Complete Rectal Prolapse.* St Louis, Mosby–Year Book, 1988.

Nichols DH, Randall CL: *Vaginal Surgery.* ed 3. Baltimore, Williams & Wilkins, 1989, pp 294–303.

Parks AG: Anorectal incontinence. *Proc R Soc Med* 1975; 68:681–690.

Chapter 16

Recurrent Breast Disease

Douglas J. Marchant, M.D.

In describing the management of reoperative breast disease, we assume that the patient has been referred following a surgical procedure, such as an open biopsy, aspiration of a cyst, or fine needle aspiration (FNA). The initial discussion will describe recurrent surgical procedures for the following benign conditions: (1) recurrent fibroadenomas, (2) recurrent squamous metaplasia, and (3) recurrent macrocyst.

The evaluation of the occult lesion and the management of the patient referred following an inadequate biopsy or incomplete surgery for breast cancer constitute an increasing number of referrals.

RECURRENT FIBROADENOMAS

The fibroadenoma is a benign neoplasm of the breast, frequently discovered by accident in the postpubertal female. Surgery is recommended, because once a patient has discovered such a mass, sooner or later she will demand removal. These lesions, though small when discovered, continue to grow and often can be removed with a smaller incision at the time of the initial diagnosis. In addition, we live in a mobile society; patients may move, become pregnant, and be examined by their obstetrician gynecologist who then "discovers" the mass. The patient indicates that it has been present for many years. What is the responsibility of the primary care physician?

A single fibroadenoma is easily removed on a day surgery basis under local anesthesia. A cosmetic incision is chosen with the patient in the sitting or standing position. The problem occurs when more than one fibroadenoma is discovered, often some months or years following the first operation. It has been my practice in young patients to order an automated ultrasound of both breasts to determine how many additional fibroadenomas are present before recommending surgical removal of the "new" lesion. This diagnostic study presents a detailed "road map" for future biopsies, and often a period of watchful waiting is in order to determine whether additional lesions occur. When the lesions are stable, a decision concerning the removal of all or some of these masses, depending on their location and size, can be made.

One final point should be made. I have reoperated on a number of patients who have had a fibroadenoma removed but who present with a "new" mass at the biopsy site. Fibroadenomas often feel quite superficial; however, they are located deep in the breast tissue, and unless one is careful during the dissection, only a small part of the lesion may be removed. The surgeon should be certain before the wound is closed that the entire lesion has been removed and submitted to pathology. The pathologist should be notified if the patient is pregnant since considerable hypertrophy occurs, erroneously suggesting the diagnosis of cystosarcoma phyllodes.

RECURRENT SQUAMOUS METAPLASIA

Squamous metaplasia, or nonpuerperal mastitis, is more common than the literature suggests. In older textbooks, the lesion is referred to as plasma cell mastitis. The characteristic history is one of recurrent drainage adjacent to the nipple or the periphery of the nipple. Drainage has been performed one or more times, usually in an emergency room or office setting. The patient is asymptomatic for several weeks or months, and the condition recurs. Antibiotics or another drainage is attempted, and again, the lesion recurs.

As the name implies, the histology is related to squamous metaplasia of the ducts. Whether this occurs as a result of infection or infection occurs following squamous metaplasia is unknown. Cultures taken at the time of surgery usually are negative. The symptom complex is not associated with pregnancy or lactation, nor does it seem to be related to trauma. There is no known relationship between this condition and the later development of breast cancer. The principal problem is recurrent pain and drainage requiring repetitive medical visits.

When a patient is referred for recurrent drainage, I take a culture. If the patient is more than 30 years of age, I obtain a mammogram and, on some occasions, an automated ultrasound to more clearly delineate the involved area. The patient is scheduled for removal of the duct system under general anesthesia on a day surgery basis. General anesthesia is preferred because of the extensive dissection required. The operation can be done under local anesthesia, but with recurrent infection, it is difficult to penetrate all of the involved areas with adequate amounts of local anesthesia.

A circumareolar incision is made in the general area of the drainage, and any sinus tract is identified and removed. The nipple areolar complex is elevated with skin hooks, and by use of sharp dissection, the duct system is removed until normal breast tissue is encountered. This may require extensive dissection toward the chest wall and beyond the nipple areolar complex. Bleeding is controlled with fine ligatures. A culture is taken, and the tissue is always submitted for rapid section diagnosis to rule out carcinoma. If the wound is dry, I do not routinely employ a drain unless the remaining cavity is quite large, in which case, a ¼-in. Penrose drain is inserted and let out through the wound with a skin suture left long, to be tied 24 hours later. I close the skin with no. 5-0 nonabsorbable sutures. The suture adjacent to the drain is tied when the drain is removed 24 hours after the surgery and all skin sutures are removed in 5 to 7 days. A pressure dressing is placed over the incision for the first 24 to 48 hours.

Even with extensive surgery, success cannot be guaranteed. I have had a few instances in which the initial cultures were negative, the pathology report confirmed the diagnosis, and wide local excision was performed. Yet, months or years later, recurrent drainage occurred. In this situation, a trial of antibiotics may be justified, but this seldom is successful. Danazol has been recommended, but it has not been successful in controlling symptomatology, and most of these patients will require reexcision.

RECURRENT MACROCYST

The etiology of the macrocyst is unknown. They are not associated with the later development of breast cancer. A number of studies have attempted to address the composition of the cyst fluid, but to date they have resulted in very little additional information concerning the etiology or the treatment of this condition. A palpable cyst probably does not increase beyond the initial size because of the atrophy of the epithelial lining produced by the pressure of the cyst fluid, and if the cyst is completely aspirated, no additional fluid will occur. In our Breast Health Center, we recommend that patients return 1 month after aspiration. If a mass is discovered at the site of aspiration, open biopsy is recommended. Evaluation of the cyst fluid seldom is helpful, although for medicolegal purposes, it may be wise to send the fluid for analysis.

Asymptomatic macrocysts should not be aspirated. We have seen a number of patients following repeated aspirations who have developed infection, and in at least one instance, mastectomy was required. It is our practice to document the presence of a recurrent cyst, and if it is symptomatic, large, or painful, to aspirate it for symptomatic relief.

REOPERATIVE TECHNIQUES FOR BREAST CANCER

Occult Lesion

With increasing utilization of screening mammography, the diagnosis of an occult lesion is common. Management depends on the expertise of the mammographer and the experience of the surgeon selected to remove the lesion. Proper handling of an occult lesion whether it represents an asymmetric density or a geographic cluster of microcalcifications requires careful interpretation by an experienced mammographer, followed by consultation with the responsible surgeon. We perform all of our localizations and biopsies under local anesthesia on a day surgery basis. The patient is seen in the radiology suite, the bent wire localization is performed, and films are reviewed by the surgeon and the mammographer. The patient is then taken to the day surgery area for the operative procedure. It is essential that a protocol be established between the operating suite, the radiology department, and pathology to expedite specimen radiography and gross inspection by the pathologist. In most instances, because of the small size of the lesion, a rapid section is not appropriate. The pathologist must ink the margins of the tissue so that when the permanent sections are reviewed, the extent of the lesion can be determined.

If the lesion is a cancer and involves one or more margins, we recommend reexcision. Alternative treatments are discussed with the patient, and if she is a candidate for wide local excision and axillary dissection, these procedures are scheduled under general anesthesia. The margins must be carefully marked by the surgeon to facilitate orientation by the pathologist. In some cases, receptor data are not available, and a newly reexcised specimen must be submitted in a fresh state for estrogen and progesterone receptor analysis.

An important consideration is the condition of the biopsy site. This point often is overlooked since the majority of patients in the past had a modified mastectomy and the location or condition of the biopsy site had little or no bearing on the outcome of the proposed surgery or the prognosis of the patient. Because of the possibility of conservative treatment, the location of the incision and the condition of the biopsy site are important. If there is a large hematoma at the biopsy site, or if there are considerable induration and erythema, it is difficult for the surgeon to determine accurately the extent of the tumor. Occasionally more tissue is removed than is absolutely necessary, compromising what might otherwise be a cosmetic closure. It is therefore essential that the open biopsy be performed by an experienced surgeon who understands the implications of the biopsy and the necessity for complete healing without undue induration and ecchymosis. All reexcisions must be carefully marked by the surgeon to facilitate evaluation by the pathologist. I mark the medial aspect, the inferior aspect, and the deep margin with appropriate sutures. These are noted on the pathology slip and also dictated as part of the operative note.

For most patients, in addition to reexcision of the biopsy site, axillary dissection is performed. I prefer to mark my incision with the patient sitting or standing. The axillary dissection is performed first with a separate set of instruments. The pectoralis major muscle and then the costocoracoid fascia are identified. Sharp dissection is performed, removing the axillary contents distal to the axillary vein and its tributaries. Only level 1 and 2 nodes can be removed in this operation, and this usually is satisfactory for diagnostic purposes. With careful evaluation by a competent pathologist, 12 or more nodes will be removed with this technique. If the wound is dry, I usually do not insert a drain. The reexcision is then performed with a separate set of instruments.

There is some debate as to whether axillary dissection is necessary for all patients, particularly older patients with normal axillae. If the receptors are positive, most of these patients will be given tamoxifen, and the axillary dissection is superfluous. Recent evidence suggests that patients with negative nodes should be offered adjuvant chemotherapy or hormonal therapy. In our Breast Health Center, we individualize the treatment of our patients. We recommend adjuvant chemotherapy in younger patients and patients who have negative receptors or those with a high mitotic index or aneuploidy demonstrated by flow cytometry. Since tamoxifen has few, if any, side effects, we recommend tamoxifen for node-negative postmenopausal patients and continue to treat them indefinitely. We do monitor estradiol levels since tamoxifen at certain dosage levels acts as an estrogen and we must be certain that there is no "estrogen flare" associated with the tamoxifen therapy.

In Situ Carcinoma

By definition, in situ carcinoma should be 100% curable. Unfortunately, there often is difference of opinion concerning the cell type and the possibility of "early invasion." There is also the possibility of extensive disease noted on the mammogram and the implication of a palpable mass associated with the lesion. For these reasons, we have developed a protocol for handling these lesions (Table 16–1).

TABLE 16–1.
Duct Cancer In Situ Treatment Guidelines

Lumpectomy
- Lesion size 2 cm in diameter (specify whether nonpalpable or palpable)
- Associated microcalcifications determined mammographically
- Microscopically normal tissue margin 0.5 cm
- If lesion is subareolar, removal of entire nipple-areolar complex

Lumpectomy plus radiotherapy or simple mastectomy
- Lesion size no more than 2 cm in diameter (specify whether nonpalpable or palpable)
- No associated microcalcifications
  - In patients treated with lumpectomy plus radiotherapy:
    - Radiotherapy to breast only
    - Excision margins to be appropriately evaluated and therapy appropriately tailored as per current Breast Health Center guidelines for invasive carcinoma

Mastectomy with level I/II lymph node dissection
- Histologically confirmed multicentric disease that is detected grossly or mammographically
- Margin positive (more than one focus or diffusely continuous) after reexcision, implying extensive disease

Patients who do not have recognizable disease by mammography and are difficult to follow and those who have lobular cancer in situ for which bilaterality is the rule rather than the exception present problems. For these patients and for those who have discontinuous areas of in situ disease noted in the biopsy specimen, we recommend modified mastectomy or reexcision and radiation therapy to the breast. We do not routinely perform mirror image biopsies for lobular carcinoma in situ. There is some debate as to whether this represents a true neoplasm or simply a marker for the later development of carcinoma.

Role of Mastectomy

With the increasing utilization of second opinion, we are seeing more and more patients in our Breast Health Center requesting a discussion of alternative treatments. This has brought into focus the role of wide local excision vs. the modified mastectomy. We provide second opinions only after a careful review of the mammograms and the microscopic slides. Often conservative treatment has been recommended, but we have noted extensive disease on the mammogram; because of this, we have chosen either total (simple) mastectomy or mastectomy with axillary dissection. The axillary dissection is recommended, because with a large area of involvement, it is possible that one or more areas in the breast will contain early invasive tumor. We do not routinely recommend axillary dissection for in situ disease that has been completely removed with adequate margins and for which there is no question of early invasion.

Another consideration concerns the location of the lesion. Often, even small lesions in the upper inner quadrant require mastectomy because of the inability to perform a cosmetic wide local excision. In some instances, with a large lesion immediately beneath the nipple areolar complex, we have recommended mastectomy, particularly for those patients with very small breasts for whom a wide local excision would leave very little tissue. In these cases, modified mastectomy with immediate or delayed reconstruction is preferable.

CONCLUSION

It is important that the surgeon understand the natural history of benign breast disease and avoid unnecessary surgery, particularly in the young patient. On the other hand, aggressive surgery is required for squamous metaplasia. For those patients suspected of having cancer, it is immediately obvious that the surgeon must understand the implications of the biopsy and participate in a multidisciplinary team that includes not only input from the medical oncologist and radiotherapist but the pathologist and radiologist as well. With this approach we can minimize the trauma to a patient already devastated by the knowledge that she has cancer and for whom the initial decision regarding treatment is most important.

BIBLIOGRAPHY

Harris JR, Hellman S, Kinne DW: Special report: Limited surgery and radiotherapy for early breast cancer. *N Engl J Med* 1985; 313:1365.

Homer MJ: Non-palpable breast lesion localization using a curved end retractible wire. *Radiology* 1985; 157:259–260.

Homer MJ, Marchant DJ, Smith TJ: The geographic cluster of breast microcalcifications—is it really intramammary? *Surg Gynecol Obstet* 1985; 161:532–534.

Homer MJ, Pile-Spellman ER: Needle localization of non-palpable breast lesions: The importance of communication. Special Report: Breast Imaging. *Applied Radiology,* November 1987.

Homer MJ, Schmidt-Ullrich R, Safaii H, et al: Residual breast carcinoma after biopsy: Role of mammography in evaluation. *Radiology* 1989; 170:75–79.

Lagios MD, Margolin FR, Westdahl ER, et al: Mammographically detected duct carcinoma in situ, frequency of local recurrence following tylectomy and prognostic effects of nuclear grade on local recurrence. *CA* 1989; 63:618–625.

Lagios MD, Westdahl ER, Margolin FR, et al: Duct carcinoma in situ, relationship of extent of non-invasive disease to the frequency of occult invasion, multicentricity, lymph node metastases and short-term treatment failure. *Cancer* 1982; 50:1309.

Peters F: Failure of danazol to prevent recurrent periareolar abscesses [letter to the editor]. *Breast Dis* 1989; 1:283–285.

Rose MA, Olivotto I, Cady B, et al: Conservative surgery and radiation therapy for early breast cancer. *Arch Surg* 1989; 124:153–157.

Rosenberg AL, Schwartz EF, Feig SA, et al: Clinically occult breast lesions: Localization and significance. *Radiology* 1987; 162:167–170.

Schuh ME, Nemoto T, Penetrante RB, et al: Intraductal carcinoma, analysis of presentation, pathologic findings and outcome of disease. *Arch Surg* 1986; 121:1303.

Chapter 17

Recurrent Gynecologic Malignancy

Stephen L. Curry, M.D.

In spite of superb diagnostic techniques, it is not uncommon for the obstetrician and gynecologist to make a diagnosis of invasive cancer via an operative procedure that is deemed to be inadequate as treatment for that particular cancer. As an example, in spite of no postmenopausal bleeding in a postmenopausal with a cystocele, after vaginal hysterectomy and anterior repair, the gynecologist rarely may be faced with a pathology report that indicates an invasive adenocarcinoma of the endometrium, and the question arises as to the appropriateness of further surgery. Should the ovaries be removed? Do the lymph nodes need to be sampled?

More common is the situation where a patient with a gynecologic malignancy has been appropriately treated and recurrence is diagnosed. Reoperation can be an important part of the curative or palliative treatment for recurring cancer. Early diagnosis of locally recurrent squamous cancer of the vulva results in a 75% cure rate with immediate local reexcision.

Finally, gynecologic surgeons are often faced with the need to carry out operative procedures for palliation. The best example here is the patient with complete obstruction of the rectosigmoid secondary to extensive recurrent cervical cancer. She may have a prolonged survival, and thus a diverting colostomy would be appropriate. In this chapter the major anatomic areas of gynecologic malignancy will be discussed, and reoperative procedures pertaining to primary curative care, recurrent cancer, and palliation will be reviewed.

VULVA

The vulva includes the labia majora, the labia minora, and the clitoris. Squamous cell carcinoma is the most common malignancy in this area. Other cancers to be considered include melanoma, Paget's disease, and metastatic cancer. The majority of patients with carcinoma of the vulva are postmenopausal and present with symptoms of itching, burning, mass, or bleeding. Aggressive biopsies of vulva lesions should always be carried out. Blue-black lesions on the vulva should be removed. Most investigators believe that classical small vulvar warts can be treated conservatively with trichloroacetic acid. However, if they persist or the patient presents with massive or atypical warts, it is critically important to carry out multiple biopsies before any therapy that will not produce a histologic specimen is initiated. Most gynecologic oncologists recommend surgical extirpation over laser therapy to produce a histologic specimen. This is especially important in patients with recurrent or persistent lesions. Recent data indicate that up to 17% of patients with what is thought to be recurrent vulvar intraepithelial neoplasia will have an invasive cancer. Of course, laser therapy is inappropriate in this situation.

Staging of vulvar carcinoma is dependent on lesion size, local spread, and lymph node metastasis. The standard route of spread for vulvar cancer is by the inguinal lymph nodes and then to the deep pelvic lymph nodes. Direct spread to the deep pelvic nodes is exceedingly rare. Until recently, the standard operative procedure for any invasive cancer of the vulva or Bartholin's gland was a radical vulvectomy with bilateral inguinal and pelvic lymphadenectomy. Recent data indicate that if the inguinal lymph nodes are not involved, the pelvic lymph nodes will not be involved, and thus in that situation pelvic lymphadenectomy is unwarranted. Still later data indicate that whole pelvic radiation therapy for the patient with metastatic nodal disease may give a higher cure rate with lower morbidity than retroperitoneal pelvic node dissection. Thus, standard treatment is now radical vulvectomy and bilateral inguinal lymphadenectomy with or without radiation therapy, depending on node status. For early lesions confined to the vulva with minimal invasion, radical local excision with unilateral superficial groin dissection is being recommended. This is also true for early melanoma. Wide local excision is more appropriately called modified radical hemivulvectomy to ensure aggressive local removal. The procedure should include 2-cm margins circumferentially and at least 2 cm of fat and muscle deep to the tumor.

Primary Cancer

For patients with invasive squamous carcinoma of the vulva, three situations portend to the need for an immediate more radical procedure. First is the patient who undergoes wide local excision of vulvar intraepithelial neoplasia or condyloma but whose final pathology report indicates an invasive squamous carcinoma. This patient should immediately undergo either a wide radical excision with superficial groin dissection or radical vulvectomy with bilateral inguinal lymphadenectomy. The choice will depend on the size, location, and depth of invasion. Individuals carrying out wide excision with superficial groin dissection must be prepared to occasionally return the patient to the operating room for radical vulvectomy and bilateral inguinal node dissection when more extensive disease is found locally, or superficial lymph nodes are abnormal.

Second, patients with a persistent Bartholin's abscess will occasionally undergo excision of the Bartholin's gland. The final pathology report may reveal an invasive adenocarcinoma of the Bartholin's gland, and in this situation the patient should immediately undergo radical vulvectomy and bilateral inguinal lymphadenectomy. Whenever persistent Bartholin's gland infection occurs, especially in patients more than 40 years of age, multiple biopsies should be taken before simple excision of Bartholin's gland.

Finally, although the majority of patients with Paget's disease of the vulva have an intraepithelial lesion that can be excised by simple vulvectomy, occasionally an underlying invasive adenocarcinoma will be discovered. This patient should be returned to the operating room for radical vulvectomy and bilateral inguinal lymphadenectomy. It is critically important to understand that although the pink velvety areas are definitely Paget's disease, normal skin can also contain pagetoid cells; thus, extremely wide margins are mandatory to decrease local recurrence. Occasionally a patient must be returned to the operating room for more extensive excision because of abnormal margins. To minimize this risk, it is recommended that frozen sections be done on all margins during the original surgery.

Recurrent Cancer

The majority of recurrences of invasive cancer of the vulva occur within 2 years of primary therapy. It is critically important to carefully follow these patients at close intervals. If the lymph nodes are normal, the majority of recurrences will be along the surgical margins on the vulva. Several authors have reported as high as a 75% long-term survival following wide local excision of early recurrences. Aggressive biopsy of any abnormality seen along the healing scar will allow for early intervention. The reexcision should be deep and wide; thus, skin flaps or grafts may be necessary. One should attempt to obtain at least 2-cm margins laterally and margins 2 cm deep. If the recurrence is in the groin or is distal, surgical extirpation can be extremely difficult and rarely beneficial.

Palliative Surgery

In vulvar cancer patients with widely metastatic disease or who are of poor operative risk, it is appropriate to carry out wide local removal as a cleansing procedure. These patients will commonly have significant necrosis and foul-smelling discharge along with severe pain. Thus, the cleansing vulvectomy can significantly palliate the remaining period of their life. Here the surgeon should remove the lesion with a small margin as rapidly as possible with the least anesthesia or analgesia necessary. Older patients will usually maintain rectal continence in spite of removal of the anterior portion of the rectal sphincter.

CERVIX

Squamous cancer accounts for 90% of all invasive cancers of the cervix. Adenocarcinoma accounts for 9%, and occasionally one sees a lymphoma or primary melanoma. The patients range in age from 18 to 80 years, with the majority being in the 30- to 50-year-old age group. The majority of patients are diagnosed by Papanicolaou smear; however, vaginal bleeding is the most common symptom. All patients with Papanicolaou smears indicating dysplasia or carcinoma in situ, now more commonly classified as cervical intraepithelial neoplasia, should undergo colposcopy with biopsy and endocervical curettage before any conservative therapy is initiated. Patients with persistent cervical discharge or presumed cervicitis should undergo colposcopy and endocervical curettage before cryotherapy or laser treatment. This is important since adenocarcinoma of the endocervix is less often visible and more difficult to pick up by Papanicolaou smear.

Cancer of the cervix spreads in a stepwise fashion with local extension into paracervical tissues, followed by lymphatic spread. Early disease is successfully treated with either radical hysterectomy and bilateral pelvic lymphadenectomy or radical radiation therapy, including external irradiation therapy and brachytherapy.

Primary Cancer

In spite of previous careful workup, it is not uncommon for a gynecologic oncologist or radiation therapist to be referred a patient with invasive squamous cancer of the cervix who has undergone a simple abdominal or vaginal hysterectomy. The literature would indicate that a delay in appropriate therapy of more than 6 months would portend a significant decrease in survival. As with primary early invasive cancer of the cervix, both radical reoperation in the form of radical upper vaginectomy and bilateral pelvic node dissection and radiation therapy have equal cure rates.

If the patient is young and the ovaries were not taken out at the original surgery, the radical surgical procedure may be more appropriate. Likewise, if upper vaginal pliability is critical, surgery can be more beneficial, depending on the original length of the vagina. By simply placing a povidone-iodine (Betadine)–soaked pack at the apex of the vagina before starting surgery, the gynecologic oncologist can carefully identify the appropriate landmarks and do a radical parametrectomy and upper vaginectomy, followed by bilateral pelvic lymphadenectomy. Since the location of the ureteral tunnels may have been disturbed by the previous surgery, the surgeon must be extra careful with this portion of the procedure. Through a generous incision and after disease in the upper abdomen has been ruled out, the perirectal and perivesical spaces are opened, and the bladder is dissected away from the anterior portion of the vagina. The uterosacral ligaments are removed. The uterers are isolated, and the cardinal ligament is removed laterally. The specimen should always include an adequate vaginal margin. The lymph node dissection should include all fat-bearing tissue surrounding the common iliac vessels, the external iliac and hypogastric vessels, and the obturator fossa, with the deep margin being the obturator nerve.

Recurrent Cancer

Patients with documented central recurrence of cancer of the cervix can have long-term survival after an exenterative procedure. Recent reviews indicate that operative mortality is less than 2%, and 5-year cure rates range from 40% to 60%, depending on patient selection. Most gynecologic oncologists would recommend that pelvic exenteration only be carried out in light of a biopsy-proved central recurrence with no evidence of pelvic sidewall or lymphatic spread on computed tomography scan. Changes in the intravenous (IV) pyelogram and symptoms such as leg or back pain portend an increased risk of cancer outside the surgical field. In selected patients with anterior recurrence, the rectum can be spared by doing an anterior exenteration.

Before an exenterative procedure, the patient should undergo an extensive workout to determine the feasibility of a successful operation. This should include an extensive medical and psychologic workout to ensure her ability to withstand the operative procedure along with the prolonged morbidity and body changes that will result from this operation. On entering the abdomen, the surgeon must carefully evaluate the entire peritoneal cavity to ensure that the recurrence is localized to the planned area of surgical extirpation. Next, the area over the aorta and vena cava should be identified and the retroperitoneal space opened. Laterally, the surgeon should identify the ureters and ensure that they are not injured. A careful dissection of all fatty tissue containing lymph nodes from the bifurcation of the aorta and vena cava to the renal vessels is done, and this tissue is sent for frozen section.

If these nodes are normal, one proceeds to the pelvis, where the retroperitoneal spaces are entered and all lymph-bearing tissue is removed from the external iliac artery and vein, the hypogastric artery and vein, and the obturator fossa. Next, the perirectal and perivesical spaces are opened, and the surgeon ensures a tumor-free margin between the biopsy-proved disease and the pelvic sidewall. Only at this point does the surgeon proceed with removal of the bladder, uterus, cervix, vagina, and rectum if a total exenteration is to be carried out. A majority of patients can undergo immediate reconstruction of the vagina. Multiple flap procedures have been described for this purpose.

Palliative Surgery

Occasionally, after a prolonged disease-free interval, a single pulmonary nodule or several unilateral pulmonary nodules will be noted, and it may be appropriate to remove these for long-term palliation. Although some authors would recommend palliative exenteration, most gynecologic oncologists would not carry out this extensive a procedure on a patient who would receive little benefit.

Great controversy exists as to the appropriateness of urinary diversion for palliation of recurrent or widespread cancer of the cervix. To date, there are no significant chemotherapeutic agents or regimens that produce long-term survival. In most patients, urinary diversion prolongs life with significant side effects, such as pain. On the other hand, uremia usually results in significant decrease in pain and even euphoria. This may allow for a more pleasant terminal period. Colostomy, ileostomy, or percutaneous nephrostomy is appropriate in carefully selected patients to palliate severe side effects such as bowel obstruction, significant enteral vaginal fistula, or severe painful pyelonephritis.

ENDOMETRIUM

Adenocarcinoma of the endometrium is the most common gynecologic malignancy. Because the cure rate is so high, there is a tendency to be conservative in the treatment of this disease. These patients are usually between the age of 40 and 70 years old, obese, and nulliparous. They most often present with abnormal vaginal bleeding. Until recently, the standard procedure was a total abdominal hysterectomy and bilateral salpingo-oophorectomy with or without radiation therapy given either preoperatively or postoperatively. Recent large studies have indicated that prognostic factors other than stage include differentiation of the tumor, depth of myometrial invasion, and pelvic and periaortic lymph node status.

The most common procedure for diagnosis is presently an office endometrial sample following an endocervical curettage. If a diagnosis of endometrial cancer is made and tissue is sufficient for grading, formal fractional dilatation and curettage (D&C) is unnecessary. However, when the curettage specimen of the office biopsy is equivocal, a formal fractional D&C is mandatory.

Two pathologic varients, papillary serous adenocarcinoma and clear cell carcinoma, behave more like ovarian cancer. It is important to evaluate the omentum and peritoneal surfaces in these situations. A good treatment regimen for these cases has not been identified yet.

The preoperative workup must include a mammography, since there is a high association with breast cancer. The standard operation is total abdominal hysterectomy with bilateral salpingo-oophorectomy, peritoneal washings, and selective periaortic and pelvic lymph node sampling. Postoperative therapy is tailored to the histologic findings. Deep myometrial invasion, spread beyond the uterus, or extension to the lower uterine segment or cervix usually indicates a need for postoperative radiation therapy.

Unsuspected Primary Cancer Diagnosed After Hysterectomy

Occasionally patients will undergo a total abdominal or vaginal hysterectomy and subsequent histologic review will reveal adenocarcinoma of the endometrium. At this point, the gynecologic surgeon is confronted with the need either to reoperate to rule out metastatic disease or to administer postoperative radiation therapy. With the extensive prognostic data collected over the last 15 years, this question has become less significant in that the risk of adnexal or lymphatic spread is exceedingly low for the patient with well-differentiated endometrial cancer and no or minimal myometrial invasion. Therefore, most clinicians would recommend careful follow-up with neither further surgery nor postoperative irradiation therapy. On the other hand, if significant negative prognostic factors such as poor differentiation, deep myometrial invasion, or extension to the lower uterine segment or cervix are present, most clinicians would recommend postoperative radiation therapy. When radiation therapy is going to be given, reoperation is generally unnecessary. In a premenopausal patient with continued ovarian function, it may be appropriate to reexplore the patient to remove the ovaries and carry out lymph node sampling if postoperative radiation therapy is not planned.

Recurrent Cancer

Numerous studies have looked at the use of total pelvic exenteration for recurrent endometrial cancer in the central pelvis. The majority of these studies have indicated a very poor prognosis because these patients routinely die of widespread disease from distant metastasis. Recent data indicate that radiation therapy alone is effective for very small central pelvic recurrences, but reductive surgery plus radiation therapy are more beneficial in patients with vaginal lesions greater than 1 to 2 cm. In this situation, an exploratory laparotomy with evaluation of the periaortic and pelvic nodes, followed by removal of the vaginal cuff mass without radical pelvic dissection, is carried out to allow postoperative radiation therapy with the least possible complications. Recurrent disease in areas other than the vaginal cuff is traditionally treated with radiation therapy, chemotherapy, or both.

Palliative Surgery

Palliative surgery is appropriate in endometrial cancer, because in many patients this is a slow-growing, prolonged illness. Colostomy, ileostomy, or urinary diversion is appropriate in selected individuals. Debulking of lymph node metastases, followed by radiation therapy or chemotherapy, is appropriate in selected patients. Occasionally a patient with recurrence will present with bowel perforation, because this cancer is known to invade through the bowel wall. This situation requires emergency bowel bypass, but the procedure should be as conservative as possible.

OVARY

There are three categories of primary ovarian cancer. Epithelial ovarian cancers arise from the surface epithelium and tend to present in middle-aged women as widespread intraperitoneal disease. These are the most common ovarian cancers and have a very poor prognosis. Serous and mucinous carcinoma are the two most common histologic patterns. Germ cell cancers present in the teenage years usually with pain and a rapidly expanding pelvic mass. These tumors are unilateral, and prognosis over the last several years has been significantly improved with the use of aggressive combination chemotherapy. Finally, stromal tumors of the ovary tend to produce hormones and grow very slowly. The majority of these tumors are treated with surgery alone, because recurrence is rare.

Over the last 20 years, a significant amount of basic science and clinical research has led to a better understanding of the epidemiology and treatment of ovarian cancer. Three significant areas require comment. First, the understanding of the spread of this cancer and the areas where microscopic metastases may be found has led to a better operative staging procedure. Second, excellent postoperative chemotherapy in combination with aggressive tumor reductive surgery has led to prolonged survival. Finally, tumor markers such as α-fetoprotein, human chorionic gonadotropin, and CA 125 assist the clinician in managing these patients.

Primary Cancer

Patients referred with apparently localized and well- or moderately differentiated epithelial ovarian cancer who have had incomplete surgical evaluation are candidates for immediate reexploration. A recent prospective study completed by the National Cancer Institute and the Gynecologic Oncology Group indicates that patients who have been properly surgically staged in the above category do not require postoperative therapy. Survival is the same for patients who receive postoperative therapy and those who do not. The initial operation or reoperation should always include a careful assessment of both hemidiaphragms with either biopsies or washings for cytology. Biopsies of both abdominal gutters (to the left of the ascending colon and to the right of the descending colon), a partial omentectomy, periaortic lymph node sampling at and above the level of the renal vessels, bilateral pelvic lymph node sampling, and multiple pelvic peritoneal biopsies, including the deep cul-de-sac, should be done. Most authors recommend removing only the infracolic omentum in a staging procedure. Occasionally, in a patient who has not completed her family, the uterus and contralateral tube and ovary may be left. This is uniformly true in patients with germ cell tumors or stromal tumors who have not completed their families. Patients with poorly differentiated lesions or any evidence of spread, including rupture of the tumor before or at the time of surgery or surface excrescence on the ovary, should receive postoperative chemotherapy or radiation therapy.

Patients who have undergone exploratory laparotomy with a finding of widespread ovarian cancer and little evidence of an aggressive attempt at maximal tumor reduction may be candidates for immediate reexploration and tumor reduction. Another option is to administer aggressive chemotherapy, followed by tumor reduction at a later date. To date, there is no evidence that either of these approaches is more appropriate; however, the majority of patients undergo immediate reexploration. Since anatomically this is usually a surface-spreading lesion, a retroperitoneal approach can allow the surgeon to aggressively debulk the tumor with minimal injury to critical organs. If it is judged that all visible tumor can be debulked, it is appropriate to resect areas of bowel with reanastamosis. Finally, if the last visible residual disease is on the right hemidiaphragm, some surgeons would aggressively remove this area.

Recurrent Cancer

It is critically important to differentiate the evaluation of the complete responder to primary chemotherapy from the patient who has a recurrence of her ovarian cancer and is reexplored for tumor debulking.

Second-Look Operation

The second-look operation in ovarian cancer has been evaluated in a large number of studies. Presently, it is reserved for patients with known persistent disease who have completed a required course of chemotherapy and have no evidence of persistent disease either on examination, radiologic testing, or CA 125. Patients who are candidates for further therapy either via protocol or as further curative therapy in the form of intraperitoneal radioactive substances or chemotherapy will undergo a second-look operation. This operation, through a generous incision, will involve a careful evaluation of the entire peritoneal cavity and the retroperitoneal spaces. Extensive biopsies should include the diaphragm surfaces, all peritoneal surfaces, all adhesions, and the retroperitoneal lymph nodes or retroperitoneal spaces if the nodes have been removed. Multiple pelvic peritoneal biopsies are mandatory. Usually this operation should result in 30 to 50 separate histologic specimens for evaluation. Simple opening of the peritoneal cavity, taking a look around and removing a couple of adhesions, is inappropriate and should not be considered a negative second-look operation. If persistent disease is found, the surgeon should attempt to remove as much cancer as possible. Numerous retrospective studies have shown a significant prolongation of survival if persistent tumor is aggressively debulked.

Debulking

Several studies have indicated a significant prolongation of survival in patients who can undergo secondary debulking after failure of cisplatin-based chemotherapy. If the patient has ascites or has never responded to primary chemotherapy, it is very unlikely that secondary debulking will be of benefit. The same principles portend in this procedure as with those of primary debulking in that a retroperitoneal approach is usually most beneficial. Unless all visible tumor can be removed, it is inappropriate to carry out extensive bowel resections or risk damage to vital organs. Follow-up intravenous or intraperitoneal chemotherapy is then used to further prolong life.

Palliative Surgery

Although epithelial ovarian cancer is a surface-spreading disease that rarely invades vital organs, partial or complete bowel obstruction is often seen. This is secondary to kinking of the small bowel or hypoperistalsis due to mesenteric implants. In most cases, nausea and vomiting can be relieved by conservative measures. However, occasionally long-term palliation can be afforded by reexploration and bowel bypass. Patients must be carefully selected, and surgery should be as conservative as possible. Preoperatively a long tube is passed, and intraoperatively the bulb of the tube is identified to find the small bowel above the obstruction. This small bowel is then anastomosed in a side-to-side fashion to the most appropriate area of colon. It is paramount to obtain a preoperative barium enema to ensure that there is no obstruction of the lower colon.

SUMMARY

Although an awareness of appropriate techniques for diagnosis and workup of gynecologic cancer has been stressed over the last 20 years, a small number of patients continue to require immediate reexploration for evaluation and/or treatment of their cancer. Every obstetrician and gynecologist should be fully aware of these situations and understand the need for further surgery. Unnecessary delay can result in decrease in survival.

More important, careful follow-up at close intervals of the recently treated oncology patient may lead to the early diagnosis of recurrence at a point where reoperation may be curative. Finally, it is critically important that each patient be afforded the best possible palliative care, which may include operative procedures that will extend life or alleviate significant symptoms without creating severe complications.

BIBLIOGRAPHY

Aalders JG, Abeler V, Kolstad P: Recurrent adenocarcinoma of the endometrium: A clinical and histopathological study of 379 patients. *Gynecol Oncol* 1984; 17:85.

Andras EJ, Fletcher GH, Rutledge F: Radiotherapy of carcinoma of the cervix following simple hysterectomy. *Am J Obstet Gynecol* 1973; 115:547.

Barber HR: Pelvic exenteration. *Cancer Invest* 1987; 5:331.

Berek JS, Knapp RC, Malkasian GD, et al: CA 125 serum levels correlated with second-look operations among ovarian cancer patients. *Obstet Gynecol* 1986; 67:685.

Bergen S, Disaia PJ, Liao SY, et al: Conservation management of extramammary Paget's disease of the vulva. *Gynecol Oncol* 1989; 33:151.

Boronow RC, Morrow CP, Creasman WT, et al: Surgical staging in endometrial cancer: Clinical-pathologic findings of a prospective study. *Obstet Gynecol* 1984; 63:825.

Buchler DA, Kline JC, Tunca JC, et al: Treatment of recurrent carcinoma of the vulva. *Gynecol Oncol* 1979; 8:180.

Castaldo TW, Petrilli ES, Ballon SC, et al: Intestinal operations in patients with ovarian carcinoma. *Obstet Gynecol* 1981; 139:80.

Chafe W, Richards A, Morgan L, et al: Unrecognized invasive carcinoma in vulvar intraepithelial neoplasia (VIN). *Gynecol Oncol* 1988; 31:154.

Chambers SK, Chambers JT, Kohorn EI, et al: Evaluation of the role of second-look surgery in ovarian cancer. *Obstet Gynecol* 1988; 72:404.

Disaia PJ, Creasman WT, Boronow RC, et al: Risk factors and recurrent patterns in stage I endometrial cancer. *Am J Obstet Gynecol* 1985; 151:1009.

Disaia PJ, Creasman WT, Rich WM: An alternate approach to early cancer of the vulva. *Am J Obstet Gynecol* 1979; 133:825.

Gallup DG, Jordan GH, Talledo OE: Extraperitoneal lymph node dissections with use of a midline incision in patients with female genital cancer. *Am J Obstet Gynecol* 1986; 155:559.

Greven K, Olds W: Isolated vaginal recurrences of endometrial adenocarcinoma and their management. *Cancer* 1987; 60:419.

Griffiths CT: Surgical resection of tumor bulk in the primary treatment of ovarian carcinoma. *Natl Cancer Inst Monogr* 1975; 42:101.

Gunn RA, Gallager HS: Vulvar Paget's disease, a typographic study. *Cancer* 1980; 46:590.

Hacker NF, Berek JS, Lagasse LD, et al: Primary cytoreductive surgery for epithelial ovarian cancer. *Obstet Gynecol* 1983; 61:413.

Hacker NF, Nieberg RK, Berek JS, et al: Superficially invasive vulvar cancer with nodal metastases. *Gynecol Oncol* 1983; 15:65.

Hatch KD, Shingleton HM, Soong SJ, et al: Anterior pelvic exenteration. *Gynecol Oncol* 1988; 31:205.

Heller PB, Barnhill DR, Mayer AR, et al: Cervical carcinoma found incidentally in a uterus removed for benign indications. *Obstet Gynecol* 1986; 67:187.

Hoskins WS, Rubin SC, Dulaney E, et al: Influence of secondary cytoreduction at the time of second-look laparotomy on the survival of patients with epithelial ovarian carcinoma. *Gynecol Oncol* 1989; 34:365.

Imachi M, Tsukamoto N, Matsuyama T, et al: Pulmonary metastasis from carcinoma of the uterine cervix. *Gynecol Oncol* 1989; 33:189.

Jones WB: Surgical approaches for advanced or recurrent cancer of the cervix. *Cancer* 1987; 60:2094.

Krebs HB, Goplerud DR: Surgical management of bowel obstruction in advanced ovarian carcinoma. *Obstet Gynecol* 1983; 61:327.

Lawhead RA, Clark DG, Smith DH, et al: Pelvic exenteration for recurrent or persistent gynecologic malignancies: A 10-year review of the Memorial Sloan-Kettering Cancer Center experience (1972–1981). *Gynecol Oncol* 1989; 33:279.

Lederman GS, Niloff JM, Redline R, et al: Late recurrence in endometrial carcinoma. *Cancer* 1987; 59:825.

Makela J, Kairaluoma MI, Kauppila A: Palliative surgery for intestinal complications of advanced recurrent gynecologic malignancy. *Acta Chir Scand* 1987; 153:57.

Morris M, Gershenson DM, Wharton JT: Secondary cytoreductive surgery in epithelial ovarian cancer: Nonresponders to first-time therapy. *Gynecol Oncol* 1989; 33:1.

Morris M, Gershenson DM, Wharton JT, et al: Secondary cytoreductive surgery for recurrent epithelial ovarian cancer. *Gynecol Oncol* 1989; 34:334.

Orr JW, Ball GC, Soong SJ, et al: Surgical treatment of women found to have invasive cervix cancer at the time of total hysterectomy. *Obstet Gynecol* 1986; 68:353.

Piver MS, Barlow JJ, Lele SB: Incidence of subclinical metastasis in stage I and II ovarian carcinoma. *Obstet Gynecol* 1978; 52:100.

Piver MS, Barlow JJ, Lele SB, et al: Survival after ovarian cancer induced intestinal obstruction. *Gynecol Oncol* 1982; 13:44.

Podczaski ES, Stevens CW, Manetta A, et al: Use of second-look laparotomy in the management of patients with ovarian epithelial malignancies. *Gynecol Oncol* 1987; 28:205.

Podratz KC, Schray MF, Wieand HS, et al: Evaluation of treatment and survival after positive second-look laparotomy. *Gynecol Oncol* 1988; 31:9.

Podratz KC, Symmonds RE, Taylor WF: Carcinoma of the vulva: Analysis of treatment failures. *Am J Obstet Gynecol* 1982; 143:340.

Rubin SC, Benjamin I, Hoskins WJ, et al: Intestinal surgery in gynecologic oncology. *Gynecol Oncol* 1989; 34:30.

Rubin SC, Hoskins WJ, Benjamin I, et al: Palliative surgery for intestinal obstruction in advanced ovarian cancer. *Gynecol Oncol* 1989; 34:16.

Runowicz CD: A critical assessment of the role of second-look surgery in ovarian carcinoma. *Cancer Invest* 1987; 5:479.

Stacy D, Burrell MO, Franklin EW: Extramammary Paget's disease of the vulva and anus: Use of intraoperative frozen-section margins. *Am J Obstet Gynecol* 1986; 155:519.

Stanhope CR, Symmonds RE: Palliative extenteration—what, when, and why? *Am J Obstet Gynecol* 1988; 152:12.

Tunca JC, Buchler DA, Mack EA, et al: The management of ovarian-cancer-caused bowel obstruction. *Gynecol Oncol* 1981; 12:186.

Walton L, Ellenberg SS, Major F, et al: Results of second-look laparotomy in patients with early-stage ovarian carcinoma. *Obstet Gynecol* 1987; 70:770.

Young RC, Deckler DG, Wharton JT, et al: Staging laparotomy in early ovarian cancer. *JAMA* 1984; 250:3072.

Young RC, Walton L, Decker D, et al: Early stage ovarian cancer: Preliminary results of randomized trials after comprehensive initial staging. *Proc Am Soc Clin Oncol* 1983; 2:578.

Chapter 18

Minor Surgery

Tim H. Parmley, M.D.

Minor surgical procedures are, of course, only relatively minor and tend to suffer because they are not treated with the appropriate degree of gravity. For example, when, as is commonly the case, the histologic interpretation of material from an endocervical curettage obtained at the time of differential dilatation and curettage (D&C) is equivocal, the interpretation, the therapy, and the patient's future may rest on the care with which the procedure was done. Too often it was done by the most junior member of the team who possessed little understanding of the degree of precision required and who was inadequately supervised. This inappropriate attitude is the single most important reason for reoperations with so-called minor surgical procedures.

THE LABIA

Biopsies

Biopsies seldom, if ever, lead to the type of surgical complication one thinks of routinely. Bleeding is easy to control, and any subsequent infection is usually easily treated. Damage to other structures is unlikely. The most common serious complication of a labial biopsy is subsequent overtreatment because of pathologic misreading due to operator-pathologist technical error. Almost all technical artifacts in histologic specimens tend to make any disease in the tissue look more advanced than it is. For this reason, invasion may be inaccurately suggested and radical surgery advised for what is truly an intraepithelial malignancy. Although often attempted, rebiopsy seldom clarifies the original confusion.

Technical artifacts arise from two sources. The first is that the biopsy is removed in a sufficiently imprecise manner using crushing instruments on the portion of tissue that must be microscopically viewed. The edges of the biopsy that subsequently will be viewed as "margins" may be crushed or "chewed," producing distortion. The second is that the biopsy is maloriented so that surface features appear deep in the tissue and are incorrectly viewed as invasive.

Appropriate handling requires the careful dissection of a biopsy specimen using fine forceps and a minimum of manipulation. Key's punches may help produce biopsies that have been minimally distorted. The biopsies should be removed from the labia with sharp instruments that do not pull or chew them repeatedly, and then the biopsy should be rapidly fixed and sent to the pathology laboratory in a manner that allows for the maintenance of orientation. If necessary, the operator should consult with the pathologist to achieve this goal.

Labial Adhesions

The classically described surgical approaches to labial adhesions are usually not necessary. The surface epithelium of the labia is quite thin in children, and when due to poor hygiene or for any reason it becomes denuded, the apposing labia may become adherent. It is usually possible to successfully treat them with daily applications of local estrogen until they separate. When estrogen application alone does not achieve this goal, daily application of gentle pressure applied with a Q-tip will successfully complete the process in almost all cases. This can be done while applying the estrogen and without hurting the child. Older children can even be taught to treat themselves in this manner. This achieves the further benefit of assuring them that no pain will occur. Only in long-standing, chronic, or recurrent cases is surgery likely to be necessary.

Surgical separation should be done under general anesthesia, and postoperatively local estrogen should be used to maintain labial separation long enough for the epithelial surfaces to reestablish themselves. Care in diagnosing and dealing with the underlying cause of the initial problem is the factor that prevents recurrence. Failure to identify this underlying cause leads to the recurrent problem that makes surgery necessary.

Condylomata

Because condylomata frequently recur, and in the acute phase of an infection new ones may appear as quickly as old ones are treated, it is common to say the initial treatment failed and that a new one must be tried. This is usually not an accurate assessment. There is a difference between rapid recurrence that outpaces the rate at which old lesions are destroyed and true failure in which the method does not even remove initial lesions. The first is appropriately treated with more aggressive management, but the latter requires a change of methodology. Some cases are extensive enough to require surgery or laser vaporization, and laser therapy of surrounding normal skin may reduce recurrences.[1] In many simple cases, however, local therapy is judged to have failed when it has not been given a fair trial. Either trichloroacetic acid or podophyllin will treat the majority of patients with condylomata. Initially the patient should be seen as often as every 2 or 3 days with repeated treatments if necessary and then careful follow-up with an immediate therapeutic response to any recurrence. More extensive examples treated surgically or by laser also should be seen frequently enough to treat recurrences promptly. Even these more aggressive methodologies are no guarantee against recurrence.[2]

VESTIBULE

The epithelium of the vestibule has a separate embryologic origin from that of either the vagina or the external skin.[3] It is derived from the urogenital sinus and is of endodermal origin. Therefore, both the epithelium and the appendages of the epithelium differ from those of the ectodermal skin and the mesodermal vagina. This has important clinical consequences. Perhaps the most important is that vestibular epithelium does not respond as well to estrogen as does the vaginal epithelium. The appendages, which consist of the minor and major vestibular glands (Bartholin's), also differ from those of the external skin and are involved in different diseases.

Local Excisions

In the vestibule, abnormalities of the minor vestibular glands or of Bartholin's may result in the need for surgical intervention. An inflammatory reaction in the minor vestibular glands that is associated with dyspareunia and contact pain is a poorly understood condition that is difficult to diagnose and treat.[4] Referred to as minor vestibular gland adenitis, or vestibulitis or urogenital syndrome, or vulvar vestibular syndrome (see Chapter 22), this condition is of unknown etiology. The occasional involvement of the lower urinary tract, the lower gastrointestinal (GI) tract, or both has prompted the suggestion that it is part of the spectrum of some more widespread disorder. Others have suggested human papillomavirus infection.

Typically, the patient is one who has developed incapacitating dyspareunia and lesser degrees of pain or burning on contact in the vestibule. The condition is resistant to multiple forms of local and systemic therapy: antibiotics, local and subcutaneous steroids, antifungals, antihistamines, anticholinergics, local 5-fluorouracil, nonspecific lubricants, and psychotherapy. Many patients are desperate when seen and are on the verge of insanity as a result of their condition rather than the reverse.

Although an examination may reveal very little, significant erythema usually can be located in the vestibule anywhere from, and including, the hymeneal ring outward to the inner surface of the labia minora or the perineum. Anteriorly erythema may include varying portions of the periurethral or anterior vestibule up to the clitoris. The erythema may be pinpoint or diffuse but if the vestibule is examined with some type of magnification, such as a colposcope, it is often possible to tell that it consists of round spots about the tiny orifices of the minor vestibular glands. The use of a cotton-tipped applicator to elicit pain is helpful both diagnostically and in planning therapy. Minimal contact with the applicator should elicit the patient's symptoms at specific sites and not at others. Failure to clearly demarcate affected and unaffected areas raises questions about the diagnosis and makes therapy difficult.

This symptom complex may also be associated with urinary or lower GI symptoms. When this is so, the diagnosis is more obscure and may or may not be identical to minor vestibular gland adenitis. Patients with Sjögren's disease or Crohn's disease may have vulvar complaints.

If the patient's symptoms can be clearly elicited by touching specific areas in the vestibule and not others and no other symptoms or disease are present, surgical excision will cure about two thirds of the patients and will help most of the latter. There is a hard core of 5% to 10%, however, who do not respond. Among those helped but not cured, the usual complaint is that "you didn't get it all." This may be due to operator error in delineating the full extent of the disease, and it may be due to true progression or recurrence at other sites. In any case, it has not been possible to avoid this problem.

A standard surgical procedure for excision in this condition has been described.[4] It consists of the removal of the vestibular skin beginning at a level just beneath the urethra. Including the hymeneal ring and extending laterally from it about 0.5 cm out on to the surface of the labia minora, the excision is carried posteriorly down to and over the perineal body. Subsequent to this excision, the vagina is mobilized for approximately 3 cm from its lower border. Any scar tissue is removed, and the vaginal epithelium is exteriorized and sutured to the skin. This procedure results in excision of the vestibule from the level of the urethra posteriorly to and including the fourchette. It may be extended anteriorly if the patient's disease extends anteriorly. Adenomas of the minor vestibular glands are not uncommon and present as bulging fatty masses in the underlying tissue.[5] They are also sources of discomfort and must be removed. Their frequent presence in the subepithelial tissue may account for the frequent failure of the superficial ablative procedures such as laser and cryotherapy to solve this clinical problem. Factors that influence the success rate include careful preoperative delineation of the extent of the problem, generous excision of the affected area, including the hymeneal ring, removal of adenomas, excision of any subcutaneous scar, and an adequate perineoplasty. The latter may be the most important part of the procedure.[6] It substitutes the vaginal epithelium and its subcutaneous tissue for the vestibular skin. The fourchette and perineum are then more responsive to estrogen.

Excised specimens reveal an inflammatory reaction underlying the epithelium of the ducts of the minor vestibular glands rather than the gland proper. This is consistent with the idea that viral infection of this epithelium is occurring. Human papillomavirus infection would also explain many of the clinical vagaries observed with this condition.

Bartholin's Gland

Abscesses of Bartholin's gland are one of the more frequent and more troublesome of those clinical entities demanding minor surgical attention. It is the common teaching that to prevent reclosure and reaccumulation of pus, the incision in a well-developed Bartholin's abscess must be adequate. This is true but an oversimplification. Under the best of circumstances, Bartholin's abscesses may close prematurely. The appropriate approach is a long vertical excision extending over the vestibular aspect of the mass from its uppermost to lowermost extent. The cavity should be fully explored and then packed. The patient should be treated with antibiotics and followed closely to change or replace the packing if it has fallen out. It may be necessary to see the patient daily, because the condition may resolve rapidly, and the cavity and the incision shrink equally quickly.

When due to prior infection a Bartholin's duct cyst is formed, it may be marsupialized or treated with the Word catheter.[7] To decrease the chances of recurrence, marsupialization should be done by removing a major portion of the vestibular wall of the cyst. If more than 50% of the wall of the cyst can be removed without doing a partial vulvectomy, this is desirable. The edges of the remaining cyst are then sutured to the external surface of the skin. If it is not possible to remove a large portion of the cyst without removing much of the vulva, an equally effective alternative is the use of the Word catheter.[8] This device possesses an inflatable bulb on its tip. A small incision is made in the vestibular aspect of the cyst at the appropriate site for the orifice of Bartholin's gland duct. The tip of the catheter is placed within the cyst. The bulb is inflated, and the external tip of the catheter is tucked into the vagina. Epithelialization of the catheter tract will then occur. Recurrences are often the result of failure to monitor the patient closely to make sure the device stays in place postoperatively. The catheter is removed after 4 to 6 weeks.

URETHRA

Prolapse

When an infant or small child presents with vaginal bleeding and "something," the "something" is often a prolapse of a distal portion of the urethral mucosa. The meatus is everted, and the prolapsed mucosa may be partially strangulated. Edema produces swelling, and engorgement of blood produces a bright red color. The result is a velvety red bleeding mass surrounding the urethral orifice. It may or may not be painful.

A surgical approach has been described. It consists of excision of the prolapsed portion of the mucosa and suturing of the urethral mucosa to vestibular skin.[9] If sutures are placed before the excision, the urethral mucosa does not retract out of view when the excision is performed. Local estrogen will also resolve most prolapsed urethras and do so promptly. With either surgical or hormonal therapy, voiding may or may not be a problem, and the child must be observed until this has been resolved.

Caruncles

Caruncles are also mucosal eversions at the urethral meatus. However, they are more localized than the eversions produced by urethral prolapse. In the postmenopausal patient, they are usually posterior because this is the portion of the urethral meatus most dependent on estrogen support. Biopsies are performed on many of them as a diagnostic procedure, which largely removes them. On the other hand, they also will respond to local estrogen.

VAGINA

Vaginal conditions sometimes viewed as minor surgical ones include cysts and septa. A major source of difficulty is that many of these are, in fact, not minor but major procedures requiring extensive intraoperative dissection and postoperative support.

Cysts

Small asymptomatic vaginal cysts need no therapy and should be ignored. If they are symptomatic and truly confined to the vaginal wall, they can often be shelled out easily by a combination of blunt and sharp dissection, or be marsupialized. Many, however, extend laterally and superiorly into the broad ligament, where they may be in relationship to both major vessels and the ureter. These are not minor procedures. They may be approached from below but may also require combined abdominal and vaginal approaches.

Transverse Septae

Vaginal septae can be similarly misleading. Transverse vaginal septae can be thin or thick. Their removal should probably not be regarded as a minor procedure. Experience is required to make even this initial judgment. It is important that they be completely excised but without damaging the vaginal wall excessively. Either error may result in vaginal stricture. Extensive postoperative support with vaginal forms may be necessary.[10] Although careful excision and primary closure may be successful in the case of thinner examples of septae, thicker ones require grafting. The need for reoperation commonly results from a too-casual approach to this clinical condition by an operator under the impression that simple excision and suturing of the base is all that is required.

Imperforate Hymen

Fortunately, the excision of an imperforate hymen seems to be much less likely to result in stricture than the excision of a transverse vaginal septum. Care, nevertheless, should be exercised in excising the membrane without producing undue scarring or residual skin tags that might produce annoying symptoms. This is achieved by first making a cruciate incision in the center of the membrane so that the vagina is entered. Then the base of the membrane can be visualized both above and below and precise excision accomplished.

Longitudinal or Vertical Septae

Vertical vaginal septae are usually less of a problem than transverse ones. They may not require excision at all, but when they are responsible for dyspareunia, it is usually possible to accurately visualize their base and excise them completely. Careful vaginal closure with fine absorbable material usually makes a vaginal form unnecessary, but patients should be observed closely at first to make sure the opposite vaginal walls are not developing any type of adherence.

CERVIX

Conization

Conizations are done for either diagnostic or therapeutic reasons and sometimes both. In either case, postoperative pathologic examination is important. This means the specimen must be removed as atraumatically as possible. Furthermore, it must be removed intact and not in pieces. No more than is necessary should be removed to avoid postoperative stenosis and excessive hemorrhage. Either one of these may result in the need for an otherwise unwarranted hysterectomy.

Careful delineation of the extent of the lesion to be excised using Schiller's reagent or preferably both Schiller's and the colposcope leads to a more precise initial incision with more adequate margins. Regardless of the instruments used, that is, knives or lasers, an effort should be made to make incisions that are carried to their completion with the initial effort so that repeated assaults on the same area of tissue are not necessary. During excision of the cone, the cervix must be stabilized without grasping the excised piece in a destructive manner. Most grasping should be directed at the unexcised portion of the cervix. If the tissue cone must be grasped, it should be done with fine forceps directed at a surface that is uninvolved with disease. After excision, the tissue cone should be carefully labeled and sent to the pathology laboratory in an oriented manner. Additional therapy is distressingly often the result of pathologic uncertainty occasioned by iatrogenic trauma to the excised tissue.

Differential Dilatation and Curettage

The extension of endometrial cancer into the endocervix is considered a reason to advance the stage of the disease and to modify the treatment.[11] This is presumably due to the fact that by advancing into the cervix, the endometrial tumor gains access to the cervical lymphatic watershed in addition to that of the uterine fundus. Thus, it is of high importance to know whether or not endometrial malignancy extends into the cervix. For this reason, many believe that almost all diagnostic D&Cs should be differential ones. It is also for this reason that the differential D&C is one of the most common gynecologic surgical procedures, and the endocervical curettage portion of the procedure is one of the most often repeated because of a lack of precision in its initial performance.

It is rare for a pathologic specimen obtained as the result of a differential D&C to show identifiable endocervix clearly involved by adenocarcinoma. Most commonly what is seen are free tumor fragments in the specimen labeled endocervical curettage. This places the entire burden of determining whether or not the tumor involves the patient's cervix on the assurance with which the surgeon can say, "I know precisely from where I obtained that tissue, and it was clearly endocervical." In contrast, what is usually the case is that when asked, the surgeon expresses uncertainty, and the endocervical curettage must be repeated. At this point, due to recent manipulation, the endocervical specimens are even more likely to contain viable tumor fragments desquamated from above.

Technique is seldom the issue. It usually is one of conscious attitude. The cervical material should be obtained first before sounding or dilating the cervix. The small sharp curette should be placed slowly and carefully up to the internal os and then brought down forcefully. A rapid to and fro motion will almost invariably result in uncertainty about how high the curettage went. The operator should so focus his or her consciousness on the procedure and so record the fact in the record that it is subsequently possible to say with considerable assurance that unless an endometrial tumor is desquamating viable, not necrotic, fragments that are freely floating in the endocervical canal, the presence of viable malignant tissue in the endocervical curettage means that the tumor is present in the patient's endocervix.

REFERENCES

1. Ferenczy A, Mitao M, Nigai N, et al: Latent papillomavirus and recurring genital warts. *N Engl J Med* 1985; 313:784–788.
2. Riva JM, Sedlacek TV, Cunnane MF, et al: Extended carbon dioxide laser vaporization in the treatment of subclinical papillomavirus infection of the lower genital tract. *Obstet Gynecol* 1989; 73:25.
3. Tuchmann-Duplessis H, Haegel P: *Illustrated Human Embryology*, New York, Springer-Verlag, 1974, vol 2.

4. Woodruff JD, Parmley TH: Infection of the minor vestibular glands. *Obstet Gynecol* 1983; 62:609.
5. Axe S, Parmley TH, Woodruff JD, et al: Adenomas in minor vestibular glands. *Obstet Gynecol* 1986; 68:16.
6. Woodruff JD, Genadry R, Poliakoff S: Treatment of dyspareunia and vaginal outlet distortions by perineoplasty. *Obstet Gynecol* 1981; 57:750.
7. Matthews D: Marsupialization of Bartholin's cysts. *J Obstet Gynaecol Br Commonw* 1966; 73:1010.
8. Word B: Office treatment of cysts and abscess of Bartholin's gland duct. *South Med J* 1968; 61:514.
9. TeLinde RW: *Operative Gynecology*, ed 3. Philadelphia, JB Lippencott Co, 1962, p 787.
10. Jones HW Jr, Rock JA: *Reparative and Constructive Surgery of the Female Generative Tract.* Baltimore, Williams & Wilkins Co, 1983.
11. Hacker NF: Uterine cancer in, Berek JS, Hacker NF (eds): *Practical Gynecologic Oncology.* Baltimore, Williams & Wilkins Co, 1989.

Chapter 19

Postoperative Hemorrhage

James L. Breen, M.D.

Julian E. De Lia, M.D.

With the exception of evisceration and hemorrhage, few surgical complications necessitate reoperation as an emergent procedure. Reviewing the literature on postoperative hemorrhage, one is impressed by the volumes of blood that are required to stabilize patients before they are brought to a successful hemostatic outcome. This may reflect the natural tendency of surgeons to initially deny the need for reoperation in the immediate postoperative period or to the difficulties encountered by the surgeon in controlling hemorrhage because of the extensive primary and collateral circulation surrounding the operative field.

Postoperative hemorrhage may occur in any patient despite the most careful of surgical techniques. Its stage, however, may be set by the following: an inappropriate abdominal incision, speed or impatience on the part of the surgeon, improper handling of tissues, poor surgical technique, and failure to closely inspect the operative field before closure.

Three specific surgical principles regarding the handling of tissue pedicles are essential to reduce the risk of intraoperative and postoperative bleeding. Recall that the purchase point of surgical clamps is limited to their distal third or half; therefore, incorporating an entire pedicle or overloading the clamp to its crotch leads to slippage of the suture or rotation of vasculature within the pedicle. Second, regardless of the suture material or the methodology of suture ligature, the surgeon should place the needle as close to the clamp as possible. This is facilitated by rolling the clamp to expose the tissue-clamp interface and placing the needle through the pedicle riding the surface of the clamp. Finally, once pedicles have been ligated, and this is particularly true of vascular pedicles, they should not be tagged because traction may cause ligature slippage or tissue tearing. Careful suturing and handling of pedicles are paramount in the prevention of postoperative hemorrhage.

The gynecologic surgeon should be prepared to recognize hemorrhagic complications early to resolve them with appropriate techniques—techniques that obviate the need to refer to other chapters in this text. One may expect, when reoperation is necessary, that the presence of large dissecting hematomas, friable tissues, disseminated intravascular coagulation, and consumption coagulopathy will further complicate the surgical picture. It is reassuring that large documented series regarding the management of postoperative hemorrhage are rare. The recommendations made in this chapter are based on personal experiences and articles that consist of case reports and limited, uncontrolled studies. These recommendations will range from simple ligation of offending vessels to newer approaches, such as interventive radiology.

ANATOMY AND PHYSIOLOGY OF PELVIC BLEEDING

Familiarity with the vascular anatomy of the pelvis is imperative not only in performing pelvic surgery but also for understanding the approaches to control intraoperative or postoperative hemorrhage. There is an intricate primary and collateral circulation to pelvic structures (Fig 19–1). Branches of the anterior division of the internal iliac (hypogastric) artery provide the major blood supply to the organs of the female pelvis. The hypogastric artery arises at the bifurcation of the common iliac artery, at a point opposite the lumbosacral intervertebral disc and in front of the sacroiliac joint. It then descends to the upper part of the greater sciatic foramen, where it divides into the anterior and posterior trunks. The latter gives off the iliolumbar and lateral sacral arteries before leaving the pelvis through the greater sciatic foramen as the superior gluteal artery. The anterior division leaves the pelvis through the lesser sciatic foramen as the inferior gluteal artery. In the process it gives off the obturator, superior vesicle, inferior vesicle, uterine, vaginal, middle hemorrhoidal, inferior hemorrhoidal, and pudendal arteries.

The initial approach to any patient with significant postoperative bleeding is to maintain or restore hemodynamic stability, followed immediately by a search for the offending vessel. The rate of blood loss from injured or unligated blood vessels can be quantitated by a simple equation:

$$\dot{Q} = S\sqrt{\frac{P_I - P_E}{e} + V^2}$$

Q is the rate of blood loss, S is the surface area of the laceration, P_E is the extravascular pressure, P_I is the intravascular pressure, e is the density of the blood, and V is the velocity of blood flow in the vessel. Clearly, a suture that reduces S to zero will cease all flow. For example, hypogastric artery ligation reduces flow by decreasing both V and P_I. P_E can be increased to equal P_I by pressure packs or military or medical antishock trousers (MAST) suits. Arterial embolization reduces S to zero in terminal vessels and is similar to a hypogastric artery ligation. Patients in shock have low P_I and V values and, therefore, may represent a problem to the surgeon trying to identify the offending vessel during extreme hypotensive periods. The latter may explain the occasional need for a second reoperation. This formula does not take into consideration the status of the patient's coagulation system.

POSTHYSTERECTOMY BLEEDING

Postoperative hemorrhage may complicate any operation whether it be a simple or extensive procedure. Postoperative hemorrhage requiring reoperation complicates approximately 0.8% of hysterectomies.[1]

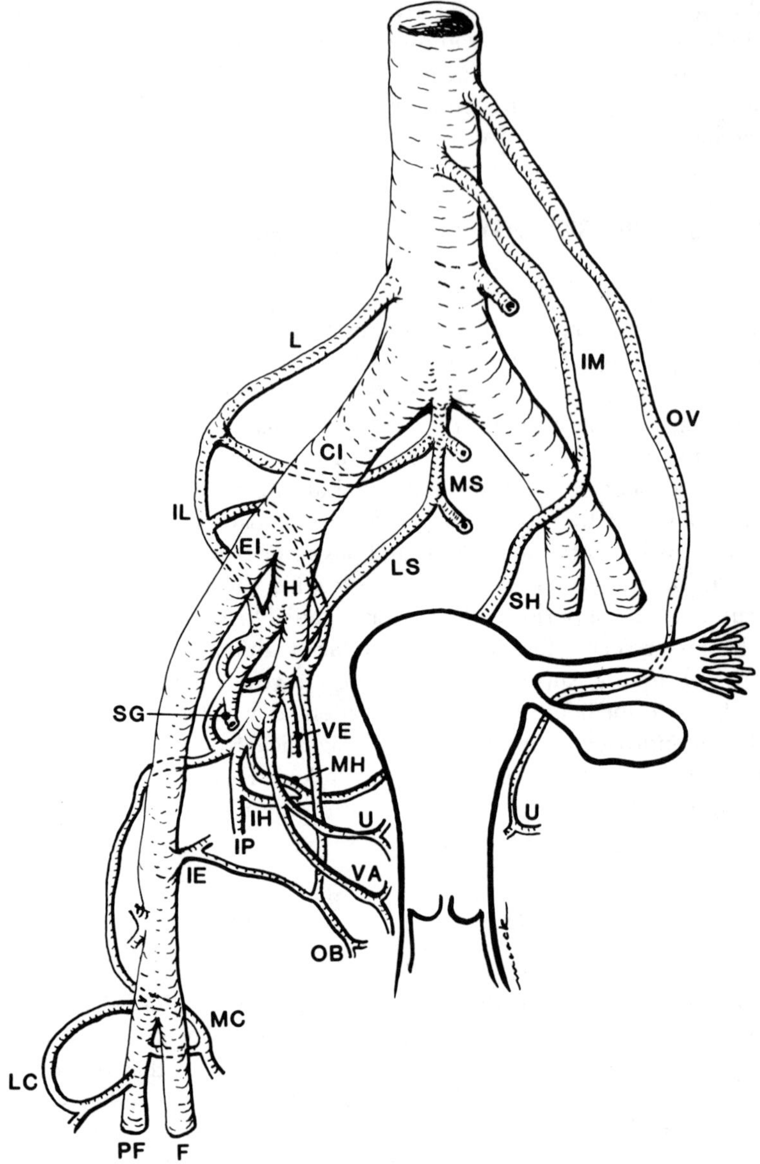

FIG 19–1.
Primary pelvic arterial circulation and pertinent collateral vessels. *IM,* inferior mesenteric; *L,* lumbar; *OV,* ovarian; *CI,* common iliac; *MS,* middle sacral; *IL,* iliolumbar; *EI,* external iliac; *LS,* lateral sacral; *H,* hypogastric (internal iliac); *SH,* superior hemorrhoidal; *SG,* superior gluteal; *VE,* vesicle; *MH,* middle hemorrhoidal; *U,* uterine; *IH,* inferior hemorrhoidal; *IP,* internal pudendal; *VA,* vaginal; *IE,* inferior epigastric; *OB,* obturator; *MC,* middle femoral circumflex; *LC,* lateral circumflex; *F,* femoral; *PF,* deep femoral.

Inapparent postoperative intra-abdominal bleeding may be difficult to diagnose. Suspicion should be aroused if any of the following occurs: excessive postoperative pain; persistent oliguria; abdominal rigidity or distention; shoulder, vaginal, or scapular pain; tachycardia; or hypotension. In these situations, serial evaluations of the hemoglobin and hematocrit values are helpful. Ultrasound, culdocentesis, or an abdominal tap may aid in the diagnosis. Once the diagnosis is made or the index of suspicion is high without supporting evidence, celiotomy with complete exploration of the abdomen is mandatory.

Hysterectomy techniques that extraperitonealize vascular pedicles and leave the vaginal cuff open increase the likelihood that postoperative bleeding will be recognized early. Bleeding that is retroperitoneal or intra-abdominal, without access to the vagina, is usually diagnosed after the patient has lost a significant volume of blood. In 1,219 vaginal hysterectomies reported by Smith and Pratt, 7 patients who required reoperation for hemorrhage developed symptoms 5 to 11 hours postoperatively.[2] Physical examination may reveal a distended abdomen with decreased bowel sounds or differential dullness on percussion, which may or may not shift (the latter is true of retroperitoneal bleeding). Ultrasound scanning may be useful in locating the site of a hematoma, but the ultimate discovery is at reoperation.

Patients who manifest postoperative bleeding early (i.e., within the first 24 hours) generally bleed from a pedicle that was inadequately sutured or from a pedicle in which suture breakage or slippage occurred. Bleeding after the first 24 hours is usually due to tissue or suture sloughing, but this etiology has decreased with the advent of synthetic absorbable sutures that retain their tensile strength for up to 30 days.

Although the most common site of significant postoperative bleeding following hysterectomies is the vaginal vault, any vascular pedicle may be implicated.

Bleeding that occurs within the first 24 hours is best managed by appropriate reexploration and resuturing of the offending vessels. Those cases where postoperative bleeding is more indolent (i.e., presenting as a hematoma, both confined and self-tamponading) may require reoperation or merely observation. The reoperative procedure—hematoma evacuation and placement of hemostatic sutures diminishes the risk of secondary infection and abscess formation. Conversely, many hematomas may self-tamponade and stabilize without additional bleeding or subsequent infection. The decision to operate on stable hematomas is highly individualized and is based primarily on how stable the patient is and what are the risks of infection. The risk of infection relates to the indication for the original surgery, the use of antibiotics, and the general metabolic status of the patient.

Postoperative hemorrhage of significance is almost always arterial in origin and must be controlled surgically. The first step in management includes the restoration of blood volume with fluid, blood, and specific blood products. An initial examination should be attempted before anesthesia and surgery, especially if bleeding from the vagina is noted. With the patient in a lithotomy position, clots are removed and the vaginal cuff is examined closely. If a bleeding vessel is identified at or near the cuff, one or more superficial sutures may suffice. If bleeding is extensive or originates above the vaginal apex, exploratory celiotomy becomes mandatory. Once the decision to explore the patient is made, a midline incision of sufficient size should be made to facilitate adequate exploration of all pelvic and abdominal structures. After all clots are evacuated, exploration of the abdomen along with careful localization of all previous pedicle sites will usually suffice and allow for religature. The cyclic spurting of blood from arteries facilitates their location and allows for precise clamping compared with a diffuse venous ooze, which does not allow for clamping. Regardless of the severity of bleeding, blind haphazard clamping and suturing of tissues is to be condemned. Direct compression with a finger or pack and releasing the compression slowly will aid in accurate clamp and suture placement. These conventional steps will resolve most cases of postoperative bleeding. If the bleeding, however, is diffuse or the bleeding vessels are located deep in the pelvis where they cannot be either located or, if located, are not amenable to suturing, direct pressure with a pack and a hypogastric artery ligation should be performed.

HYPOGASTRIC ARTERY LIGATION

Once the surgeon exhausts the conventional means of controlling postoperative hemorrhage without success, the ultimate resolution of bleeding may be accomplished by ligating the internal iliac (hypogastric) artery.[3] Bilateral ligation of these arteries is an integral part of the management of massive obstetric and gynecologic hemorrhage, and all surgeons should be familiar with its technique. The procedure, while decreasing the mean uterine artery pressure and blood flow by only 24% and 48%, respectively, produces its most significant physiologic effect by reducing the arterial pulse pressure by 85%.[4] Hypogastric artery ligation does not control hemorrhage from branches of the ovarian artery, which if bleeding must be ligated separately, or from generalized venous oozing.

Hypogastric arteries may be exposed either extraperitoneally or intraperitoneally, the latter being the preferred approach if there is extensive intraperitoneal bleeding. The common iliac artery and its two main branches are easily palpable and visualized along the pelvic sidewall. Care should be taken to retract the ureter and its peritoneum medially during the procedure. An attempt should be made to ligate the hypogastric artery distal to its posterior division, but many times it is easier to tie the hypogastric near its origin from the common iliac artery. The origin of the division is not always obvious but generally occurs within the first 2 to 3 cm from the iliac bifurcation. Once the site for ligation is determined, the loose areolar tissue and adventitia are dissected from the artery. In an effort to avoid injury to the hypogastric vein, a Babcock clamp is used to elevate the artery. A right angle or

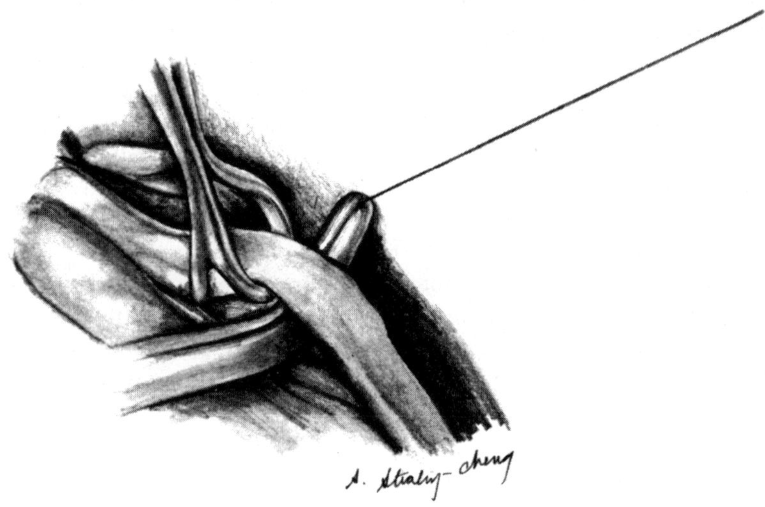

FIG 19–2.
Right hypogastric artery ligation. Hypogastric artery held by a Babcock and a suture placed on tip of Mixter clamp, ready to be passed under the artery.

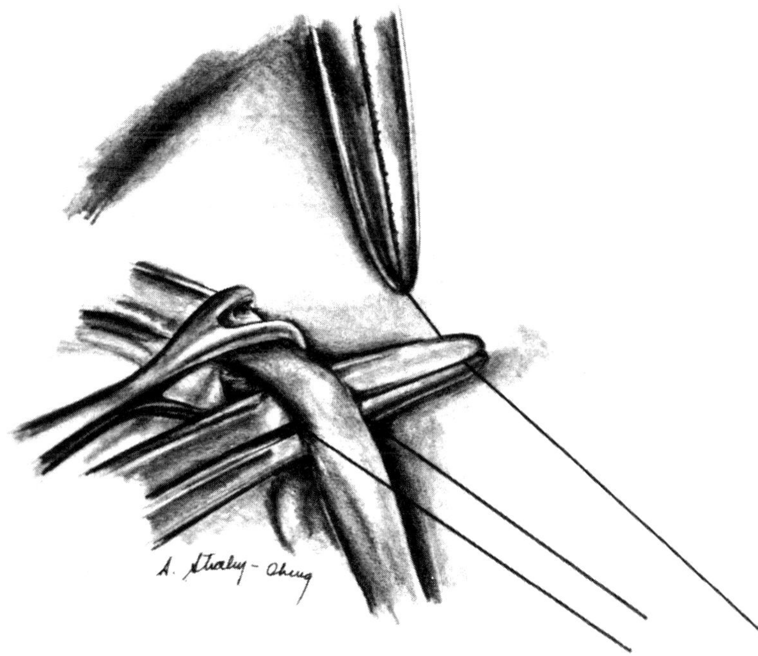

FIG 19–3.
Hypogastric artery ligation. Mixter clamp is repositioned below hypogastric artery and suture on tonsil clamp is brought down and grasped by Mixter clamp for second pass below hypogastric artery.

Mixter clamp is passed beneath the artery, hugging its surface (lateral to medial clamp may add additional protection to the underlying vein). A no. 2 synthetic polyglycolic suture is passed to the tip of the right angle clamp and drawn up for tying (Fig 19–2). The vessel should be doubly ligated, but transection is never recommended (Figs 19–3 and 19–4). Technical problems associated with hypogastric artery ligation include ligating the external iliac artery or the ureter and lacerating the hypogastric vein. The operator should palpate the femoral pulses, identify the ureter both before and after the ligation, and use extreme care around the hypogastric vein. The most common error associated with this procedure, however, is waiting too long to perform it.

The success rate of hypogastric artery ligation in postoperative hemorrhage is difficult to assess. Approximately one half of the patients with hemorrhage will respond successfully.[5] Table 19–1 lists the indications for hypogastric ligation at the Saint Barnabas Medical Center over a 20-year period. Note that the leading indication was for teaching. It is better to learn under a controlled situation rather than when truly indicated. Should this procedure fail, additional surgical and nonsurgical options remain.

ANGIOGRAPHIC ARTERIAL EMBOLIZATION

For serious postoperative pelvic hemorrhage, many proclaim that angiographic embolization should be undertaken if a vaginal examination fails to reveal the

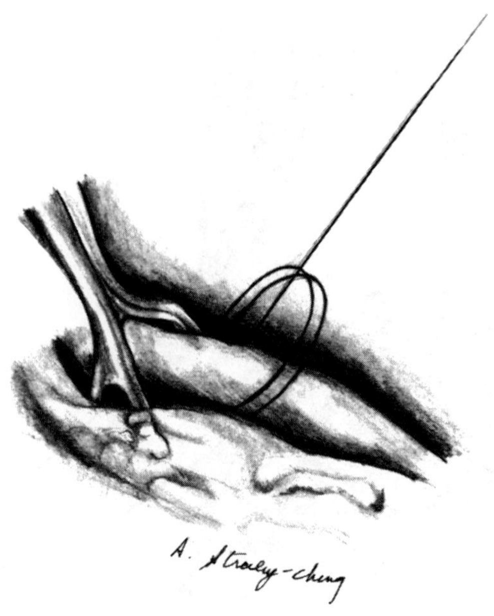

FIG 19–4.
Hypogastric artery ligation. The doubly passed suture is ready to be tied.

bleeding site. In some circumstances, angiographic access to a bleeding artery may be easier than a surgical approach. Embolization has been described as being successful for controlling hemorrhage from pelvic tumors, trauma, radiation, postpartum hemorrhage from uterine and vaginal sources, abdominal pregnancy, and postabortal hemorrhage.[6–8] Its use for posthysterectomy bleeding not controlled by

TABLE 19–1.
Hypogastric Artery Ligation Indications*

Procedure	No. of Patients
Radical gynecologic surgery	
Therapeutic	5
Prophylactic	35
Teaching	358
Total abdominal hysterectomy	7
Uterine rupture	6
Vaginal hysterectomy	4
Hot knife conization of the cervix	4
Cold knife conization of the cervix	3
Cryosurgery of the cervix	3
Placenta accreta	3
Uterine atony	3
Anterior colporrhaphy	1
Total	432

*Data from Saint Barnabas Medical Center, Livingston, NJ, 1969–1989.

reoperative procedures is well documented.[9] It may also be appropriate in patients with a coagulopathy that has not been corrected.

Angiographers recommend that the surgeon request an angiographic consultation early. A patient who is reasonably stable and has not undergone reoperation is preferred because of the added technical simplicity and higher success rate. The key to successful embolization is accurate identification of the bleeding vessel. Previous hypogastric artery ligation makes embolization more difficult. Conversely, radiographic failure does not compromise the possibility of subsequent surgery. Remember, however, that embolization requires 1 to 2 hours, so that in severe hypotensive shock, this is not appropriate.

A wide selection of agents are available for transcatheter embolization, and the choice is determined by the duration of desired occlusion, the size of the vessel to be occluded, the rate of blood flow through the vessel, and whether or not the vessel tapers or branches.[10] Absorbable gelatin sponge (Gelfoam), as small pledgets, are used to occlude small tapering vessels for short-term (10–30 days) occlusion. Larger, nontapering vessels are occluded with a detachable balloon or Gianturco coil. If angiographic embolization is not immediately available to the patient, reoperation is the obvious course. Should the second operation fail (with or without hypogastric artery ligation), the following techniques may prove useful.

PELVIC PACKS

The surgeon is occasionally faced with controlling hemorrhage from large raw surfaces, venous plexuses, or inaccessible areas within the pelvis, often with the added problem of a coagulopathy. In these situations, one may employ a pack to produce a pelvic tamponade. The variably known umbrella, or mushroom pack, was described by Logothelopulos in 1926 to control bleeding, primarily after radical surgical procedures.[11–13] He demonstrated its effectiveness by placing the pelvic pack to control bleeding in a patient who had a hysterectomy without vessel ligation! The pack consists of a square, fine-mesh gauze laparotomy pad of cotton or nylon 24 in. to a side. Fifteen to 20 yards of 2-in. gauze tape or 6 yards of 4-in. head-roll gauze is layered into the center of the pack, taking care to prevent tangling, which may prevent removal. A funnel-shaped sling is then formed when the four corners of the pad are brought together, with a short tail of the gauze left free and tagged with a suture. The diagonal corners of the pack are brought over the pack and tied (Fig 19–5). This bolus of gauze is then placed in the true pelvis with the tail exiting the vagina. If bleeding points are observed near the pelvic brim, additional gauze may be necessary. This pack may also be applied through the vagina and formed inside the pelvis. Here the pad is held in front of the vulva by the corners, and the center is pushed through the vagina into the pelvis by inserting gauze with a ring forceps. The four corners are brought together and pulled down to seat the pack.[11] Approximately 2 to 5 kg of traction weight is applied to the tails of the pack for 48 to 72 hours, with the tension released every 8 hours to prevent pressure necrosis of pelvic tissues. Passing the tails through a no. 80 doughnut pessary and cross-clamping the tails with a Kelly clamp after applying sufficient traction to seat the pack are satisfactory. A Foley catheter is placed in the bladder so that the bulb is above the pack. Decreased urine output after restoring circulating volume may indicate excessive traction. Broad-spectrum antibiotics are advisable

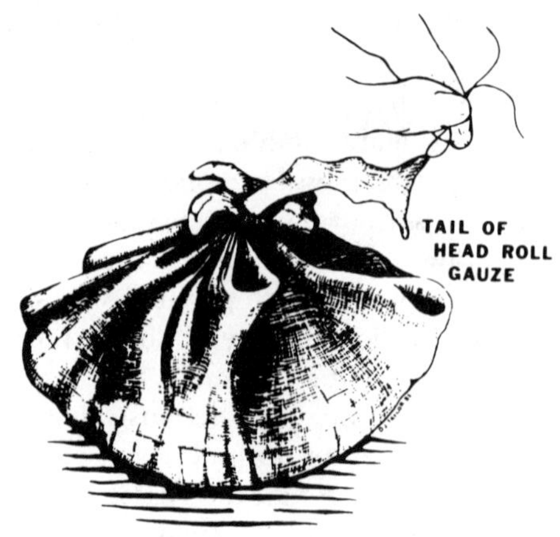

FIG 19–5.
Umbrella pack ready for pelvic tamponade. Diagonal corners of the laparotomy pad are brought together and secured after carefully filling with layered gauze. The tagging suture should be placed through the cuff into the vagina. (From Cassels JW, Greenberg H, Otterson WN: *J Reprod Med* 1985; 30:689. Used by permission.)

during its use. Regardless of the technique of insertion, the pack is removed vaginally. Before its removal, the ends are soaked in saline and hydrogen peroxide. The pack may be removed under analgesia on the following day.

More conventional packing, however, may be appropriate. In a patient with broad surface bleeding or bleeding in areas inaccessible to conventional suturing or clamping, transabdominal placement of 2-in. packs in the pelvis is highly effective.[3] The technique is to take a 2-in. pack, and moving it from right to left, place it over the entire pelvis, bringing it out through a stab wound in the groin. When bleeding is extensive, it is usually necessary to use five or six 2-in. packs. The second pack is placed over the first and brought out through a separate stab wound. Never tie two packs together, because they have to be removed through the incisions in the groin. If six packs are used, there will be six exit sites within the groin.[5] It is important to tag each pack with either a safety pin or a suture, so that you know which pack is on the bottom and which is on the top. This is important, because it is embarrassing to start removing what you think is the top pack the day after surgery and find that you are pulling on the bottom packs instead. The top-most packs should be moved on the day after surgery and the bottom packs removed 72 hours after surgery. It is important to cover the patient with broad-spectrum antibiotics during this period.

GRAVITY (MAST) SUIT

Similar to angiographic embolization, the use of the MAST suit is highly successful. The MAST suit is generally employed in catastrophic events where traditional measures have failed or where the patient must be stabilized before surgery. These situations include rupture of the liver in pregnancy, abdominal pregnancy, postcesarean hysterectomy, disseminated intravascular coagulation, intractable intraoperative bleeding, bleeding following radical pelvic surgery, and shock from tubal pregnancies. The suit may occasionally be an option to hysterectomy and severe postpartum hemorrhage in women desiring future childbearing.[14]

Patients placed in MAST suits respond with a decreased blood loss and a rise in blood pressure as a consequence of increased peripheral resistance in the vessels within the suit. These effects allow for improved perfusion of critical organs such as the heart, lungs, brain, and kidneys. Irreversible shock, adult respiratory distress syndrome, and tubular necrosis may be prevented. Reoperated patients in whom surgical intervention has failed to control bleeding and those with secondary coagulopathies are prime candidates. In some patients it may obviate the need for further surgical intervention and provide time to correct coagulation-related bleeding disorders if additional surgery is needed.

Once the suit is applied, it is inflated from the legs to the abdominal compartment with 10 to 40 mm Hg pressure to establish a stable perfusion and decreased bleeding. The suit is removed 12 to 24 hours after the bleeding has stopped by deflating the abdominal compartment first, followed by the legs, in 5 mm Hg increments every half hour.[15] Gynecologic surgeons should familiarize themselves with the proper application of the MAST, because it may prove to be a life-saving technique. Most hospitals will have a MAST suit in their burn units, emergency rooms, and intensive surgical care units.

SUMMARY

Every gynecologic surgical procedure, regardless of how well planned and skillfully executed, is characterized by a certain irreducible loss of blood that is commensurate with the magnitude of the operation, the vascularity of the surgical field, and the capabilities of the surgeon. In most operations, blood loss may be kept to an acceptable minimum by applying the basic principles of hemostasis. Even a moderate amount of uncontrolled bleeding, involving in some situations up to 30% of the circulating blood volume, may not seriously alter circulatory dynamics. However, uncontrolled, unanticipated, excessive blood loss may be catastrophic.

Hemorrhage during or after surgery is usually not anticipated, but few gynecologists have not had a routine procedure abruptly transformed into a life-threatening drama. Under these circumstances, the attitude of the surgeon may be the deciding factor in the outcome of the situation. Though a degree of alarm is a normal reaction, the surgeon must keep a clear head, even in the presence of massive hemorrhage. One important factor is the surgeon's realistic appraisal of his or her personal limitations; it is a wise individual who accepts these limitations and seeks assistance.

REFERENCES

1. Fehrman H: Surgical management of life-threatening obstetric and gynecologic hemorrhage. *Acta Obstet Gynecol Scand* 1988; 67:125–128.
2. Smith RD, Pratt JH: Serious bleeding following vaginal or abdominal hysterectomy. *Obstet Gynecol* 1965; 26:592–595.
3. Breen JL, Kindzierski J, Gregori C: Surgical hemorrhage and infection, in *Current Therapy in Surgical Gynecology*. Philadelphia, BC Decker, 1987.
4. Burchell RC: Physiology of the internal iliac artery ligation. *J Obstet Gynaecol Br Commonw* 1968; 75:642–651.
5. Clark SL, Phelan JP, Yeh S, et al: Hypogastric artery ligation for obstetrical hemorrhage. *Obstet Gynecol* 1985; 66:353–356.

6. Brown BJ, Heaston DK, Poulson AM, et al: Uncontrollable postpartum bleeding: A new approach to hemostasis through angiographic arterial embolization. *Obstet Gynecol* 1979; 54:361–365.
7. Greenwood LH, Glickman MG, Schwartz PE, et al: Obstetric and nonmalignant gynecologic bleeding: Treatment with angiographic embolization. *Radiology* 1987; 164:155–159.
8. Kivikoski AI, Martin C, Weyman P, et al: Angiographic arterial embolization to control hemorrhage in abdominal pregnancy: A case report. *Obstet Gynecol* 1988; 71:456–459.
9. Rosenthal DM, Colapinto R: Angiographic arterial embolization in the management of postoperative vaginal hemorrhage. *Am J Obstet Gynecol* 1985; 151:227–231.
10. Marx MV, Picus D, Weyman PJ: Percutaneous embolization of the ovarian artery in the treatment of pelvic hemorrhage. *Am J Radiol* 1988; 150:1337–1338.
11. Cassels JW, Greenberg H, Otterson WN: Pelvic tamponade in puerperal hemorrhage. *J Reprod Med* 1985; 30:689–692.
12. Guerre EF, O'Keefe DF, Elliot JP, et al: Uncontrollable intraabdominal hemorrhage treated with packing and use of a MAST suit. *J Reprod Med* 1987; 32:230–232.
13. Logothetopulos K: Eine absolut sichere Blutstillungs methode bei vaginalen und abdominalen gynakologischen operationen. *Zentralbl Gynaekol* 1926; 50:3202–3204.
14. Hall M, Marshall JR: The gravity suit: A major advance in management of gynecologic blood loss. *Obstet Gynecol* 1979; 53:247–250.
15. Kaback KR, Sanders AB, Meislin HW: MAST suite update. *JAMA* 1984; 252:2598–2603.

Chapter 20

Postoperative Infection

David L. Hemsell, M.D.

Surgical procedures and the likelihood of postoperative infection have been classified with regard to contamination by operative site flora and preservation of appropriate operative technique. There are four separate categories of surgical procedures, each associated with a range of postoperative infection. *Clean* operative procedures are those performed for nontraumatic indications, and inflammation is not encountered. Surgical technique is maintained, and the respiratory, alimentary, and genitourinary tracts are not entered. Infection without antimicrobial prophylaxis ranges from 1% to 5%, and perioperative antimicrobial administration does not decrease the incidence of infection. Most laparoscopic and adnexal surgical procedures qualify for this category.

The majority of gynecologic surgical procedures are classified as *clean-contaminated* cases since the vagina is entered or operated through in the absence of obvious clinical infection. Minor break in surgical technique is allowed without changing category. The observed infection rate is between 5% and 15% for patients whose procedures are in this category. Antimicrobial prophylaxis is indicated for high-risk procedures and/or populations only; all do not require prophylaxis, but risk identification is mandatory. For example, dilatation and curettage (D&C) and cervical conization are rarely followed by infection; antimicrobial prophylaxis is usually contraindicated. The opposite is true for vaginal hysterectomy. Abdominal hysterectomy, however, may fall into either a high-risk or a low-risk category in different hospitals or in different patient populations in the same hospital, so individual determination is mandatory. Risk factors potentially increasing the pelvic infection rate following hysterectomy are presented in Table 20–1. Immune system deficiencies are uniformly associated with an increased incidence of postoperative infection, regardless of surgical classification. This deficiency may be the result of chemotherapy for malignancy, glucocorticosteroid therapy, or immunotherapy for transplant patients and may be a significant underlying factor contributing to a higher infection rate in socioeconomically deprived indigent populations. Antimicrobial prophylaxis is indicated when patients are immunocompromised and undergo gynecologic surgical procedures.

Contaminated procedures are those in which there is a major break in surgical technique or gross spillage from the gastrointestinal (GI) tract. Entrance into the genitourinary or biliary tract in the presence of infected urine or bile results in placement in this category, but no mention was made in the original classification

TABLE 20–1.
Potential Risk Factors for Pelvic Infection After Hysterectomy

Lower socioeconomic status
Patient age
Patient weight
Diabetes
Excessive blood loss
Prolonged surgical procedure
Menstrual cycle phase
Operator experience
Recent pelvic surgery
Catheter placement
Concomitant surgical procedure or procedures
Preoperative anemia
Postoperative anemia

description regarding surgery in the acutely infected upper reproductive tract.[1] For example, laparoscopy or laparotomy for acute salpingitis should be included in this category. Infection rates in this category range between 10% and 25%; at least perioperative antibiotic administration is required, and delayed wound closure may be appropriate, as is the case when procedures qualify for the classification of *dirty* or *infected* procedures. Such procedures are followed by infection 30% to 100% of the time; antimicrobial administration is therapeutic and not prophylactic, as is the case with contaminated procedures.

Operative site infections continue to account for about 40% of hospital-acquired infections, and they account for almost one fourth of adverse events in California leading to litigation. Morbidity and monetary impact are significant. In our indigent patient population undergoing hysterectomy, pelvic operative site infection at least doubles the hospital stay and hospital bill; infection in the abdominal wall may triple those variables. Actual infection rates have been decreasing during the last several decades, however. Emphasis on decreased preoperative stay, improved surgical techniques, appropriate utilization of perioperative antimicrobial, improved suture material, improved anesthesia techniques, early ambulation, and early return to the home environment all contribute to the reduction in postoperative infection. The importance of surgical technique and its contribution to infection prevention was stressed by Richardson and co-workers, who reported a decrease in operative site infection after abdominal hysterectomy from 22% to 2.4% by technique alteration only.[2] Gentle handling of tissue, small pedicles, and accurate hemostasis are imperative. Active rather than passive drainage is associated with a lower infection rate in those situations when drainage is indicated. Improved patient nutrition has undoubtedly contributed to diminished infection in indigent populations.

HYSTERECTOMY

Febrile Morbidity

The incidence of asymptomatic temperature elevation, or febrile morbidity, after hysterectomy differs by surgical approach in our patients. It has been observed in up to 40% of women after abdominal hysterectomy and in as high as 27% of women after vaginal hysterectomy. This recurrent oral temperature elevation to 38° C or above occurs a mean of about 50 hours after either surgical approach. A retrospective review of the charts of women undergoing abdominal and vaginal hysterectomy revealed that in the early and mid-1970s, most women with this phenomenon were treated with parenteral antimicrobial, frequently without a diagnosis. A progress note would reflect no identifiable problem, recurrent temperature was recorded on the vital sign graphics sheet, and there was an order for parenteral antimicrobial on the hospital order sheet. An infection diagnosis did not usually appear on the chart face sheet of these asymptomatic patients. Febrile morbidity is rarely observed after most other gynecologic procedures. Recurrent temperature elevation may certainly be one sign of infection, but it should not be the only one present before therapy for pelvic or abdominal incision infection. Operative site examination and an infection diagnosis are mandatory before antimicrobial therapy is initiated.

The exact origin of this early and asymptomatic temperature elevation is infrequently identified. Extremity phlebitis occurs rarely following elective gynecologic surgical procedures because intravenous (IV) lines are removed early. Intravenous sites should always be investigated when the source of postoperative temperature elevation is sought. Microatelectasis is certainly a contributor; an x-ray film of the chest is usually normal even in the presence of decreased basilar breath sounds and crackles at auscultation, however. In the absence of pyelonephritis, the urinary tract is not a contributor to temperature elevation in our patients, including those with an indwelling transurethral catheter after surgical repair for urinary stress incontinence. Thus, a chest x-ray film, blood culture, urinalysis, and urine culture are not cost effective in the identification of the source of asymptomatic postoperative pyrexia in our patients. Leukocytosis is the rule after surgery, so a complete blood cell count with differential does not usually guide one to the source. A thorough history and a careful physical examination are the appropriate evaluators for asymptomatic and symptomatic temperature elevation that occurs during the immediate or late postoperative period. The upper respiratory tract and middle ears must also be evaluated but are rarely the cause, with the possible exception of "viral upper respiratory tract infection." A pelvic examination is infrequently necessary if gentle, deep palpation of the lower abdomen over the surgical site is "normal," with "expected tenderness." Administration of perioperative antimicrobial to prevent operative site infection after vaginal and abdominal hysterectomy did not alter the incidence of asymptomatic temperature elevation when compared with placebo.

Cellulitis

The most common postoperative infection is a cellulitis in pelvic tissues. It is observed almost exclusively after hysterectomy. I believe that all women develop cellulitis at the vaginal surgical margin after hysterectomy. It is characterized by small vessel engorgement resulting in erythema and heat, stasis, and endothelial leakage with interstitial edema, which cause induration, and an inflammatory polymorphonuclear infiltrate. It is truly a cuff cellulitis, and it is more of a histologic diagnosis than it is a clinically important diagnosis, at least in our indigent patient population. Antimicrobial therapy is infrequently required for this diagnosis during the immediate postoperative period; it is observed most frequently in women who have been discharged from the hospital after an uneventful postoperative course.

They present before their appointed clinic follow-up visit complaining of central lower abdominal, pelvic, and/or lower back pain and excessive and frequently foul-smelling vaginal discharge. At bimanual examination, an indurated, erythematous, vaginal margin is identified, and it is more tender than anticipated. Purulent secretions are in the vagina. A low-grade temperature elevation may also be present. These findings are the rule during the immediate postoperative period, but at that time, they are not symptomatic and quickly disappear. After discharge from the hospital, these are abnormal findings and will not disappear without antimicrobial therapy. Readmission to the hospital is unnecessary in most instances, and oral antimicrobial therapy as an outpatient is appropriate therapy. The broadest spectrum of bactericidal coverage is afforded by amoxicillin and clavulanic acid (Augmentin). If the only complaint is vaginal discharge and the only finding is purulent vaginal secretions, local therapy such as povidone-iodine or vinegar douche usually result in resolution without requiring antimicrobial administration.

If host cellular and humoral mediated defense mechanisms are unable to control the normal inflammatory process at the vaginal surgical margin, the process extends into the parametrial regions. This infection usually develops during the immediate postoperative period and before discharge from the hospital. It does not usually affect both parametria equally, but rather it is predominantly a unilateral phenomenon. Symptoms of increasing unilateral lower abdominal and pelvic pain precede or accompany recurrent temperature elevations and appear a mean of about 80 hours after hysterectomy, regardless of surgical approach. New-onset lower abdominal and pelvic pain are present, and the underlying parametrial area is thickened and tender, but no mass is usually present. Peritonitis and ileus are absent, but anorexia is common. This is a true pelvic cellulitis.

Adnexitis

If adnexae are retained at hysterectomy, adnexitis may also develop, and presentation is very similar to that of pelvic cellulitis. There is a difference in findings at pelvic examination; tenderness is absent in the lateral parametrial areas but, rather, is cephalad thereto or central and above the vaginal cuff. This infection is also usually unilateral and may be associated with a palpable mass. Suturing adnexae to the areas adjacent to the vaginal cuff may increase the potential for subsequent infection. Postoperative pain secondary to adnexal attachment to the vaginal cuff area can also be avoided by not extraperitonealizing the round ligament or utero-ovarian ligament. The predominant reason given for extraperitonealizing those pedicles is for identification and accessibility should bleeding occur postoperatively. In my experience, bleeding has been intraperitoneal even when these pedicles were extraperitonealized. For those two reasons, I do not extraperitonealize the round or utero-ovarian ligament. Some gynecologic surgeons extraperitonealize those ligaments at vaginal hysterectomy but not at abdominal hysterectomy; if such were advantageous, the procedure should be performed regardless of approach.

The Supravaginal Space

There is a collection of 40 to 200 mL of serum, lymph, and/or blood between the vaginal margins and the pelvic peritoneum. This is an excellent medium for the growth of bacteria inoculated during surgery. Before we began to evaluate antimicrobial prophylaxis in our patient population, the open cuff technique was associated with a significantly lower pelvic infection rate than was observed if the vagina were sutured closed. Evaluation of cuff management after the initiation of antimicrobial prophylaxis at hysterectomy revealed no difference in infection rates. Active drainage of that space to reduce the postoperative infection rate has been evaluated by several investigators. For some investigators, drainage was as effective at preventing postoperative infection as was perioperative antimicrobial. For others, it was ineffective in preventing postoperative pelvic infection. These conflicting results underscore the importance of individual determination of factors contributing to postoperative pelvic infection and the most efficient means of preventing that infection. Of course, if one could avoid the perioperative administration of antibiotic and have low infection rates by the use of mechanical measures, then potential complications of prophylaxis such as an allergic or even an anaphylactic reaction, suprainfection, induction of antimicrobial resistance, and flora alteration at the operative site and other sites would be avoided. Compared with no prophylaxis, administration of a single dose of antimicrobial at hysterectomy does not adversely affect the postoperative lower reproductive tract flora or resistance patterns in those bacteria when prospectively evaluated. Multiple doses over even as short a period as 8 hours does alter the flora qualitatively and is associated with an increase in species that are resistant to the prophylactic regimen.

Prophylaxis

We prospectively evaluated a 1-gm parenteral dose of cefazolin in 746 women undergoing vaginal and abdominal hysterectomy. The overall postoperative infection rate was 7.2%.[3] By historical comparison, that is significantly less than the rate of 45.1% observed with placebo in earlier prospective studies.[4, 5] A single 1- to 2-gm dose of cefazolin was the recommended prophylactic regimen for hysterectomy in a recent review.[6] A list of antibiotics approved by the Food and Drug Administration (FDA) for single preoperative dosing at vaginal or abdominal hysterectomy is presented alphabetically in Table 20–2.

Endocarditis Prophylaxis

If antimicrobial is required to protect an abnormal or damaged heart, other antimicrobial administration is unnecessary. Types of abnormalities requiring such protection include valvular heart disease, prosthetic valves, congenital heart disease (excluding uncomplicated secundum atrial septal defect), idiopathic hypertrophic subaortic stenosis, and mitral valve prolapse with regurgitation. Regimens recommended to prevent valvular damage or endocarditis appear in Table 20–3. A one-time administration is proposed by some; others recommend a second dose 8 hours later.

Abscess

With antimicrobial prophylaxis, the development of pelvic abscess after gynecologic surgery is currently a rare infection. Before antimicrobial prophylaxis, the most common location for a pelvic abscess was in the space between the pelvic peritoneum and the vaginal margin. The overall incidence of postoperative pelvic

TABLE 20–2.
FDA-Approved Single-Dose Antimicrobial Regimens for Prophylaxis at Hysterectomy

Generic Name	Product Name	Manufacturer
Cefonicid	Monocid	Smith Kline & French Laboratories
Ceforanide	Precef	Bristol Laboratories
Cefotaxime	Claforan	Hoechst-Roussel Pharmaceuticals
Cefotetan	Cefotan	Stuart Pharmaceuticals
Cefoxitin	Mefoxin	Merck, Sharp, & Dohme
Ceftriaxone	Rocephin	Roche Laboratories
Cefuroxime	Zinacef	Glaxo Laboratories

infection in retrospective studies was as high as 60%, and between 5% to 10% of women developed a cuff abscess. Mechanical drainage was established by opening the central portion of vaginal margins in the examination or treatment room. Abscess formation causes temperature elevation and lower abdominal and pelvic pain, and it may cause back pain. It is central rather than lateral discomfort, and a tender mass can be palpated above the vaginal apex. These women do not appear more ill clinically than women with pelvic cellulitis. In fact, they may have less symptomatology.

An abscess can also develop in an adnexa following surgery. Classically, adnexal abscesses do not develop during the initial hospitalization, but rather, occur 1 to 2 weeks after discharge from the hospital. The immediate postoperative course in women who develop this life-threatening infection is uncomplicated, as is the postoperative period at home until the abscess, which is almost always ovarian, ruptures about 18 days after the surgical procedure. Patients deteriorate quickly and require immediate stabilization and surgery. It is assumed that the genesis of this infection following hysterectomy is ovulation adjacent to the normal inflammatory response in the pelvis. The corpus luteum becomes a perfect culture medium for

TABLE 20–3.
Endocarditis Prophylaxis at Gynecologic Surgical Procedures

Antimicrobial	Dose
Ampicillin plus	2 gm intramuscularly or intravenously 30 min before procedure
Gentamicin	1.5 mg/kg intramuscularly or intravenously 30 min before procedure
Vancomycin (penicillin allergy)	1 gm slowly infused intravenously over 1 hr beginning 1 hr before procedure

the inoculated bacteria, which can be avoided by scheduling surgery just before anticipated ovulation in the ovulatory woman, and the adnexa should be as far away from the area of normal inflammatory response as possible. It is not just a break in ovarian integrity, because ovarian cystectomy at vaginal or abdominal hysterectomy is not a risk factor for infection.

Hematoma

An infected hematoma developing extraperitoneally above the vaginal cuff or in the lateral pelvis is an infection that has a relatively late onset during the hospital course or soon after discharge from the hospital. It is not associated with symptoms or abnormal physical findings in the majority of patients. Temperature elevation in a patient who has no symptoms, who has a normal abdominal examination, and who wants to go home is the common presentation when manifestation occurs before discharge. There is usually disparity between the patient's hemoglobin concentration and what it should be based on the preoperative hemoglobin concentration and the estimated blood loss during the surgical procedure. Pelvic examination should be performed, but it may not result in detection of a mass because of the soft consistency of the hematoma. Ultrasonography will identify these structures, and it is more cost effective than computed tomography (CT) or magnetic resonance imaging (MRI). Broad-spectrum antimicrobial therapy should be instituted, and drainage through the vagina should be performed if it can be done in a treatment room. If therapy is withheld, patients will eventually become symptomatic, and physical evidence of infection will become clinically apparent. When the infection develops after discharge from the hospital, a tender mass is usually palpable, and patients are symptomatic and febrile.

Abdominal Wall Infection

The diagnosis of abdominal incision infection is easier to make because of observational capability and the ability to more thoroughly evaluate the area. Erythema and tenderness at skin edges are usually associated with purulence in the incision, increasing pain, and temperature elevations that develop late on the third or fourth postoperative day. This infection may develop in conjunction with pelvic infection, or it may be the only infection that develops. The incidence of abdominal incision infection is significantly lower than pelvic infection after hysterectomy, and it is rarely observed after other procedures. Perioperative antimicrobials do not appear to alter the already low incidence of abdominal incision infection. Rather, mechanical factors seem to be more important in preventing wound infection. Shaving of the skin other than just before the procedure, occlusive drapes, excessive use of cautery, passive drains, and drains exiting through the incision all have been shown to be associated with an increased incidence of infection. Incision placement is also important; a transverse incision in the abdominal wall crease of a woman with a large panniculus will develop infection.

Drainage is the foundation of therapy for abdominal wall infections. Mechanical care with wet to dry dressing changes three times daily is usually sufficient, although parenteral antimicrobial therapy may be necessary. Fine mesh gauze stimulates fibroblastic proliferation and granulation tissue development and should be carefully applied to wound margins. It can be held against the margins with gauze, which should be moistened with sterile saline after dressing change. Its use with hydrogen peroxide or povidone-iodine before the next debridement will make removing the fine mesh gauze much less uncomfortable for the patient.

Hematoma or seroma formation in an abdominal incision may have the same impact on hospital stay because the incision separates. The tissue should be cultured, as should the purulent material in an infected incision. One must be certain that infection is not present before reclosure of such wounds. Many times the entire incision is not involved by a seroma or hematoma as is the case when clinical infection occurs.

PATHOGENS

The pelvic and abdominal incision infections that develop after hysterectomy are polymicrobial, as are the other occasional postoperative infections. Inoculation of the operative site occurs at vaginal transection. The fact that bacterial contamination occurs at the beginning of and throughout vaginal hysterectomy may explain why infection rates without prophylaxis are higher after that procedure. The contamination at abdominal hysterectomy occurs close to the end of the procedure, and the vaginal preparation agent has been in place until the vagina is entered. Contaminating bacteria are the normal flora of the lower reproductive tract; isolates recovered from pelvic and abdominal incision infection sites after hysterectomy in Parkland Memorial Hospital are presented in Table 20–4. A mean of four species is recovered from an infection site, and 60% of the isolates are aerobic. Sixty-five percent of those bacteria are gram-positive, and *E. faecalis* (enterococcus) accounts for almost one half. *Escherichia coli* is the predominant gram-negative aerobe (61%). *Proteus* and *Enterobacter* species account for about 17% each. *Peptostreptococcus* species comprise about one half of the anaerobic isolates, and *B. bivius* is the predominant gram-negative anaerobe recovered. *Bacteroides fragilis* group isolates are

TABLE 20–4.
Bacteria Recovered From Infection Sites After Gynecologic Surgical Procedures

Staphylococcus aureus
Staphylococcus epidermidis
Enterococcus faecalis
Streptococcus, group B
Escherichia coli
Enterobacter species
Klebsiella species
Proteus species
Pseudomonas species
Peptostreptococcus species
Clostridium species
Bacteroides species
Bacteroides fragilis group
Bacteroides bivius
Fusobacterium species

recovered from less than 5% of patients with postoperative pelvic-abdominal incision infection. A mixture of aerobic and anaerobic bacteria are isolated from most infection sites; aerobes only or anaerobes only may be recovered.

Antibiotic Therapy

A broad-spectrum therapeutic regimen is necessary to eradicate the majority of the important potential pathogens from operative site infections following gynecologic surgical procedures. Combination regimens are infrequently required for successful therapy of most postoperative infections not associated with abscess formation. Combination therapy has a greater likelihood of success when an abscess or infected hematoma is present. Frequently used empiric regimens are presented alphabetically in Table 20–5. Duration of antibiotic administration is not well established. Ten to 14 days of therapy were recommended at one time. In most instances, prolonged therapy has been proved to be unnecessary. Our practice is to administer parenteral antimicrobial until the patient without an abscess has been afebrile at least 24 hours. The parenteral antimicrobial is discontinued, and the patient is discharged without oral antimicrobial. If an abscess or infected hematoma is present, the parenteral regimen is administered until the patient has been afebrile for at least 48 hours. Prolonged administration invites suprainfection, induced resistance, toxic side effects, and allergic reaction. Stopping therapy too early, however, invites recurrence, so clinical evaluation is mandatory.

Controversy exists regarding the necessity to culture before therapy for postoperative pelvic infection, primarily because of the contamination potential. Care must be taken to disinfect the area through which the sample is obtained. A protected sample obtained from cephalad to the vaginal margin would identify the most likely pathogens of extraperitoneal cellulitis. Any intraperitoneal infection site cannot be cultured without risk for potentially significant morbidity. Culture of pu-

TABLE 20–5.
Commonly Used Therapeutic Regimens for Operative Site Infections After Gynecologic Surgical Procedures

Single-agent cephamycin/cephalosporin
Cefotetan
Cefoxitin
Cefotaxime
Ceftizoxime
Single-agent penicillin
Mezlocillin
Piperacillin
Ticarcillin
Penicillin/β-lactamase inhibitor
Ampicillin/sulbactam
Ticarcillin/clavulanic acid
Combination regimens
Clindamycin plus aminoglycoside (plus penicillin)
Metronidazole plus aminoglycoside (plus penicillin)

rulent material that is drained from a space will accurately identify pathogens present. A sterile needle and a glass syringe should be used whenever possible. The needle should be plugged with a rubber stopper after the air is expelled from the syringe. Air can diffuse through a thin film of pus on a swab, killing most anaerobes; certain plastics may oxidize aspirated material. To just culture the vaginal cuff will not predictably result in clinically useful information. Microbiologic information currently available is certainly more useful than what existed even 5 years ago. Anaerobic isolates were not reported by many laboratories. Later, species were identified, but sensitivity data were not provided. Now with automation, more and more laboratories are able to provide such data, but not for about 72 hours. If laboratories cannot provide suitable answers, there is certainly no need to perform cultures. When positive, blood cultures do yield invaluable information. The incidence of positive blood cultures accompanying postoperative infections in women undergoing gynecologic surgical procedures may be as high as 1%, certainly not high enough to justify routine blood culturing before parenteral antimicrobial therapy is initiated for all patients.

OTHER INFECTIONS

Necrotizing Soft Tissue Infection

Several very rare but devastating and potentially life-threatening infections can develop following elective gynecologic procedures. One such infection is necrotizing soft tissue infection. This infection can be divided into clostridial and nonclostridial or synergistic gangrene, and its location can be superficial or deep. The superficial infection of the skin and subcutaneous tissues does not involve the fascia. Clinical presentation is markedly different from clostridial infection that is associated with gas production, muscle involvement, and marked symptomatology. The latter requires immediate drainage and surgical removal of damaged tissue. Myonecrosis may develop in pelvic or abdominal wall muscles. Large doses of parenteral penicillin G are required to eradicate the organisms not surgically removed. The infection not associated with *Clostridium* species is a very slowly progressive infection caused by microaerophilic streptococci, Enterobacteriaceae, hemolytic streptococci, *S. aureus*, and other mixed bacteria. Early care is not sought by the patient because of the indolent nature of the infection.[7] Parenteral antimicrobial and resection are necessary for cure, however.

Necrotizing Fasciitis

Necrotizing fasciitis was named by a University of Texas Southwestern Medical Center/Parkland Memorial Hospital surgeon.[8] This rapidly progressive infection has been also referred to as β-hemolytic streptococcal gangrene, synergistic necrotizing cellulitis, gangrenous erysipelas, hospital gangrene, Meleney's gangrene, gram-negative anaerobic cutaneous gangrene, or nonclostridial gas gangrene. It has acute onset, and systemic involvement is apparent early. Predisposing factors include diabetes, arteriosclerotic heart disease, age more than 50 years, and debilitating disease of any type. Clinical clues as to its existence are the development of dermal blisters, ecchymotic areas, or both in an area of cellulitis or gas in the tissues (crepitus). Excessive edema exists beyond the area of apparent mild cellulitis. A thin gray fluid may seep through the skin, which slips over underlying tissue and does not bleed when cut. Superficial vessels become occluded, thereby depriving the area of oxygen and making it impossible to deliver antibiotics to the affected area. *Staphylococcus aureus*, Enterobacteriaceae, *E. faecalis*, hemolytic streptococci, *Bacteroides* species, *Peptostreptococcus* species, and *Fusobacterium* species have been recovered from tissues involved with this infection. They produce large quantities of proteolytic enzyme, which allow rapid spread to contiguous tissues along fascial planes. Even massive doses of multiple antibiotics are ineffective; only frequently disfiguring but life-saving surgical removal of affected areas and to tissues exhibiting vigorous bleeding will halt the progress and result in the cure of this infection. Broad-spectrum antimicrobial therapy should be administered preoperatively and continued until the area is covered with a good base of granulation tissue. This infection has been observed after abdominal hysterectomy,[9] tubal sterilization,[10] and around a suprapubic catheter.[11]

Septic Pelvic Thrombophlebitis

Septic pelvic thrombophlebitis very infrequently complicates a postoperative infection. The presentation that we observe is almost identical to that of a woman with an infected hematoma on the fourth postoperative day; she is asymptomatic and has a normal abdominal and pelvic examination but has a mild tachycardia and recurrent temperature elevations. The woman with phlebitis, however, has responded to and is still receiving parenteral antimicrobial therapy for a postoperative pelvic infection. Sonography does not detect a mass, and in most instances, CT scan does not detect thrombi. Perhaps this entity is just inflammatory phlebitis. Septic embolization is not observed. Altering the antibiotic regimen is not beneficial, but heparin administration results in normocardia and disappearance of temperature elevations. As little as 5,000 units every 8 hours may be effective. Drug fever is in the differential diagnosis; eosinophilia and a positive result of a direct Coombs test are commonly present with this rare complication of antimicrobial therapy in the asymptomatic, febrile patient who is clinically cured by antimicrobial therapy.

This presentation is quite dissimilar to presentations observed when this entity was initially described in the early 1950s, before the introduction of the excellent antibiotics that we now have available. Hectic alterations in temperature were observed in women who were clinically septic with headache, malaise, and chills. As septic embolization occurred, tachypnea, cough, and hemoptysis developed, and patients became anxious and restless. Chest x-ray films were abnormal in up to almost 50% of cases in some earlier reports when surgery was the only means of diagnosing this potentially fatal complication; mortality rate was about 50%. Diagnosis and therapy have changed from invasive surgery to noninvasive methods. The pelvic event is most accurately diagnosed by CT or MRI, and embolization is indicated by arterial blood gas determination and isotopic lung scan. Surgical ligation of the inferior vena cava and possibly the ovarian veins has been replaced by heparin therapy unless embolization occurs or persists after heparinization. Umbrella placement has replaced vena cava ligation in most instances.

Heparin therapy is not without the potential for sequelae. Careful attention must be given to dose and response as measured by the prothrombin time. If more heparin is required to achieve the same degree of anticoagulation, or if the platelet count falls, the white clot syndrome[12] should be suspected. Although it occurs in less than 1% of those given bovine or porcine heparin by any route, a 20% major limb amputation rate can result, and the mortality rate may be as high as 50%. Broad-spectrum antimicrobial therapy should be continued until the patient has been afebrile for at least 48 hours.

Toxic Shock Syndrome

One last potentially devastating syndrome should be discussed since it relates to postoperative infections, although it is not an infection in the strictest definition but a response to a toxin produced by *S. aureus*. That is the toxic shock syndrome. Clinical symptomatology, physical findings, and laboratory results of nonmenstrual-related toxic shock are identical to those observed in women with menstrual-related syndrome; the median interval between surgical procedure and onset of symptoms is about 2 days. Signs of wound infection are usually minimal, but wound cultures are positive for *S. aureus*. Patients with chronic nonhealing surgical incisions are at risk for late development of the syndrome; such has been reported up to 65 days after a surgical procedure.[13] Gynecologic surgical procedures that have been followed by toxic shock are presented in Table 20–6.[13]

Patients complain primarily of fever and malaise and have experienced diarrhea. Conjunctival and pharyngeal hyperemia without purulent exudate are present, and the tongue is “strawberry” or “raspberry.” There is a nonpainful and nonpruritic erythema of the skin that is more prominent over the trunk. Orthostatic hypotension or overt shock may be present, and the temperature reading is equal to or greater than 38.8°C. There are laboratory signs of poor organ system perfusion and leukocytosis with a left shift. A collaborative definition for severe toxic shock syndrome is presented in Table 20–7. One must have all major criteria and at least three minor criteria to meet criteria for the strict definition. Those who receive therapy early may not manifest the fully developed syndrome. Bacterial sepsis, scarlet fever, enterovirus infection, meningococcemia, measles, Rocky Mountain spotted fever, leptospirosis, and Stevens-Johnson syndrome must be ruled out.

Therapy for this response to staphylococcal toxin is supportive and must be initiated before other diagnoses have been excluded. The cornerstone of therapy is large volumes of IV fluid and electrolytes to replace losses through diarrhea, insensible loss, and capillary leakage to the interstitial space. Severe edema may result, representing the latter event rather than vascular volume overload. To differentiate and guide management, one must monitor central venous pressure and urinary out-

TABLE 20–6.

Gynecologic Surgical Procedures Following by Toxic Shock Syndrome

Tubal ligation
Ovarian cystectomy
Marshall-Marchetti-Krantz
Urethral suspension
Laparotomy
D&C
Hysterectomy
Laser vaporization of condyloma

TABLE 20–7.
Toxic Shock Syndrome: Definition Criteria*

- Major criteria
  - Temperature ≥ 38.8°C
  - Diffuse macular erythroderma
  - Late skin desquamation, particularly hand palms and soles of the feet (1–2 wk)
  - Hypotension
    - Orthostatic syncope
    - Systolic blood pressure <90 mm Hg for adults
- Minor criteria—organ system involvement
  - GI (vomiting or diarrhea)
  - Muscular (myalgia or CPK value > twice normal)
  - Mucous membrane involvement (conjunctival, oropharyngeal, vaginal)
  - Renal (BUN and creatinine values > twice normal or >5 WBCs/HPF without infection)
  - Hepatic (bilirubin, SGOT, SGPT levels > twice normal)
  - Hematologic (platelets <100,000/mm^3)
  - Central nervous system (disorientation or consciousness alteration without focal localizing signs)
- Negative results (if obtained)
  - Blood, CSF, and throat cultures
  - Serologic tests for measles, leptospirosis, Rocky Mountain spotted fever

*CPK = creatine phosphokinase; BUN = blood urea nitrogen; WBCs = white blood cells; HPF = high-power field; SGOT = serum glutamic oxaloacetic transaminase; SGPT = serum glutamic pyruvic transaminase; CSF = cerebrospinal fluid.

put. Dopamine administration may be necessary. A careful search must be made in incisions for the staphylococcal focus so that mechanical drainage can be accomplished and the toxin source eliminated. Antistaphylococcal antibiotic must also be administered and continued for perhaps up to 10 days. When it is administered early, there is evidence, albeit retrospective, that administration of corticosteroid significantly decreases the severity of and shortens the duration of the toxin-induced syndrome. In spite of appropriate resuscitation and management of the infected site, up to 5% of those with this syndrome are at risk for death, usually because of adult respiratory distress syndrome, disseminated intravascular coagulopathy, or unresponsive hypotension with myocardial failure.

SUMMARY

Fortunately, the infrequent postoperative infections that do develop after gynecologic surgery are not serious and respond promptly to the broad-spectrum anti microbials currently available. Gynecologists must be aware of risk factors in their patient population, and they must use antimicrobial prophylaxis as indicated. Antimicrobial therapy should not be initiated without operative site examination and a diagnosis that will be placed on the cover sheet of the patient's chart. Careful surveillance of response to therapy and awareness of devastating conditions will allow early diagnosis, appropriate therapy, and potential prevention of these rare postoperative infections and syndromes.

REFERENCES

1. Ad Hoc Committee of the Committee on Trauma, Division of Medical Sciences, National Academy of Sciences, National Research Council: Postoperative wound infections: The influence of ultraviolet irradiation of the operating room and of various other factors. *Ann Surg* 1964; 160(suppl):1–81.
2. Richardson AC, Lyon JB, Graham EE: Abdominal hysterectomy: Relationship between morbidity and surgical technique. *Am J Obstet Gynecol* 1973; 115:953–961.
3. Hemsell DL, Johnson ER, Hemsell PG, et al: Cefazolin for hysterectomy prophylaxis. *Obstet Gynecol* 1990; in press.
4. Hemsell DL, Cunningham FG, Kappus S, et al: Cefoxitin for prophylaxis in premenopausal women undergoing vaginal hysterectomy. *Obstet Gynecol* 1980; 56:629–634.
5. Hemsell DL, Reisch J, Nobles B, et al: Prevention of major infection after elective abdominal hysterectomy: Individual determination required. *Am J Obstet Gynecol* 1983; 147:520–528.
6. Van Scoy RE, Wilkowske CJ: Prophylactic use of antimicrobial agents in adult patients. *Mayo Clin Proc* 1987; 62:1137–1141.
7. Borkawf HI: Bacterial gangrene associated with pelvic surgery. *Clin Obstet Gynecol* 1973; 16:40–65.
8. Wilson B: Necrotizing fasciitis. *Am Surg* 1952; 18:416–431.
9. Henderson WM: Synergistic bacterial gangrene following abdominal hysterectomy. *Obstet Gynecol* 1977; 49(suppl):24–27.
10. Badendoch DF: Meleney's gangrene following sterilization by salpingectomy. *Br J Obstet Gynaecol* 1981; 88:1061–1062.
11. Bearman DM, Livengood CH III, Addison WA: Necrotizing fasciitis arising from a suprapubic catheter site. *J Reprod Med* 1988; 33:411–413.
12. Stanton PE Jr, Evans JR, Lefemine AA, et al: White clot syndrome. *South Med J* 1988; 81:616–620.
13. Petitti O, D'Agostino RB, Oldman MJ: Nonmenstrual toxic shock syndrome. *J Reprod Med* 1987; 32:10–16.

Chapter 21

Foreign Bodies Left Behind

Bruce H. Drukker, M.D.

Sponge and pad counts have been a ubiquitous part of surgery for years. Needle and instrument counts are new measures to assure quality in the surgical theater. The institution of these "counts" is mandated by the occasional foreign body inadvertently left behind at surgery and discovered surreptitiously at a later date. These accounts, although infrequent, continue to permeate the substance of our specialty and can lead to disturbing interventions on behalf of the patient, as well as obvious concerns for the provider of care (i.e., physicians, nursing personnel and hospitals). The purpose of this chapter is to review the implications of both purposeful and nonpurposeful foreign bodies that are left behind.

PURPOSEFUL PLACEMENT OF FOREIGN BODIES

In gynecologic surgery, a number of foreign bodies can deliberately be incorporated into a surgical field and left for a brief or extended period. In some situations, permanency of the foreign body is the goal.

Catheters and Drains

Short-term foreign bodies, that is, those left in place a few days to 2 to 3 weeks, include latex rubber or silicone catheters and latex rubber or silicone drains, generally with suction. These structures are left in situ with an external point of egress or access. The traditional rubber urinary drainage catheter (Foley, Malecot), although a foreign body, is rarely left behind for extended periods in gynecologic surgery. However, as a foreign body, they provide superb points of entrance for microorganisms to the urinary tract. Urinary tract infection is directly related to the duration of indwelling catheter use, location and its manipulation. Rubber catheters have been found as foreign bodies in the peritoneal cavity in gynecologic patients, usually as a complication of an illegal pregnancy termination. Silicone catheters are surmised to be less reactive but generally are fraught with the same types of problems associated with rubber catheters. Rubber and silicone catheters handled correctly do not break away or separate with a portion of the catheter left in the bladder. Thus, retained portions of these surgical appliances is uncommon. If they do break and a portion is left behind, they can easily be retrieved at cystoscopy.

The ureteral stent, another form of catheter, is left behind purposefully for 6 to 8 weeks. Stents can be placed by the more common percutaneous route or by retrograde insertion. Stents are generally used for situations related to ureteral injury, which may be due to vascular problems, trauma, or iatrogenic interference. Urinary extravasation and urinoma formation are not acceptable and must be drained. The stent will preserve renal function, prevent urinoma formation, and encourage healing.

If severe infection occurs and antibiotic therapy is not helpful, the stent must be removed to permit clearing of the problem. Replacement can then be considered.

T-shaped or straight drains have been used in gynecologic surgery for decades, initially with trepidation, then with selective uniformity, and presently with discretion. They have been irrigated or left to drain independently for a few days. They are then advanced for arbitrary distances and at arbitrary times until they have been removed. They should be considered as short-term foreign bodies. Currently the majority of drains are tubes or perforated flat devices attached to negative suction reservoirs. They are usually sewed in place until removal. Plain latex drains may initially be sewed in place with the classic safety pin on its outer end. As the drain is removed, the safety pin prevents the drain from moving back into its drainage track, truly a rather unusual occurrence. Drains can cause problems from a retention standpoint if they are trapped inadvertently by a suture, particularly a permanent suture. If suture entrapment occurs, one can wait a few days if absorbable suture is used and again attempt removal. Eventually the drain will move, and the problem will be resolved. On the other hand, if the operator knows permanent suture was used, there is no alternative other than reoperation and removal if a sharp tug does not remove the drain and it is visualized to be intact after removal. In general, the scrupulous gynecologic surgeon rarely has any difficulty with drains. Gore-Tex drainage systems thought to be quite inert should be handled in a similar fashion.

Meshes

Various forms of mesh are also purposefully left behind. Meshes can be nonpermanent, such as those made from polyglactin or polyglycolic acid. Permanent mesh used most commonly is knitted polypropylene. Polyglactin absorbable mesh has recently been considered a useful item to install at the pelvic brim for patients who may require radiation therapy to the pelvis, particularly following total abdominal hysterectomy and bilateral salpingo-oophorectomy for adenocarcinoma of the endometrium. Polypropylene mesh, on the other hand, usually has been used to repair extensive fascial defects or less frequently to support the urethrovesical junction in patients with recurrent and debilitating stress urinary incontinence. If the mesh erodes into the vagina, it can become infected, and removal would be necessary. Polypropylene mesh has also been used for retroperitoneal placement in sacrovaginal suspensions for extensive vaginal prolapse. In this instance, it is appropriate to be sure there is no continuity between the polypropylene or sutures used to place the mesh at the apex of the vagina and the vaginal epithelial mucous membrane. Should such point of access for vaginal microorganisms exist, a serious potential for infection and retroperitoneal abscess does exist.

Lyophilized dura mater has also been used for these suspensions. Tissue reactivity is minimal, and there have been few complications.

Gauze Packing

The use of gauze packing in abdominal gynecologic surgery purposefully placed and left behind with intent is extremely uncommon. It is usually associated with emergent situations related to hemostasis where all other means of control have failed. It is by far the least desirable means of obtaining vascular control. Not only does it require secondary intervention for removal, but it has a notoriously poor track record with respect to maintenance of a sterile environment. It is a perfect culture site, superbly bathed in tissue fluid, and microorganisms flourish. This technique should truly be identified as a last resort. It is in the realm of surgical heroics when all else fails.

On the other hand, long gauze packing strips are used with some frequency following both minor and major vaginal surgery. Again, the theory relates to pressure with concomitant hemostasis of small vessels not visualized at surgery or those on the edges of transected tissue planes that are anticipated to spontaneously coagulate and not be troublesome. Occasionally the patient's vascular physiologic verve exceeds these coagulation expectations. Hemostasis achieved by suture or electrocoagulation is superior to packing. Generally, vaginal packing, regardless of the configuration of the gauze, is removed within 24 hours. After this brief "locum tenens in vaginum" even the less discriminating physician can appreciate the unique culture resource for vaginal organisms provided by this foreign body. Olfactory sensations critically reinforce this observation. Vaginal packing should be avoided and not made a standard part of a particular vaginal surgical procedure. On the other hand, it can occasionally be used to solve a hemostasis problem. In these situations it should be used carefully, slightly moistened by a solution of normal saline and dilute povidone-iodine. Prophylactic antibiotics used appropriately and with increasing frequency with some major vaginal procedures may reduce egress of deleterious organisms into open tissue planes. However, the best treatment of vaginal packing is timely removal.

In my estimation, if the sun rises or sets twice on a pack, the subsequent problems of potential pelvic cellulitis or vaginal infection, regardless of antibiotics, are substantial. An exception relates to the necessity of vaginal packing associated with intravaginal and uterine intracavitary irradiation. Often this must be left in place for 48 to 72 hours. Since there are no open tissue planes during this procedure, serious infection is usually not a problem despite occasional vaginal mucosal abrasions that can occur during placement of the afterloading devices. Here again, moistening of the pack in a solution of normal saline and dilute povidone-iodine reduces to a degree bacterial growth. Symptoms developing are often subtle, with pelvic discomfort, pressure, and eventually pain and a febrile response. If any of these symptoms occur and do not respond to conservative treatment, removal is required.

Surgical Clips

Originally introduced by Harvey Cushing[1] and for years confined to intracranial procedures, surgical clips have been used with much more frequency following Samuel's introduction of metallic hemostatic clips in 1960.[2] In gynecologic surgery, metallic clips, both small and large, are frequently used for hemostasis in the abdomen, pelvis, omentum and retroperitoneal, periaortic, and pelvic areas.[3] These clips are also used for bowel anastomosis and maintenance of hemostatic control for some vessels, as well as in general surgical procedures on the stomach, pancreas, and biliary tract. The inert characteristics of the metal have led to no serious problems with infection. On the other hand, the clips have been known, on occasion, to migrate. Reports of deleterious effects of such migration in gynecologic patients are not available.

FOREIGN BODIES ACCIDENTALLY LEFT BEHIND

Fiber Products

Retained foreign bodies inadvertently left behind following gynecologic surgery are most frequently surgical sponges (gosypiboma), laparotomy pads, and occasionally towels. This does not occur with great frequency, and retention of towels is very infrequent. If the retained foreign body substance is small, often an aseptic granuloma will form, and the patient has little or no discomfort.[4] In other situations, particularly when the foreign substance is larger, adhesions may form, with subtle symptoms of partial intestinal obstruction. The patient may experience minimal to moderate abdominal cramping, change in stool pattern, and generalized lower abdominal discomfort. Occasionally a sponge may even be extruded via the gastrointestinal tract.

Other patients may develop symptoms of mild to moderate pelvic or abdominal inflammation. Fever, leukocytosis, point tenderness, and rebound all may be present. The patient may be able to localize pain or perceive an area of fullness. These symptoms herald the presence of a pelvic or abdominal intraperitoneal or retroperitoneal abscess secondary to infection of a foreign body.

The diagnosis of a retained fiber-containing foreign body can be difficult, often requiring traditional abdominal and pelvic radiographic assessment or ultrasound and computed tomography (CT). Diagnosis is particularly difficult if the foreign body has no radiopaque stripe or marker.

When plain radiographs are used, a whorl-like image may be produced, both for gauze with or without markers. This appearance is attributed to "gas" trapped in the fibers of the gauze. Unfortunately the whorl-like appearance of the foreign body is not uniformly encountered. In fact, it is quite infrequent. Thus, traditional radiographic imaging has not consistently aided in diagnosis.[5]

Ultrasound has also been used to demonstrate the presence of fiber-containing foreign bodies.[6] Sonographic imaging of sponges is intense, with sharply described acoustic imaging. This acoustic shadowing may be inappropriately large in the presence of air or calcifications within the foreign body. On occasion some masses may have an alternate sonographic characteristic, with markedly diffuse and irregular internal echoes. Unfortunately this is a rather nondescript and nonspecific appearance. Ultrasonography appears to assist definitely with diagnosis of a foreign body in less than 50% of patients with a retained fiber-containing foreign body.

Computed tomography appears to be the most useful tool for diagnosis of the fiber-containing foreign body. In most studies, CT scans image well-demarcated round or oval masses. Imaging characteristics most commonly were low density (approximating water or between water and blood). Low and medium complex masses (blood attenuation) have also been identified. High-density masses (greater than liver attenuation) have also been noted, but infrequently. Occasionally focal peripheral or central calcification is noted, or gas bubbles can be seen. The use of intravenous contrast material at time of CT is particularly helpful since it can create an image enhancement at the periphery of the fiber foreign body. On occasion, but with considerably less frequence, the inner component of the mass will image as enhanced. Apparently the longer a fiber-containing foreign body remains in place, the greater the frequency of calcification. This has been documented in unusual situations, as when a diagnosis was made on CT but the patient refused operative intervention and remained asymptomatic. A repeat CT subsequently in approximately 6 to 12 months demonstrated new calcifications in the identified mass.

If a fiber-containing foreign body (sponge, laparotomy pad, or towel) is identified, it should be removed regardless of absence of symptoms. At the time of surgery, adhesions should be anticipated. Bowel preparation also is important to permit complete surgical extirpation of the foreign body with completion of any indicated bowel surgery at that time. Following removal of the foreign body, the area should be copiously irrigated before closure of retroperitoneal and peritoneal spaces. There are no strict guidelines for drainage, but if the area of removal is clean and there is no abscess formation, routine drainage does not appear to be indicated.

Metal Products

Inadvertent retention of metallic surgical instruments such as clamps or scissors is infrequent (Fig 21–1). The current concept of operative instrument counts will virtually eliminate this problem. If any instrument is left behind, symptoms are not usually those of infection or abscess formation. In fact, patients may be asymptomatic or may have minimal vague abdominal pains.[7] Interestingly, these pains, however, may be accentuated by certain postural changes, such as bending forward or backward. One has to have a very high degree of suspicion to make this diagnosis, which is verified by an abdominal or pelvic radiograph. In all situations, surgical removal is mandated.

Surgical needles are an additional problem. They can break, be misplaced, or fly off the needle holder. This occurs particularly when it is being returned to the person passing instruments. A broken needle with a small portion missing may be very difficult to locate with or without radiographs or magnets. If it is a small piece (<1 cm) and cannot be located, it is better to leave it in place than to create a large amount of surgical morbidity with blind dissection. The metal can be treated like a retained clip with minimal anticipated difficulty. The patient should be informed of the situation and advised of the rationale for the decision not to pursue a small fragment. On the other hand, a complete needle should be sought using all routine means and only as a last resort allowed to remain in the pelvic or abdominal cavity, as might occur rarely when a tiny microsurgical needle has been lost and cannot be retrieved even though it can be visualized on a radiograph.

Despite counts of sponges, laparotomy pads, needles, and instruments, a few surgeons still consider a routine plain abdominal and pelvic radiograph as standard procedure in the surgical suite when closure has been completed and before transfer to the postoperative recovery area.[8]

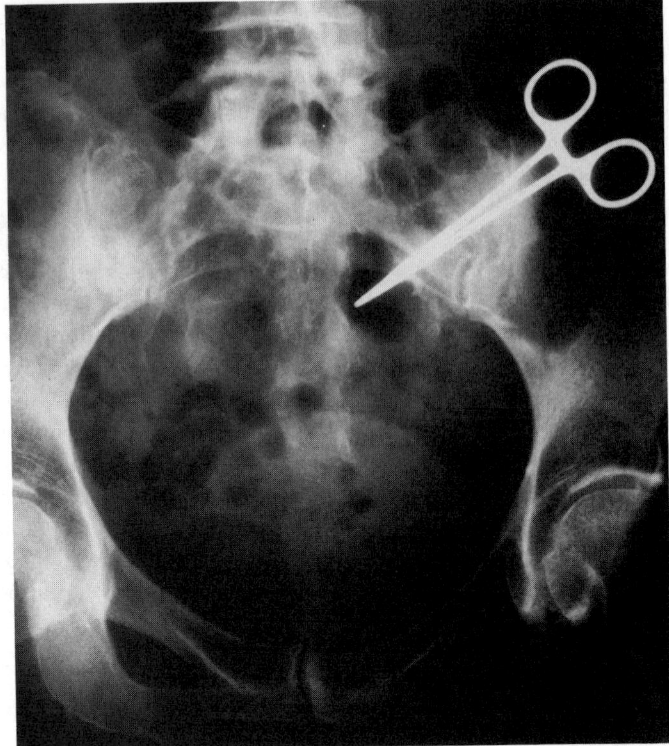

FIG 21–1.
Hemostat inadvertently left in place during major gynecologic surgery. Removal required a second surgical procedure.

SUMMARY

Foreign bodies purposefully left behind should not be a problem. Those placed on a temporary basis should be removed within the anticipated prescribed time. Those left on a permanent basis must be removed if they become infected or are in other ways deleterious.

On the other hand, foreign bodies noted in an abdominal or pelvic location that were inadvertently left behind should be removed if they are deemed of concern. These include all items except a small portion of needle, which should be innocuous. Before and after removal of such items, careful explanation to the patient is mandatory.

REFERENCES

1. Cushing H: The control of bleeding in operations for brain tumors with the description of silver "clips" for the occlusion of vessels inaccessible to the ligature. *Ann Surg* 1911; 54:1–19.
2. Samuels PB, Roedling H, Katz R, Cincotti JJ: A new hemostatic clip: Two year review of 1007 cases. *Ann Surg* 1966; 163:427–431.
3. Morgenstern L: Surgical shrapnel. *Am J Surg* 1982; 144:597–598.
4. Kokubo T, Itai Y, Ohtomo K, et al: Retained surgical sponges: CT and US appearance. *Radiology* 1987; 165:415–418.

5. Olnick HM, Weens HS, Rogers JV Jr: Radiologic diagnosis of retained surgical sponges. *JAMA* 1955; 159:1525–1527.
6. Chau W, Lai K, Lo K: Sonographic findings of intra abdominal foreign bodies due to retained gauze. *Gastrointest Radiol* 1984; 9:61–63.
7. Morrison L, Homesley H: Carcinoma of the cervix complicated by a soup spoon. *Obstet Gynecol* 1978; 51(suppl 1):55–65.
8. Jones S: The foreign body problems after laparotomy. *Am J Surg* 1971; 122:785–786.

Chapter 22

The Recurrent Small and Painful Vagina

David H. Nichols, M.D.

Few things are as annoying to the patient and disquieting to her surgeon as a finding that the patient's vagina is too small postoperatively for coital comfort. If the vaginal wall retains some elasticity and the patient is optimistically confident and prepared to invest some time in its mechanical enlargement, the vagina may be stretched by frequent coitus or the wearing of graduated dilators. The latter should first achieve depth and may then be replaced by progressively wider obturators to increase width. This process requires from 3 to 9 months of sustained effort in which the dilator is generally worn for a minimum of 2 hours daily. If desired, the time may be divided between morning and evening. If, on the other hand, the patient is uncomfortable with this approach, surgical relief should be promptly considered.

If the vagina is inelastic, supplemental estrogen, especially by the vaginal route, may restore both elasticity and blood supply. A proper dose of estrogen cream for most patients would be the vaginal installation of 1 to 2 gm at bedtime two or three times each week. After 2 or 3 months, if elasticity is preserved, the dosage may be reduced to 1 or 2 gm once each week but must be continued indefinitely.

VULVAR VESTIBULAR SYNDROME

Another cause of coital discomfort is the vulvar vestibular syndrome. This syndrome should be recognized by the characteristic history of sudden onset, dyspareunia, and difficulty inserting a vaginal tampon, often in a patient who has been taking birth control pills. Point tenderness limited to the area of the vestibule can be demonstrated by mapping the area with a Q-tip. There is usually an accompanying vestibular erythema without coincident vaginitis or purulent discharge. There may be a focal inflammatory process, occasionally with small ulcers. The lesions are best visualized through a magnifying glass, and most are in the posterior portion or the fourchette, though they may be found less commonly in the vestibular tissues lateral to the urethra. Almost all patients are white (see Chapter 18).

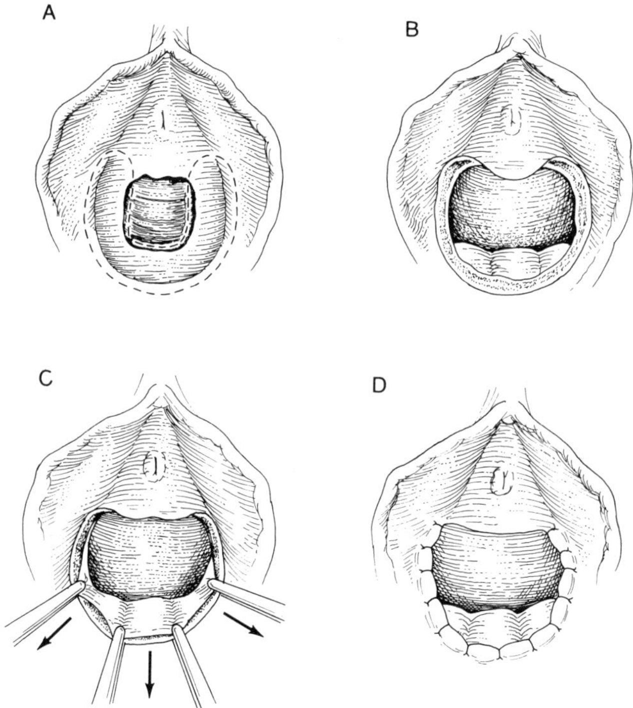

FIG 22–1.
Vestibulectomy. **A,** the painful area of vestibular epithelium is carefully demarcated preoperatively, the subepithelial tissues infiltrated by a liquid tourniquet (0.5% lidocaine in 1:200,000 epinephrine), and an incision made *(dashed line).* **B,** the appearance after this excision. The posterior vaginal wall is undermined and mobilized, **C,** so that its edge may be sewn to the residual perineal skin, **D.** (Redrawn from Nichols DH, Randall CL: *Vaginal Surgery,* ed 3. Baltimore, Williams & Wilkins Co, 1989.)

Nonspecific management includes discontinuance of oral contraceptives and the application of a 4% topical aqueous lidocaine (Xylocaine) solution for 5 minutes three or four times daily. In perhaps one third of instances, this program appears to be curative, and after some 6 months of therapy, no additional treatment may be necessary. For those in whom it is not curative, a surgical vulvar vestibulectomy and vestibuloplasty are required, which are best done in the hospital under anesthesia. All of the areas of painful tenderness in the vestibule are excised. The posterior vaginal wall is mobilized cranially for a distance of 3 cm, then sewn to the cut edge of the remaining perineal skin (Fig 22–1). The procedure seems to produce long-lasting results superior to the use of laser vaporization. If additional areas of vulvar vestibular syndrome develop in the future, the treatment can be repeated as necessary.

INTROITAL STRICTURE

A mechanical stricture of the introital perineum may be remedied by a midline perineotomy closed transversely. One should remember that this will shorten a vagina by an amount equal to half of the length of the incision. The proper length of

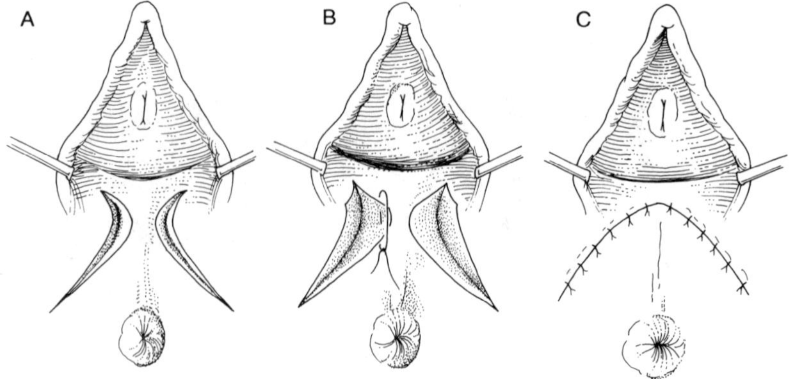

FIG 22–2.
Bilateral perineoplasty is performed to enlarge a constricted outlet in a patient with an already shortened vagina. Bilateral incisions are made, **A.** They are closed with interrupted sutures, **B.** Notice that in the end result, **C,** point *a* is no longer adjacent to point *b,* enlarging the outlet by two times the distance between the *a* and *b.* (Redrawn from Nichols DH, Randall CL: *Vaginal Surgery,* ed 3. Baltimore, Williams & Wilkins Co, 1989.)

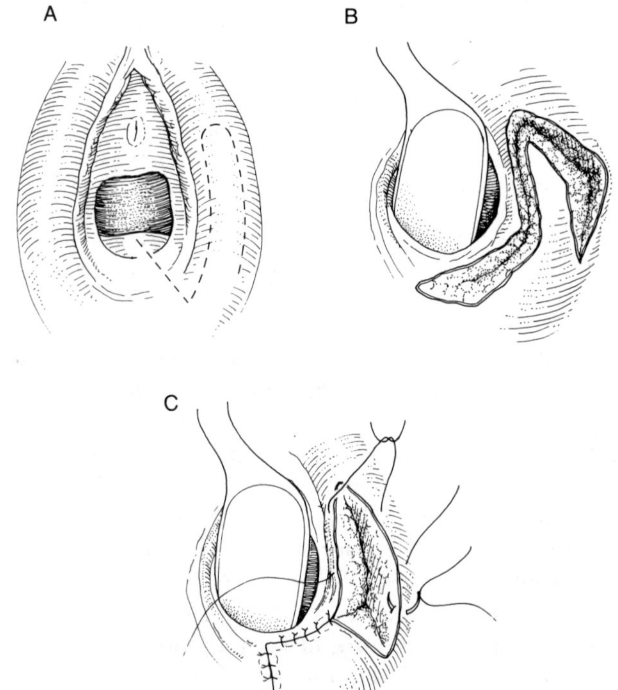

FIG 22–3.
Labial cutaneous graft. The tissues are thoroughly infiltrated by a liquid tourniquet, and an incision made as shown by the *dashed line* **(A).** This is made through the full thickness of the skin and the underlying connective tissue **(B).** The flap is undermined and swung into the defect created by the perineotomy, then fixed in place by a few interrupted sutures **(C).** The labial defect is closed. Notice the transposition of the tissue *(a).* (Redrawn from Nichols DH, Randall CL: *Vaginal Surgery,* ed 3. Baltimore, Williams & Wilkins Co, 1989.)

an adult vagina for a sexually active woman is relative, however. From a functional point of view, it should be of sufficient length to contain the sexual partner's phallus during coitus. For preserving an already compromised vaginal depth, a Z-plasty flap is helpful.

For the postvulvectomy patient with introital stricture, the bilateral episiotomy is most effective (Fig 22–2). When this is not feasible, a fibroepithelial flap rotation is useful (Fig 22–3). Although the latter may include the risk of including some of the vulvar hair-bearing area from the labia majora in the transplanted flap, the risk of troublesome hair growth in the vagina is negligible. The hair usually undergoes subsequent atrophy. In a patient requiring still more vulvar space, swinging of a flap from the medial thigh is useful. One should try to keep the length of the flap no more than one and one half times the width to lessen the risk of compromising its distal blood supply and producing subsequent necrosis.

MIDVAGINAL STRICTURE

For the patient with midvaginal stricture observed either at the completion of a colporrhaphy or at some future postoperative time, lateral relaxing incisions through the full thickness of the vaginal at the 3 or 9 o'clock position (or both) may salvage the situation (Fig 22–4). The incisions are best made under anesthesia in the operating room. Infiltration at the site of incision with 20 mL of 0.5% lidocaine

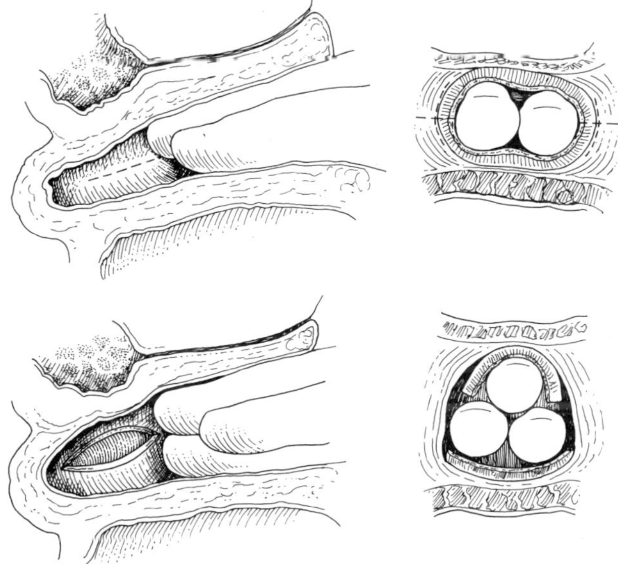

FIG 22–4.
Digital examination discloses a midvaginal stricture as noted in the upper drawings in which the vagina will admit but two fingerwidths. An incision is made along through the full thickness of the lateral vaginal wall at the 3 and usually 9 o'clock positions and the vagina undermined for about 1 cm in each direction, so that the caliber will admit three fingerbreadths comfortably. It should be kept open by frequent wearing of an obturator during the healing process until reepithelialization has begun. (Redrawn from Nichols DH, Randall CL: *Vaginal Surgery,* ed 3. Baltimore, Williams & Wilkins Co, 1989.)

with 1:200,000 epinephrine will produce a liquid tourniquet. Bleeding points may be coagulated or ligated, but the incisional edges need not be stitched. The patient must wear a postoperative vaginal obturator until a firm base of granulation tissue has been established. If a conventional plastic or glass obturator is not available, one may use the barrel of a disposable plastic 60-cc conventional syringe or an Asepto syringe from which the projecting distal nipple has been removed. The ob-

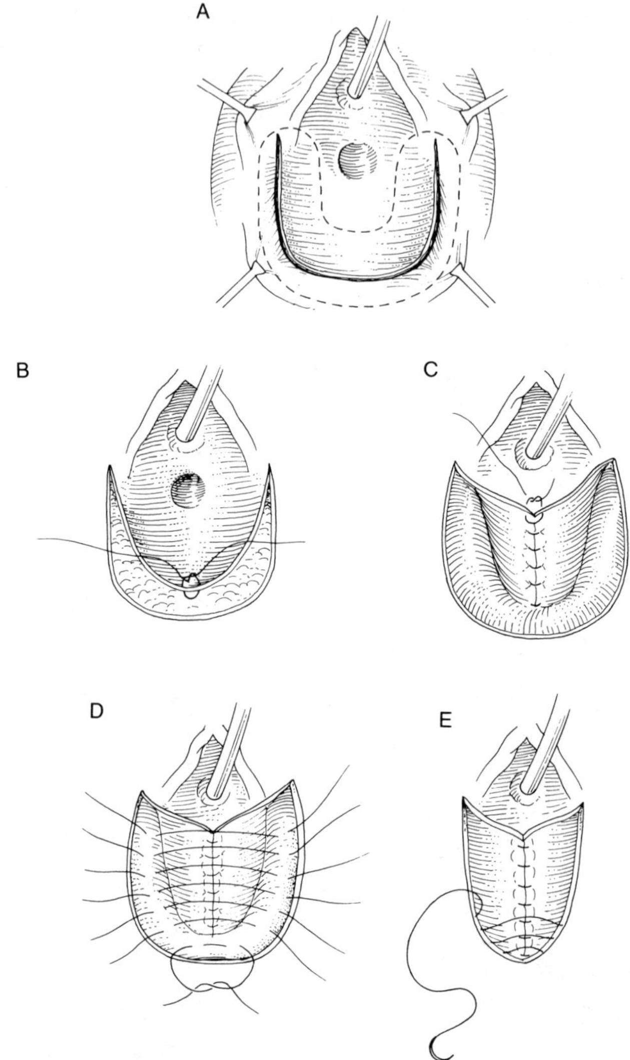

FIG 22–5.
Williams vestibuloplasty. After the subepithelial tissues have been thoroughly infiltrated by a liquid tourniquet, a U-shaped incision beginning approximately 4 cm lateral to the external urethral orifice is made **(A),** and the tissues are undermined *(dashed line).* The edges of the new vaginal pouch are brought together by interrupted stitches **(B),** placed so that the knots are tied inside of the pouch. This is continued until the level of the anterior hymenal site is reached **(C).** A second layer of interrupted stitches brings the subepithelial tissue together, and a modest perineorrhaphy may be added **(D).** The skin of the perineum is closed from side to side by a running subepithelial stitch **(E).** (Redrawn from Nichols DH, Randall CL: *Vaginal Surgery,* ed 3. Baltimore, Williams & Wilkins Co, 1989.)

turator, which should be taken in and out frequently, should be lubricated with an estrogen cream.

When the vagina appears to be of adequate diameter but is too short for coitus, depth may be added at the distal end with a Williams vulvovaginoplasty (Figs 22–5 and 22–6). When the patient is sexually active, or by the use of progressively longer obturators if she is not, the depth of the vagina can be progressively increased, and a gradual change to a more normal axis brought about. With time and sustained sexual use, the normal vaginal depth and axis can be approximated.

The construction of a neovagina by the Abbe-Wharton-McIndoe operation is a particularly useful procedure (Fig 22–7). The patient must, however, wear an obturator postoperatively to guard against scarring and contraction, which would subsequently diminish vaginal width. When from one reason or another the vagina is massively fibrosed and undilatable, usually as the result of previous surgery, a vaginectomy can be performed (Fig 22–8) followed by placement of a split-thickness skin graft to line the cavity of the fresh deep wound.

One or two rectangles of donor skin 0.0019-in. thick and large enough to cover the outside of the obturator are harvested from the buttock (from an area generally covered by the patient's undergarments), from the medial surface of the thigh, or from the suprapubic area. Xeroform dressing is placed over the donor site and is removed only when the process of healing has separated it, usually after 2 to 3 weeks, from the surface of the new skin.

For the patient in whom a donor site is unacceptable, human amnion from a recent but sterile cesarean section may be used provided that the donor mother has been tested negative for HIV. The chorion is separated from the amnion and discarded. The amnion is placed mesenchymal side out over a condom-covered sponge rubber or urethane foam obturator.

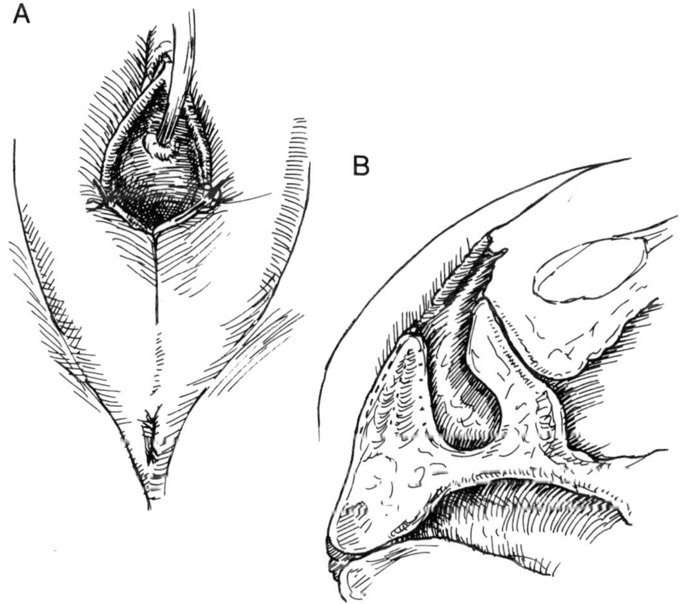

FIG 22–6.
Vulvovestibuloplasty at the completion of the operation **(A)** and in sagittal section **(B).** (Redrawn from Capraro VJ, Capraro EJ: *Obstet Gynecol* 1972; 39:544.)

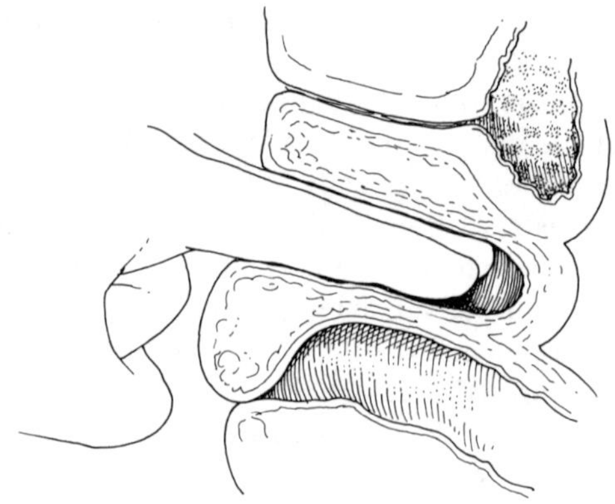

FIG 22–7.
The newly created tunnel of the neovagina in sagittal section with the operator's fingers demonstrating its depth and axis. An obturator covered by split-thickness skin or amnion can now be inserted. (Redrawn from Nichols DH, Randall CL: *Vaginal Surgery,* ed 3. Baltimore, Williams & Wilkins Co, 1989.)

When adequate hemostasis has been obtained, the obturator is placed into the newly created vaginal cavity. It may be secured either by temporarily sewing together the labia over the obturator with several interrupted large sutures or, in the case of a skin graft, by tacking the free edge of the graft to the epithelium of the new introitus and the labia majora loosely stitched together to hold the obturator in place.

The bladder may be drained by a suprapubic catheter to reduce the remote possibility of pressure necrosis of the urethra with subsequent fistula formation. In 5 to 7 days, the labial stitches are cut, and the soft obturator is replaced by a firm mold fashioned from balsa wood or preformed plastic. For the first 6 months, the mold should be removed only during voiding or defecation. After that, it should be

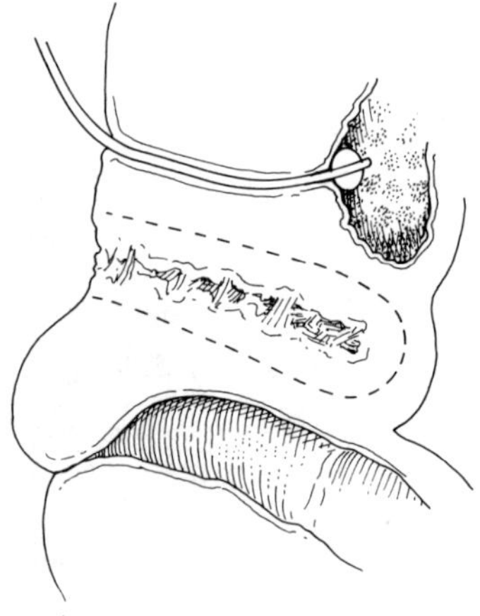

FIG 22–8.
A massively scarred vagina in sagittal section. The entire vagina and much of the scar tissue are excised by sharp dissection along the planes *(dashed line),* starting laterally on each side, then posteriorly, and finally anteriorly beneath the urethra and bladder. A suitably covered obturator will be placed in the new tunnel. (Redrawn from Nichols DH, Randall CL: *Vaginal Surgery,* ed 3. Baltimore, Williams & Wilkins Co, 1989.)

worn regularly at night for several months and, thereafter, periodically inserted to assure maintenance of a vagina of adequate size. If discomfort is noted, the obturator should be worn again daily until no longer uncomfortable or until there is again no discomfort with its insertion.

When amnion has been used to cover the initial obturator, it is removed on the fifth or sixth postoperative day, and the obturator is washed and covered with a new layer of fresh amnion. Although it is not essential to line the newly created cavity by either a graft or amnion since a bed of granulation that forms will ultimately become epithelialized, but choosing not to do so requires the patient to endure additional months of a chronic blood-tinged discharge during the prolonged healing phase.

For the patient unable or unwilling to wear the postoperative obturator, another alternate surgical choice exists in the use of transplantation of a loop of sigmoid colon to the top of the vagina. This double operation requires a transabdominal bowel resection and anastomosis, however, and the patient must be prepared to accept the additional surgical risks involved. A two-team approach in this procedure will save much operating time. One team works from the perineal side during the procedure and the other from the abdominal side.

POSTCOITAL CYSTITIS

An occasional patient will demonstrate repetitive postcoital cystitis. In many instances, the gynecologist may observe that during pelvic examination the external urethral meatus is drawn into the vagina with vaginal penetration. Paraurethral hymenectomy is often a simple solution to this problem (Fig 22–9). Coincident perineotomy may be added if the introitus is too tight for comfort.

PHYSICAL EXAMINATION

When a patient experiences postoperative vaginal pain and tenderness, particularly after standing for a while, the surgeon should examine her carefully for the presence of a previously undiagnosed eversion of the upper vaginal vault. She may complain that the discomfort grows worse as the day progresses and is relieved by lying down. Consequently, the defect is best demonstrated when the patient is examined while standing and bearing down in a Valsalva maneuver. Similar symptoms may occur when the patient has a previously undiagnosed enterocele or a defect in the supports of the anterior vaginal wall. The latter may present as a cystocele, either anterior or posterior, or occasionally result from a lateral or paravaginal defect (see Chapter 6).

Painful ridges may sometimes be found beneath the posterior vaginal wall, usually the result of fibrosis from stitches that were placed directly into the belly of the levator muscle. Although these ridges can sometimes be gently stretched, they usually will require surgical incision to produce more effective relief.

Posthysterectomy dyspareunia will occasionally be seen as a consequence of fixation of the ovary to the vaginal vault. When conservative management with suppression of ovarian function as by oral contraceptives for a few months fails to provide relief, the treatment becomes surgical. The ovaries must be freed from the

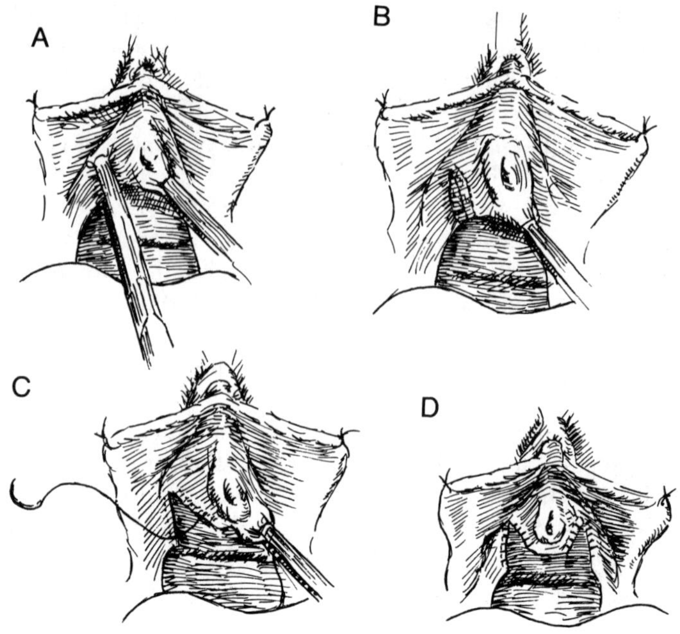

FIG 22–9.
Paraurethral hymenotomy in which a crushing hemostat is applied lateral to the external urethral meatus **(A).** An incision is made along this crushed area **(B),** and the cut edges are approximated by a running suture **(C).** End result **(D).** (Redrawn from Wood C, The Mason Clinic, Seattle, Wash.)

vault of the vagina and suspended to a higher position along the lateral pelvic side walls if they are still functional or removed if they are not.

An occasional patient will be the victim of a situation of psychosexual stress reflected as a psychosomatic vaginal discomfort. This patient will usually divulge a history of long-standing marital distress and interpersonal marital discomfort. She may be anorgasmic. Such persons are often reluctant to consider this etiology, and obtaining consultation with a psychiatrist or psychologist sympathetic to the patient's difficulties is highly recommended.

For the patient with otherwise unexplained chronic vaginal pain, often described as a stabbing or pulling sensation, one must exclude by appropriate examination the possibility of peritoneal herniation. An obturator hernia, for example, by internal pressures against the obturator nerve may provoke some referred pain to the thigh and knee (Howship-Romberg sign), which is intermittent and sometimes accompanied by abdominal pain. Occasionally when a patient complains of pain in the levator ani, examination will reveal significant tenderness in this muscle, resulting from sustained spasm in the pubococcygeus. Relief may be sought by massage of the pubococcygeus, local injections of cortisone and an anesthetic into the muscle itself, and daily heat to the area by warm douching or ultrasound. Occasionally, muscle relaxants are helpful. This so-called levator syndrome can be at times most difficult to treat because it tends toward chronicity as a vicious cycle of discomfort and spasm becomes established.

A palpable and painful neuroma rarely may develop beneath the posterior vaginal wall at the site of a previous episiotomy or posterior colporrhaphy. Its contribution to vaginal pain may be identified by the relief provided with anesthetic infiltration. The treatment is surgical excision.

For the postmenopausal patient with vaginal atrophy and loss of elasticity, long-term estrogen supplementation is useful, particularly by the transvaginal route with an estrogen cream. Gentle coital dilation with adequate lubrication can result in progressively increasing comfort.

EVERTED SHORTENED VAGINA

One will occasionally encounter the multioperated patient with total eversion of a shortened vagina. This vaginal may be too short to reach the sacrospinous ligament when reposited into the pelvis. There are several surgical treatment alternatives from which to choose:

1. Sacrospinous colpopexy may be performed using deliberate suture bridges of nonabsorbable synthetic monofilament material, such as polypropylene (Prolene, Surgilene) or polytef (Gore-Tex). If the labia are of sufficient size, a Williams vulvovaginoplasty may be added as an additional procedure to provide a supplemental distal vaginal depth of 4 to 5 cm.
2. Transabdominal sacrocolpopexy may be performed using an intermediate bridge of fascia lata or of a synthetic plastic material.
3. Ingram-Frank dilators lubricated with estrogen cream may be used to lengthen the vagina over a period of months until it will reach the sacrospinous ligament, at which time sacrospinous colpopexy may be performed.

BIBLIOGRAPHY

Berek JS, Hacker NF, Lagasse LD, et al: Delayed vaginal reconstruction in the fibrotic pelvis following radiation or previous reconstruction. *Obstet Gynecol* 1983; 61:743–748.

DiSaia PJ, Rettenmaier MA: Vaginectomy, in Sanz LE (ed): *Gynecologic Surgery.* Oradell, NJ, Med Economics Co, 1988, pp 151–157.

Feroze RM, Dewhurst CJ, Welply G: Vaginoplasty at the Chelsea Hospital for Women: A comparison of two techniques. *Br J Obstet Gynaecol* 1975; 82:536.

Goligher JC: The use of pedicled transplants of sigmoid or other parts of the intestinal tract for vaginal reconstruction. *Ann R Coll Surg Engl* 1983; 65:353–355.

Ingram JM: The bicycle seat in the treatment of vaginal agenesis and stenosis: A preliminary report. *Am J Obstet Gynecol* 1981; 140:807.

Morton KE, Davies D, Dewhurst J: The use of the fasciocutaneous flap in vaginal reconstruction. *Br J Obstet Gynaecol* 1986; 93:970–973.

Ober KG, Meinrenken GH: Allgemeine und spezielle chirurgische operationslehre, in Krischner M: *Gynäkologische Operationen.* Berlin, Springer, 1964. Quoted in Käser O, Iklé FA, Hirsch HA: *Atlas of Gynecological Surgery,* ed 2. New York, Georg Thieme Verlag, 1985.

Pratt JH: Use of the colon in gynecologic surgery, in Sturgis SH, Taymor ML (eds): *Meigs and Sturgis Progress in Gynecology*. Orlando, Fla, Grune & Stratton. 1970, vol V. pp 435–446.

Tancer ML, Katz M, Veridiano NP: Vaginal epithelialization with human amnion. *Obstet Gynecol* 1979; 54:345–349.

Williams EA: Congenital absence of the vagina: A simple operation for its relief. *J Obstet Gynaecol Br Commonw* 1964; 71:511.

Chapter 23

Ovarian Remnant and Residual Ovary Syndromes

Giglia A. Parker, M.D.

Among the interesting benign ovarian syndromes that can result in the need for reoperation after previous gynecologic surgery are the ovarian remnant syndrome, the residual ovary (adnexal) syndrome, accessory ovary, and supernumerary ovary. This chapter deals with the first two in some detail. The latter two are rare findings but need to be discussed briefly to differentiate them from the former.

Accessory ovary and supernumerary ovary both refer to ectopic ovarian tissue. In the case of accessory ovary, the ovarian tissue is located in close proximity to the normally placed ovary. It is usually attached to the broad ligament and is often connected to the normal ovary. In fact, the ectopic accessory ovary may actually have arisen when a small portion of ovarian tissue split off from the developing ovarian primordium.

A supernumerary ovary, on the other hand, is entirely separate from the normally placed ovary. The clearest cases are those in which the supernumerary ovary lies in the retroperitoneal region.[1] The ectopic ovarian tissue may be found in the omentum or in the mesentery of the bowel. It may have arisen as a result of arrested embryologic migration of germ cells en route from the yolk sac to the genital ridges or from detachment and transplant of a portion of the ovarian primordium from the genital ridge to the dorsal mesentery.[2] In either case, the supernumerary ovary would have arisen separately from the anlage of the normally placed ovary and would probably have a different blood supply. Since it would have arisen as a result of developmental abnormality, one should not be surprised to find other associated genitourinary anomalies. Renal and ureteral agenesis, bladder diverticulum, accessory fallopian tube, and müllerian fusion defects such as unicornuate, bicornuate, or septate uterus all have been found in association with a supernumerary ovary.[1]

The residual ovary syndrome, sometimes called residual adnexal syndrome, results when ovaries conserved at the time of hysterectomy subsequently become diseased. In the ovarian remnant syndrome, on the other hand, both ovaries have been previously removed.

Confusion between the residual ovary syndrome and the ovarian remnant syndrome and between the accessory ovary and supernumerary ovary arises because of the similarity of the names. Supernumerary ovary, although it is an extremely rare gynecologic condition, deserves mention in the context of the residual ovary syndrome and the ovarian remnant syndrome because it may present in a manner that mimics either. A supernumerary ovary may become symptomatic or develop neoplasia, leading to its diagnosis when there has been no previous gynecologic disease. However, if there has been a prior hysterectomy at which time the supernumerary was not discovered, the surgeon is more likely to consider a subsequent ovarian problem to lie in a residual ovary rather than in a supernumerary ovary. On the other hand, if previous bilateral oophorectomy has been performed, subsequent evidence of ovarian function will probably lead the gynecologist to suspect the presence of an ovarian remnant, but the possibility of a supernumerary ovary should not be forgotten.

Although the astute gynecologist should, therefore, be attuned to the differences in these uncommon entities, confusion on occasion is understandable. Indeed, in his classic discussion of supernumerary ovary, the first case Wharton[1] presents may be an example of ovarian remnant syndrome developing at the sites of two previously removed supernumerary ovaries.

OVARIAN REMNANT SYNDROME

Case History

B.B.W., a 42-year-old black woman, para 1,001, status post–left salpingooophorectomy for an ovarian cyst and subsequent total abdominal hysterectomy and right salpingo-oophorectomy at the time of intraperitoneal hemorrhage from a ruptured ovarian cyst, presented complaining of right pelvic pain of several months' duration. The pain was constant but with periodic severe exacerbations. Severe dyspareunia made coitus extremely difficult. The patient also gave a history of multiple episodes of pelvic inflammatory disease, and at the time of hysterectomy, extensive pelvic adhesions were noted.

Physical examination revealed a tender cystic mass in the right lower quadrant. Pelvic ultrasonogram confirmed a 3 by 4 cm cystic mass in the right pelvis (Fig 23–1). Serum follicle-stimulating hormone (FSH) level was 7.6 mIU/mL (postmenopausal normal level is 35–151 mIU/mL), serum luteinizing hormone (LH) level was 2.2 mIU/mL (postmenopausal normal level is 11–61 mIU/mL), and serum estradiol level was 186 pg/mL (postmenopausal normal level is 5–18 pg/mL).

At exploratory laparotomy a 4 by 3 cm multicystic mass was found densely adherent to the right pelvic side wall and ureter (Fig 23–2). After lysis of extensive abdominal and pelvic adhesions, retroperitoneal dissection with removal of the peritoneum of the right pelvic side wall, including the mass and remnants of the round and broad ligaments, was accomplished. A similar dissection was carried out on the left side of the pelvis.

The pathologic examination of the cystic mass revealed ovarian tissue with a corpus luteum, multiple corpora albicantia, and ovarian stroma. Six weeks after surgery, the patient had an FSH level of 61.2 mIU/mL, an LH level of 18.7 mIU/mL, and an estradiol level of less than 10 pg/mL.

Etiology

The patient just described represents a case of the ovarian remnant syndrome. Although first reported as a cause of ureteral obstruction by Kaufman in 1962,[3] the problem probably dates into the last century. In 1875, prior to the common performance of hysterectomy, Goodman noted that women occasionally continued to

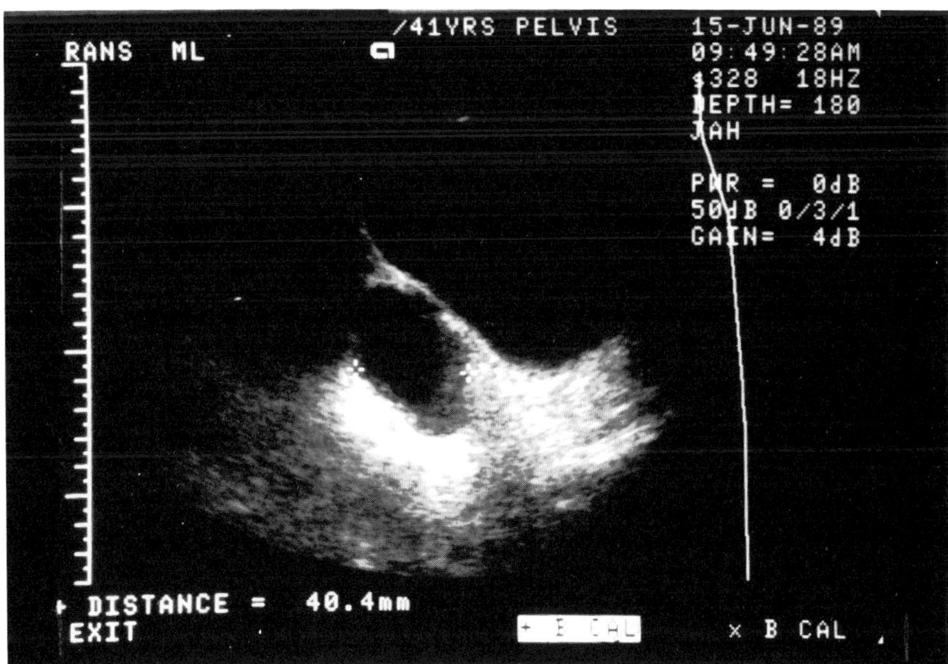

FIG 23–1.
Preoperative pelvic ultrasonogram of 3 by 4 cm cystic pelvic mass in patient with ovarian remnant syndrome.

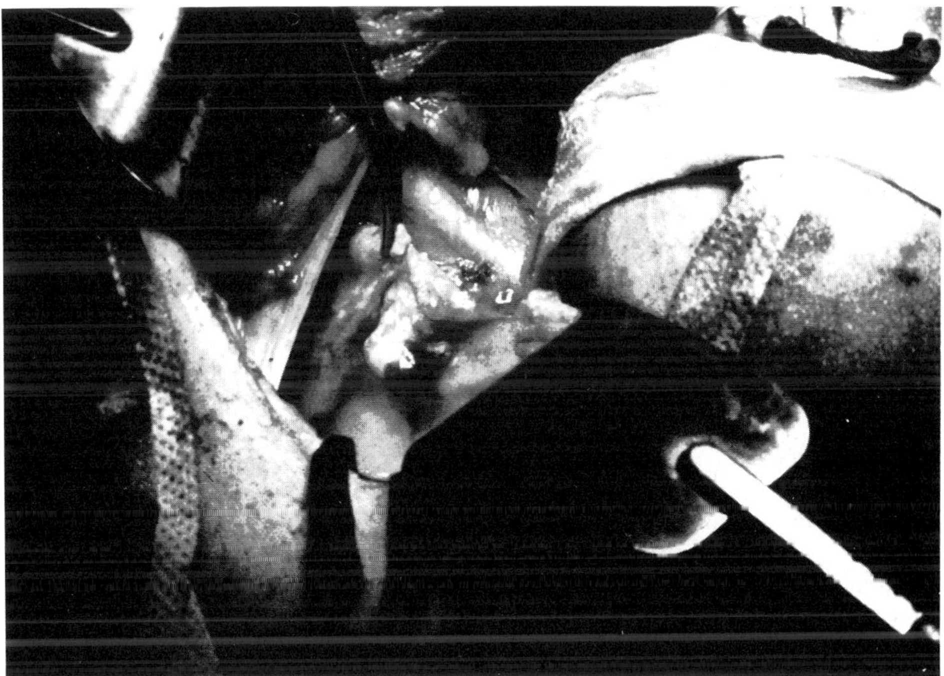

FIG 23–2.
Intraoperative photograph of cystic pelvic mass demonstrated histologically to be an ovarian remnant.

menstruate following bilateral oophorectomy. The occurrence was attributed to "supplementary ovaries," but given the rarity of that gynecologic entity, the more likely explanation is that advanced in 1903 by Malcolm, who believed the persistent menstruation after bilateral oophorectomy was attributable to an incomplete removal of ovarian tissue.[1]

Confusion on the topic persisting to the present day is evidenced by the divergent views on the etiology of ovarian remnant syndrome. The ovarian rest explanation, though it receives less support that the incomplete removal view, is based on the understanding of how the ovaries develop. In the human embryo, the primordial germ cells develop among the endodermal cells close to the allantois in the wall of the yolk sac. They then migrate along the wall of the hindgut and dorsal mesentery into the genital ridge,[4] a distance of about 0.5 mm.[2]

Witschi, in studying the migration of germ cells in the human embryo, found that occasionally there was a delay or failure of some of these cells to migrate. Although some of the cells that failed to reach the genital ridge degenerated, Witschi noted that others appeared normal. Should these germ cells induce the primitive mesenchyme of the mesentery or retroperitoneal area to undergo differentiation into ovarian stroma, functioning extragonadal ovarian tissue could result.[1]

Although this explanation describes a probable etiology for supernumerary ovaries, it is a less likely explanation for the ovarian remnant syndrome than the incomplete removal theory. Support for the latter stems from the observation that ovarian remnant syndrome frequently arises in such settings as endometriosis or pelvic inflammatory disease, where the initial dissection for removal of the ovaries proves difficult. Support for the plausibility of this explanation is provided by data from animal studies. Parkes and Smith demonstrated the viability of homografts of ovarian tissue no bigger than 1 mm^3.[5, 6] Shemwell and Weed sutured the raw surface of feline ovarian cortex to the peritoneum of the lateral abdominal wall in four adult female cats and subsequently demonstrated functioning of the transplants in all four cats.[7] Consequently, in cases where extensive disease, adhesions, increased vascularity, or alteration of normal anatomy create the possibility of leaving behind even a tiny remnant of ovarian tissue, the cells may survive, reestablish a blood supply, and begin to function with the production of follicles, cysts, or even corpora lutea. If, as is often the case, this functioning tissue is retroperitoneal or is encased in adhesions, pressure from an expanding cyst or bleeding from a corpus luteum frequently results in pain.

Diagnosis

The diagnostic workup of suspected ovarian remnant syndrome is often in part that of pelvic pain. The history may elicit complaints varying from pelvic pressure to a dull ache to a sharp stabbing pain. Dyspareunia is frequently present. The pain is usually located in the pelvis or perineum, may vary from side to side, or may be cyclic in nature. Endometriosis, pelvic inflammatory disease, diverticulitis, or adhesions may have complicated the previous surgery. Postoperatively, the patient may have experienced menopausal hot flashes that subsequently disappeared.

The symptoms usually occur within 5 years of the removal of both ovaries.[8] They are not usually present immediately after the initial surgery probably because some time must elapse for the lack of estrogen feedback to the central nervous system to cause a rise in FSH and LH levels significant enough to stimulate development of the dormant remnant. Similarly, ovarian remnant syndrome would not ordinarily develop after unilateral oophorectomy as long as the opposite ovary functions. If a mass develops at the site where the previously removed ovary was located, it would almost certainly be neoplastic. By the same token, a pelvic mass that develops from an ovarian remnant in a postmenopausal woman must be considered malignant until proved otherwise by surgical removal. Any nonneoplastic ovarian tissue remaining in a postmenopausal woman after bilateral oophorectomy would be resistant to functional or dysfunctional stimulation by FSH or LH.

On physical examination, a tender pelvic mass is often found. Occasionally, no mass will be felt or the patient may have a mass without pain. A pelvic ultrasonogram may be helpful in delineating the mass.

If gastrointestinal complaints are present, barium enema, sigmoidoscopy, or both may be appropriate. If low back pain is a symptom, consultation to rule out an orthopedic component may be worthwhile. Intravenous (IV) pyelogram is almost always appropriate. Because ovarian remnants are frequently located near the ureter, the IV pyelogram is helpful whether abnormal or normal. The presence or absence of preexisting compromise of the urinary tract is documented, and the decision regarding ureteral catheterization is facilitated. Depending on the nature of any urinary tract symptoms, one may wish to consider cystoscopy if the location of a mass or obstruction warrants ruling out bladder pathology.

Measurement of FSH, LH, and estradiol levels are definitely in order. Premenopausal levels indicate the presence of functioning ovarian tissue. Studies by Utian and colleagues never recorded FSH levels less than 70 mIU/mL and LH levels less than 30 mIU/mL in postoophorectomy patients.[9] Even if a postoophorectomy patient has been on oral menopausal replacement therapy, her estradiol level should be low, and her FSH and LH levels should be incompletely suppressed.[10, 11] On the other hand, estradiol, FSH, and LH levels in the menopausal range do not rule out an ovarian remnant. The amount of functioning ovarian tissue may be insufficient to suppress the gonadotropins.

At this point in the investigation, in contrast to the usual workup of pelvic pain, laparoscopy is probably not useful. In fact, it may be especially risky in light of the previous surgery. Similarly, computed tomography (CT) or magnetic resonance imaging (MRI) would probably add little to the diagnosis already made reasonably certain by the previous procedures.

Treatment

In the treatment of ovarian remnant syndrome, consideration may be given to three approaches: removal, suppression, or ablation. The advantages and disadvantages of each should be carefully weighed relative to the particular case under consideration.

Ablation

Ablation of the ovarian remnant by castration doses of deep radiation have the advantage of avoiding the technical difficulties and morbidity associated with a surgical treatment as well as avoiding the possibility of recurrence. However, the adhesive disease that may make surgery difficult also poses significant risk to immobilized small bowel. The dosage of radiation required for castration of the premenopausal woman is usually in the range of 2,000 rad. A smaller dose in the range of 500 to 700 rad may be sufficient for a perimenopausal castration.[12] Small bowel injury occurs at a high incidence with dosages near 4,000 rad. These figures may make radiation appear to be a safe therapeutic regimen for the treatment of ovarian remnant syndrome, but one must remember that radiation dosages are usually reported as midline dosages. Structures adherent to the anterior abdominal wall may, in fact, receive 15% to 20% more radiation than the intended treatment area.[13]

A second caveat of castration by radiation is that an unexplored pelvic mass may represent a neoplasm. Shemwell and Weed have reported a case in which a woman presumed to have an ovarian remnant and treated with castration dosages of radiation subsequently died from adenocarcinoma that developed in an area of residual endometriosis.[7] Thus, the decision to choose ablative radiation therapy for ovarian remnant syndrome must be accompanied by reasonable certainty that a mass does not represent a neoplastic process. The patient must be followed carefully. If the mass does not regress promptly, surgical exploration is mandatory.

Suppression

Suppressive therapy for an ovarian remnant may take one of several forms, the rationale behind these being to eliminate ovulatory surges of LH and/or to consistently suppress FSH. Again, the gynecologist must be satisfied that a patient does not have a neoplasm. A benign serous cystadenoma developing in a remnant of ovarian tissue, for example, would not be expected to respond to suppressive therapy. In a woman with premenopausal levels of FSH, LH, and estradiol, however, an attempt at suppression may be reasonable. Nelson and Avant have reported the successful treatment of a patient with long-standing progesterone in the form of 150 mg of intramuscular medroxyprogesterone acetate suspension (Depo-Provera) monthly.[14]

In patients with endometriosis documented by previous surgery, danazol (Danocrine) therapy has been attempted for symptom relief. Exogenous estrogen and progestin replacement regimens have also been used. However, the commonly prescribed menopausal replacement dosages may be inadequate to suppress functioning remnant tissue stimulated by endogenous gonadotropins, as evidenced by the fact that FSH levels in castrated women remain in the low "postmenopausal" range of 50 to 75 mg/mL until replacement levels as high as 2.5 mg of conjugated estrogen/day are used.[9] Supporting this contention is the report by Steege of 13 patients, 10 of whom were unsuccessfully treated with hormonal manipulation and subsequently required surgical intervention for cure.[15]

A trial of oral contraceptives or progestin-only regimes may be given to young women, but often these will be clinically contraindicated or unacceptable for long-term use. Another suppressive therapy only recently available for consideration is the use of gonadotrophin-releasing hormone analogues combined with cyclic estrogen and progesterone. If an acceptable regimen is demonstrated to sabbotage endogenous gonadotrophic stimulation of the ovarian remnant, some patients may be able to avoid surgical treatment.

Removal

To date, the most widely used treatment of ovarian remnant syndrome is surgical removal. The important principle for the gynecologic surgeon to bear in mind is that not only any identifiable mass but all tissue in which an ovarian remnant even of microscopic size could be located must be removed. This principle becomes apparent on reviewing the operative histories of many of these patients. Patients who have been taken to surgery for the removal of a mass often come back again and again for removal of the subsequent masses. The recurrence rate has been reported as between 8% and 30%.[15] Removing all tissue in which a remnant could be located should take into consideration both of the proposed etiologies of the syndrome: the previous incomplete removal of ovarian tissue as well as stimulation of previously quiescent ovarian rests. The latter should remind the surgeon to search for the rare supernumerary ovary that can mimic ovarian remnant syndrome.

Remembering this possibility, the surgeon will be led to recall the development and migration of the ovaries and, thus, to examine carefully the bowel and its mesentary, the omentum, and the course of the ovarian vessels. Adequate excision of the ovarian remnant and contiguous adherent tissue may require removal of bowel serosa and appendices epiploicae, the broad ligaments and underlying areolar and vascular tissues, and careful dissection to free an adherent ureter or pelvic vessel. The technical difficulty of the surgery in addition to frequent involvement of vital structures and the need for extensive dissection is often exacerbated by the distortions of anatomy from previous surgery and extensive adhesions, increasing the risk of bowel injury.

Decisions about attendant problems, such as stress urinary incontinence, that may also require surgical correction should be given careful thought, because the definitive procedure for ovarian remnant syndrome may itself take several hours, with an estimated blood loss of 600 to 700 mL.[15] On the other hand, if no definite remnant is discovered and operative findings do not totally explain the pain component of a patient's symptoms, presacral neurectomy may be considered.

Some surgeons prefer preoperative placement of ureteral catheters to help avoid ureteral injury during dissection of an adherent mass. Others who do not place them preoperatively may not hesitate to perform an extraperitoneal cystotomy to pass retrograde a no. 5 ureteral catheter if opening the peritoneum above the pathologic process and tracing the ureter inferiorly using sharp dissection as necessary has not solved the problem. Undue manipulation of a ureter containing a semirigid catheter may add to the potential for ureteral injury. The decision on whether to place ureteral catheters preoperatively is best made on an individual basis according to the nature and location of the mass in relation to the course of the ureter.

Surgical Procedure

The surgical procedure itself may proceed according to the following general outline. An excellent placement of the patient for operation is afforded by the modified lithotomy position in which the patient's lower legs are placed in Allen stirrups with the thighs flexed about 10 to 20 degrees. This position allows access to the urethra, vagina, and rectum should intraoperative manipulation, especially of the vagina, be deemed helpful in defining obscured surgical anatomy. Also, should ureteral catheters not be placed initially, they can be placed with ease at any point during the procedure without the necessity of cystotomy. In addition, the second assistant standing between the patient's legs has a better vantage point from which to provide a more substantial contribution to the surgery.

The patient is catheterized, and a careful but gentle pelvic examination and bimanual rectovaginal-abdominal palpation is performed. The patient is then prepared and draped for laparotomy. A transurethral Foley or ureteral catheter is inserted, if desired.

If additional pathology dictating the need for access to the upper abdomen is absent, ideal exposure to the pelvic side walls and depths is afforded by the low transverse abdominal muscle cutting incision of Maylard. After entry into the abdominal cavity, identification and restoration of normal anatomy often require extensive lysis of adhesions. Any mass thought to represent an ovarian remnant is evaluated in relation to the ureters, vessels, bowel, bladder, and vaginal vault. Complete extirpation of the mass usually requires a retroperitoneal approach. The round ligament or its remnant provides a useful landmark. Its transection near the pelvic side wall allows entry into the retroperitoneum. The ureter is identified. If it is not catheterized, a Penrose drain may be placed around it for gentle manipulation in tracing and exposing its course with sharp dissection in relation to the mass. The external iliac artery and vein are exposed. Development of the paravesical, pararectal, rectovaginal, and obturator fossa spaces may be helpful. The hypogastric artery is identified, and its anterior division may be ligated and transected, if necessary. Awareness of the inferior mesenteric vessels should be maintained to avoid interruption of the blood supply to the colon.

Good exposure, traction, and countertraction with the aid of the assistants and attention to hemostasis sometimes via packs and surgical clips facilitate the removal of the remnant along with the peritoneum of the pelvic side walls and attached tissues, which may include bowel serosa, the sheath of pelvic vessels and ureter, or bladder muscularis. Following an adequate dissection, reperitonization of the pelvis will rarely be possible and should not be unduly pursued. Before completing the procedure, the surgeon should check to be sure he or she is satisfied with the integrity of the obturator nerve, the pelvic vessels, the ureter, the bowel, and the bladder. Hemostasis should be ensured before closure, but the extensive dissection may make the placement of a negative pressure drain in the retroperitoneal space desirable.

Postoperatively, the gynecologist should be particularly attuned to the detection of such complications as ileus or bowel obstruction, anemia, hematoma, or lymphocyst formation, and urinary fistula. Adequate removal of a functioning ovarian remnant will usually result in a rise in FSH levels to more more 100 mIU/mL within 1 week of surgery, and menopausal symptoms may appear.[15]

Prevention

Of course, the ideal approach is to prevent ovarian remnant syndrome rather than subject patients to numerous or morbid procedures for its treatment. Consequently, in situations in which one is likely to encounter difficulty in removing the entire ovary, the gynecologic surgeon should be prepared for more than a simple procedure. Some of the same principles applied in the definitive treatment of ovarian remnant syndrome can be applied prophylactically as needed in preventing it. In the presence of endometriosis, pelvic inflammatory disease, extensive adhesions, inflammatory bowel disease, and other pathologies that alter normal pelvic anatomy, the surgeon performing oophorectomy should take steps to ensure that all ovarian tissue is removed. If the disease process is thought to involve adherence to bowel, preoperative bowel preparation will allow the surgeon to dissect the lesion off the bowel with less fear of entering it. A retroperitoneal approach will often facilitate the removal of pelvic pathology. If the patient is placed in Allen stirrups, ureteral catheters may be placed intraoperatively with ease if they become desirable, and the vaginal apex can be elevated with a ring forcep or Lucite mold to facilitate dissection of the rectovaginal space for removal of disease in the cul-de-sac. If the ovary is adherent to the pelvic side wall, cul-de-sac, or posterior broad ligament, the peritoneum of the area should be excised along with the specimen. With these precautions, the patient's primary procedure hopefully will be curative, and she will be spared the trauma of reoperation for ovarian remnant syndrome.

RESIDUAL OVARY SYNDROME

Case History

D.M., a 27-year-old white woman para 3 0 0 3, presented complaining of cramping lower abdominal pain "about 12 days out of the month." Dyspareunia was so severe that following a recent attempt at coitus, she came to the emergency room complaining of incapacitating pain accompanied by nausea and vomiting. Her significant past surgical history included laparoscopic diagnosis of pelvic inflammatory disease, subsequent bilateral salpingectomy, and later a vaginal hysterectomy for menometrorrhagia and uterine prolapse. On two occasions since hysterectomy, large ovarian cysts were noted at the time of laparoscopy for pelvic pain.

A markedly tender 4-cm cystic mass just posterior and caudal to the left vaginal fornix was found on pelvic examination. The pelvic ultrasonogram revealed a 4.8-cm left adnexal mass containing a 3.1-cm cyst. The patient was unable to tolerate attempted ovarian suppression with oral contraceptives, and pain was uncontrolled by nonsteroidal anti-inflammatory agents.

Diagnosis

The presence of pain, a pelvic mass, and dyspareunia represent the three most common findings in the 1% to 3%[16] of posthysterectomy patients who subsequently return to their gynecologist with the residual ovary syndrome. Although this syndrome is merely one of a number of considerations in the continuing debate over ovarian conservation at the time of hysterectomy, it deserves thoughtful attention. Although the controversy over "normal ovariotomy" dates back at least to Robert Battey in the 1870s and 1880s, more recent articles such as those by Grogan[17] in 1958 and 1967 have added fuel to the debate by stimulating interest in the residual ovary syndrome. Among 122 patients who required subsequent removal of the ovaries after previous hysterectomy, Grogan found the most common presenting symptom to be pelvic or lower abdominal pain. The pain that patients with residual ovary syndrome experience may be continuous or intermittent, frequently representing continued or abortive attempts at ovarian function. It varies in intensity from a bothersome ache to incapacitating cramps. Radiation of the pain into the legs, back, or both can occur. Some patients report vasomotor symptoms, nausea, and vomiting.

Associated urinary tract disturbances such as frequency, urgency, dysuria, and recurrent infections are reported by some patients. Interestingly, 30% to 50% of patients have had a pelvic surgical procedure before their hysterectomies. Dysfunctional uterine bleeding, leiomyomas, and pelvic pain are the three most frequent indications leading to the hysterectomy itself.

A mass is found in more than one half of the patients. Most commonly, it is located adjacent to the vaginal cuff, and frequently it is greater than 5 cm in diameter. Sometimes it is asymptomatic, but more often it is exquisitely tender and contributes to the dyspareunia, which, in Christ and Lotze's series, was found in 67% of patients.[16]

Delineation of a pelvic mass before laparotomy may be helped by sonogram, CT scan, or MRI. Adhesions and perioophoritis, as well as a retroperitoneal location of the ovary, may prevent follicular rupture into the peritoneal cavity and give rise to an expanding polycystic mass, which, on sonogram, shows solid and cystic areas[18] difficult to distinguish from neoplasia. A barium enema may be appropriate if neoplasia is a strong consideration.

Depending on the nature of the ovarian mass and the age of the patient, a blood sample may be drawn to test for tumor markers such as carcinoembryonic antigen, CA 125, human chorionic gonadotropin, and α-fetoprotein. An IV pyelogram is often appropriate if for no other reason than to rule out urinary tract damage from previous surgery.

Pathologic findings at surgery include a perioophoritis in essentially all patients and extensive pelvic adhesions involving not just the ovary but also the sigmoid, bladder, small bowel, omentum, and/or peritoneum in most. If the ovarian mass is retroperitoneal, the ureter and other retroperitoneal structures may be encased by the process. The ovary is cystic in more than one half of the cases. The cysts may be functional (corpora lutea) or dysfunctional (multiple follicular cysts, hemorrhagic cysts). Grogan reported a 10.3% incidence of endometriosis in his series.[17] Benign neoplasia was present in 13.7%, and malignant neoplasia in 8.2%.

Treatment

In contemplating an approach to the management of patients thought to have the residual ovary syndrome, the gynecologist should consider a number of questions:

What was the reason for the patient's previous surgery? Did she have pelvic inflammatory disease, with her pain being a chronic sequel of that process? If so, castration may not be the appropriate initial approach to her problem. Did she have endometriosis, which may respond to medical management? Is her pain cyclic in nature and merely one component in a complex of symptoms representing the premenstrual syndrome (PMS)? If the other PMS symptoms that exaggerate the pelvic pain and decrease her ability to cope with it can be controlled, the patient may decide that living with some monthly pelvic discomfort is more acceptable to her than surgery.

Questions concerning the degree of disability the patient experiences lead to consideration of whether the adverse effect on her quality of life significantly outweighs the risks of surgery and castration. If a pelvic mass is present, it should be managed as a pelvic mass would be in any other woman of comparable age. The usual criteria for surgical exploration apply. On the other hand, if a mass is not present or is thought very unlikely to represent a neoplastic process, one must consider the consequences for this particular patient of lost ovarian function. Are there contraindications to hormonal replacement therapy should she not tolerate an abrupt surgical menopause or be remote from the age of natural menopause?

Philosophically and practically, the management of residual ovary syndrome is not unlike the management of the ovarian remnant syndrome (see previous section). If the possibility of neoplasia is remote, a trial of ovarian suppression with long-acting progesterone, a combination estrogen-progestin regimen, or gonadotropin-releasing hormone analogues may be in order. Rarely, ablation of the ovaries by castrating doses of radiation may be considered. More commonly, the treatment is surgical.

In a young woman whose primary complaint is severe dyspareunia, the gynecologist may be hesitant to deprive her of ovarian function. If the ovaries themselves are not markedly diseased, ovariopexy rather than oophorectomy may be performed. A careful surgeon will employ principles of microsurgical technique (possibly requiring surgical loupes) to free the ovary from surrounding adhesions with minimal trauma. The ovaries may be suspended out of the pelvis by suturing them intraperitoneally to the psoas muscle. They should be marked by radiopaque surgical clips for subsequent identification should that ever prove necessary. Extreme care should be exercised to avoid torsion of the infundibulopelvic ligament. If there is a question of compromise to the ovarian blood supply, the viable ovary will demonstrate a timely greenish fluorescence under Wood's light after rapid IV injection of 3 to 4 mL of a 20% solution of fluorescein dye.

In most cases of residual ovary syndrome, salpingo-oophorectomy will be the procedure of choice. Because of previous surgery and the almost ubiquitous presence of perioophoritis and adhesions, an approach similar to that used in ovarian remnant syndrome may be helpful (see previous description). Operative benefits may be gained from positioning the patient's legs in Allen stirrups. Consideration may be given to preoperative bowel preparation and to the placement of ureteral catheters with the same provisos mentioned previously.

Lysis of adhesions will probably be necessary to restore the landmarks of pelvic anatomy and render them recognizable. A retroperitoneal approach will often be helpful and will become necessary if the ovarian mass is itself retroperitoneal and encasing the ureter or other structures.

The round ligament usually can be identified, isolated, ligated, and transected. The incision in the peritoneum is then extended cephalad along the pelvic side wall parallel to the infundibulopelvic ligament (Fig 23–3). The retroperitoneal space is developed using blunt and sharp dissection. The ureter is identified attached to the medial leaf of the peritoneum. The surgeon can trace the course of the ureter through the pelvis and, using sharp dissection, free it from the ovarian mass. With the ureter under direct visualization (Fig 23–4), the ovarian vessels can then be isolated, ligated, and cut. Proceeding caudally, the surgeon can use blunt and sharp dissection to free the adnexa from the pelvic side wall, from remaining portions of the broad ligament, from the bladder, and from the vaginal cuff (Fig 23–5). If the ovary is densely adherent to other pelvic structures, an attempt to remove the serosal layer of these organs along with the ovary should be undertaken to prevent subsequent development of the ovarian remnant syndrome. The peritoneal defect may be closed as desired. If reperitonization is not possible, the sigmoid may be used to cover the defect. Small bowel is layered into the pelvis in an orderly fashion so that, when adhesions reform, obstruction will be less likely.

Prevention

Ideally, the gynecologist undertaking a hysterectomy wishes to spare the patient reoperation for residual ovary syndrome. If the initial procedure is being performed abdominally, the operative morbidity for total abdominal hysterectomy vs.

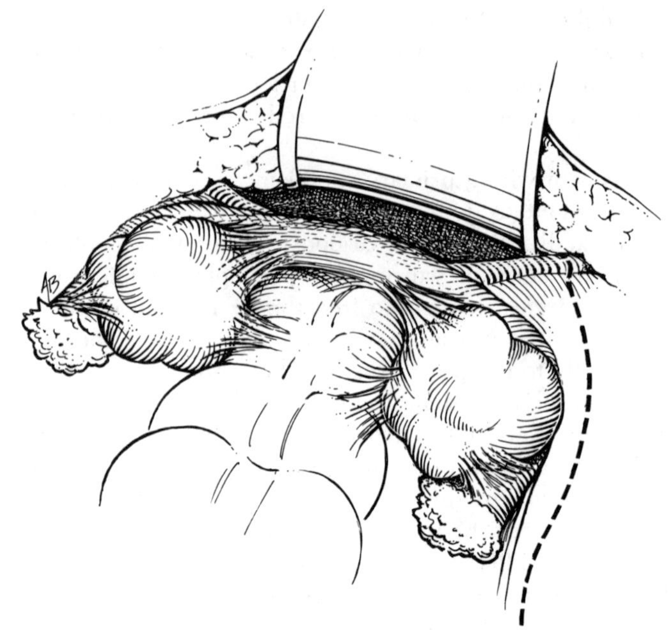

FIG 23–3.
Residual ovary syndrome. Line of peritoneal incision over round ligament and pelvic side wall to remove a diseased residual adnexa.

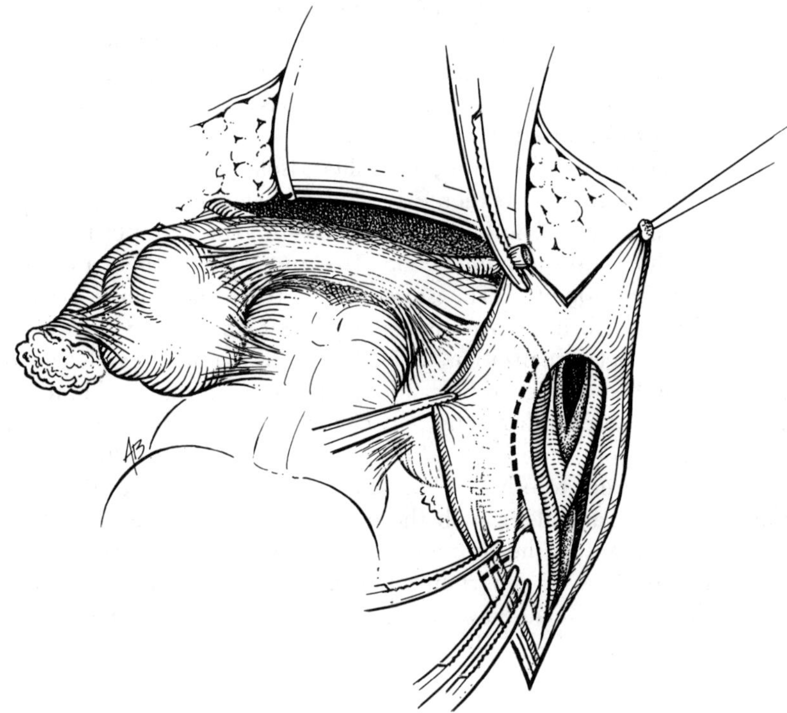

FIG 23–4.
Residual ovary syndrome. Retroperitoneal dissection identifies the course of the great vessels and ureter. The round ligament has been ligated laterally. With the ureter under direct visualization, the infundibulopelvic ligament is triply clamped.

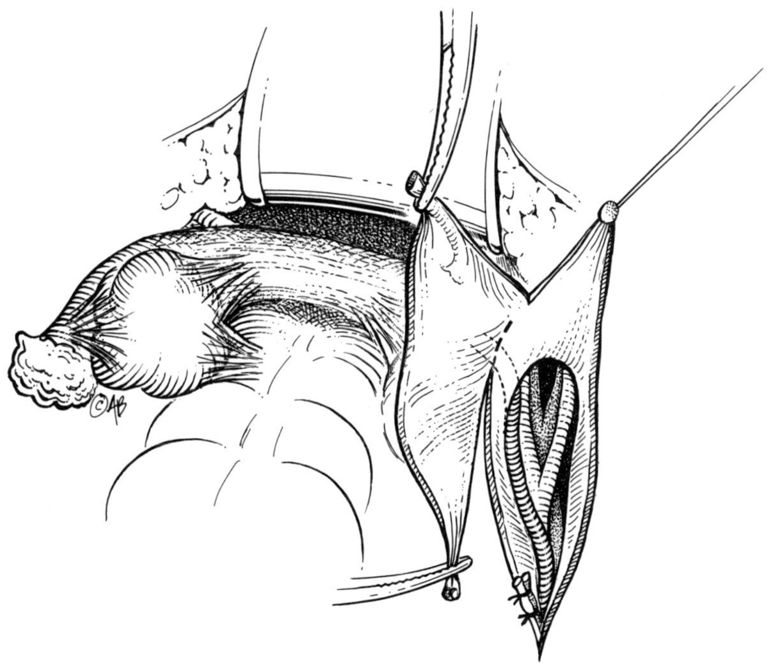

FIG 23–5.
Residual ovary syndrome. The infundibulopelvic ligament has been doubly ligated with a proximal free tie and a distal suture ligature. The course of the ureter has been traced through the pelvis so that the adnexa can safely be dissected free from the pelvic side wall, bladder, and vaginal cuff.

total abdominal hysterectomy with bilateral salpingo-oophorectomy is the same. One merely decides whether to place the clamp across the infundibulopelvic ligament or across the utero-ovarian ligament and tube. Proponents of prophylactic oophorectomy look not only toward preventing residual ovary syndrome but, more importantly, toward reducing the risk of ovarian cancer as reasons for removing normal ovaries at hysterectomy. Opponents sight DeNeef and Hollenbeck's estimate that to save three women from ovarian cancer, prophylactic oophorectomy must be routinely performed in 10,000 women at the time of hysterectomy.[19] They sometimes invite surgeons to consider for comparison the infrequency with which normal testes are removed and point out that if surgery is going to be performed to prevent cancer, greater inroads on mortality could be made by prophylactically removing the female breasts.

Rhetoric aside, careful and considerate information regarding the advantages and disadvantages of retaining the ovaries should be given to each patient as an individual. The impact of menopausal symptoms, the risks of osteoporosis and cardiovascular disease, psychologic factors, age, family history, personal history, and the patient's preference all should be thoroughly discussed and weighed. Not all patients can take hormonal replacement therapy, and the degree to which pills, pellets, and patches can mimic the complex endocrinologic function of the human ovary is debatable.

Although an in-depth discussion of the pros and cons of ovarian conservation is beyond the scope of our present subject, consideration of some of the possible etiologies of the residual ovary syndrome have a bearing on the decision to retain or remove the ovaries in a particular patient. Since nearly all ovaries requiring removal in the residual ovary syndrome are found to have perioophoritis and adhesions, ovaries found to be so involved at the time of hysterectomy might be viewed with greater suspicion, particularly if the patient has significant pelvic pain. If a decision is made to retain such ovaries, they should be freed of adhesions as far as possible, often using microsurgical techniques, and Interceed patches may be placed at the conclusion of the surgery.

Grogan has suggested two other at-risk groups: patients who have experienced conservative pelvic surgery before hysterectomy and patients coming to hysterectomy with the diagnosis of dysfunctional bleeding.[17] The first group is of concern because 35% to 50% of patients with residual ovary syndrome give such a history. The second group is of concern because the uterus being removed is merely the target organ. The dysfunction lies further upstream in the hypothalamic-pituitary-ovarian axis and may reside in the ovary itself.

An ovary cannot function properly if its blood supply is compromised. Variation in ovarian blood supply[12] ranges from sole dependence on the ovarian artery to sole dependence on the uterine artery. Generally, the medial half of the ovary and the medial two thirds of the fallopian tube are supplied by the uterine artery; the remaining lateral portions are supplied by the ovarian artery.

If the ovaries are to be retained at the time of hysterectomy, the clamps containing the utero-ovarian ligaments should be placed as close to the uterus as possible. Even this maneuver will not spare the occasional ovary that derives essentially its entire blood supply from the uterine artery. If the surgeon has any doubt regarding ovarian blood supply, it may be tested with fluorescein dye as described previously, or one may listen for arterial pulsations with a sterile Doppler.

Unless diseased, the tube should be retained with the ovary just in case its removal interrupt the arcade of vessels running through the mesosalpinx and mesoovarium. Care should be taken not to stretch or twist the ovarian vessels during reperitonization.

The ovary should not be left against an unperitonized pelvic side wall, allowing the possibility of its becoming retroperitoneal after spontaneous reperitonization. Pedicles containing the ligated utero-ovarian ligaments should not be tied together in the midline, especially in a premenopausal woman. The resulting adhesions to the vaginal vault may cause dyspareunia. At abdominal hysterectomy, consideration may even be given to elevating the ovaries out of the pelvis. Surgical clips on the utero-ovarian ligament will identify their location on subsequent radiographic studies. Finally, if a decision has been made to remove the ovaries, care should be taken that they be removed in entirety lest, in preventing the residual ovary syndrome, the surgeon set the patient up for the ovarian remnant syndrome and thus merely substitute the risk of one reoperative benign ovarian syndrome for the other.

REFERENCES

1. Wharton LR: Two cases of supernumerary ovary and one of accessory ovary, with an analysis of previously reported cases. *Am J Obstet Gynecol* 1959; 78:1101–1119.
2. Printz JL, Choate JW, et al: The embryology of supernumerary ovaries. *Obstet Gynecol* 1973; 41:246–252.
3. Kaufman JJ: Unusual causes of extrinsic ureteral obstruction, part I. *J Urol* 1962; 87:319–327.

4. Sadler TW: Urogenital system, in *Langman's Medical Embryology.* Baltimore, Williams & Wilkins Co, 1985, pp 258–259.
5. Parkes AS, Smith AU: *Proc R Soc Lond* 1953; 140:455–470.
6. Smith AU, Parkes AS: *Preservation and Transplantation of Normal Tissues.* Ciba Foundation Symposium. New York, Churchill Livingstone, 1954; pp 76–85.
7. Shemwell RE, Weed JC: Ovarian remnant syndrome. *Obstet Gynecol* 1970; 36:299–303.
8. Lee RA: Ovarian remnant syndrome, in Nichols DH (ed): *Clinical Problems, Injuries and Complications of Gynecologic Surgery.* Baltimore, Williams & Wilkins Co, 1988, p 16.
9. Utian WH, Katz M, et al: Effect of premenopausal castration and incremental dosages of conjugated equine estrogens on plasma follicle-stimulating hormone, luteinizing hormone, and estradiol. *Am J Obstet Gynecol* 1978; 132:297–302.
10. Schiff I, Tulchinsky D, et al: Oral medroxyprogesterone in the treatment of postmenopausal symptoms. *JAMA* 1980; 244:1443–1445.
11. Simon JA, diZerega GS: Physiologic estradiol replacement following oophorectomy: Failure to maintain precastration gonadotropin levels. *Obstet Gynecol* 1982; 59:511–513.
12. Mattingly RF, Thompson JD: Leiomyomata uteri and abdominal hysterectomy for benign disease, in *TeLinde's Operative Gynecology.* Philadelphia, JB Lippincott Co, 1985; pp 203–255.
13. Brown CB, Go RT: Diagnostic radiographic techniques in gynecologic oncology, in Sciarra JJ (ed): *Gynecology and Obstetrics.* Philadelphia, Harper & Row, Publishers, 1985, vol 4, chapter 54, p 12.
14. Nelson DC, Avant GR: Ovarian remnant syndrome. *South Med J* 1982; 75:757–758.
15. Steege JF: Ovarian remnant syndrome. *Obstet Gynecol* 1987; 70:64–67.
16. Christ JE, Lotze EC: The residual ovary syndrome. *Obstet Gynecol* 1975; 46:551–556.
17. Grogan RH: Reappraisal of residual ovaries. *Am J Obstet Gynecol* 1967; 97:124–129.
18. Gray R, St. Louis E, et al: Postoperative residual ovary syndrome: An uncommon cause of pelvic mass. *J Can Assoc Radiol* 1983; 34:56–58.
19. DeNeef JC, Hollenbeck ZJR: The fate of ovaries preserved at the time of hysterectomy. *Am J Obstet Gynecol* 1966; 96:1088–1097.

BIBLIOGRAPHY

Berek JS, Darney PD, et al: Avoiding ureteral damage in pelvic surgery for ovarian remnant syndrome. *Am J Obstet Gynecol* 1979; 133:221–222.

Bukovsky I, Liftshitz Y, et al: Ovarian residual syndrome. *Surg Gynecol Obstet* 1988; 167:132–134.

Dmowski WP, Radwanska E, Rana N: Recurrent endometriosis following hysterectomy and oophorectomy: The role of residual ovarian fragments. *Int J Gynecol Obstet* 1988; 26:93–103.

Hajj SN, Mercer LJ: Retrograde dissection of the adnexa in residual ovary syndrome. *Surg Gynecol Obstet* 1987; 165:451–452.

Horowitz MI, Elguezabal A: Obstruction of the ureter by recent corpus luteum located in the retroperitoneum: Report of two cases. *J Urol* 1966; 95:706–710.

Major FJ: Retained ovarian remnant causing ureteral obstruction, report of two cases. *Obstet Gynecol* 1968; 32:748–753.

Phillips HE, McGahan JP: Ovarian remnant syndrome. *Radiology* 1982; 142:487–488.

Randall CL, Hall DW, Armenia CS: Pathology in the preserved ovary after unilateral oophorectomy. *Am J Obstet Gynecol* 1962; 84:1233–1241.

Symmonds RE, Pettit PDM: Ovarian remnant syndrome. *Obstet Gynecol* 1979; 54:174–177.

Chapter 24

Anesthesia Considerations for the Reoperated Patient With Associated Diseases

Augustine M. McNamee, M.D.

Although the surgeon's main focus will be on the complexities of the surgical task, the anesthesiologist will want to know what is to be done to whom. Whether for the initial surgical procedure or at reoperation, the anesthesiologist will be concerned with the physiologic disturbances and associated diseases that the patient brings to the operating room. Advances in anesthesia knowledge and techniques have expanded our ability to offer a safe anesthesia passage to a wider range of surgical risks. The guidelines developed for the management of complex procedures have had a tendency to evolve into standards of care that, in our ever more litigious society, weigh heavily on all members of the surgical team. This chapter is orientated to help surgeons see patients with associated nonsurgical problems from the anesthesiologists' viewpoint and to anticipate what they may require and what they are trying to accomplish. It is not intended to be a manual for the practicing anesthesiologist.

The diseases I will consider are by no means complete. More complete reference texts are recommended for the more unusual diseases.[1, 2] This section will highlight the anesthesia implications of some of the conditions that quite frequently cause unanticipated aggravation for the surgeon and disappointing, if not expensive, delays for the patient.

HEMORRHAGIC SHOCK

The initiating factor in hemorrhagic shock is blood loss with its effect on the balance of the basic physiologic equation BP = CO × PVR. The fall in venous return reduces cardiac output, and if the baroreceptors sympathetic efferents and receptors are intact, the peripheral vascular resistance increases to maintain perfusion of the heart and brain but at the cost of diminished renal, splenic, and peripheral perfusion. As the delivery of molecular oxygen is decreased, pyruvate cannot generate high-energy adenosine triphosphate via the mitochondrial citric acid cycle but is converted to lactate acid with its ensuing metabolic acidosis.

The surgeon will address the source of hemorrhage, whereas it falls to the anesthesiologist to resuscitate the patient. The residua of the anesthesia will have a variable effect on the hemodynamic status of the patient. Normally the supine patient can maintain a satisfactory blood pressure with an 800-mL blood loss. Hypotension will occur earlier if the patient has had spinal or epidural anesthesia with persistance of sympathetic blockade. Hypotension remote from an inhalation or IV narcotic anesthesia is a reasonable index that the blood loss is considerably in excess of 800 mL. Restoration of blood volume is fundamental and usually straightforward in an otherwise healthy patient. In those with preexisting problems, the therapeutic interventions will be more involved. In addition to arterial blood pressure, central venous pressure monitoring, urinary output, and arterial blood gases, a Swan-Ganz catheter would be indicated in the presence of significant existing coronary or valvular disease. Interpretation and manipulation of the hemodynamic data from central balloon catheters would require a chapter in itself. Information from the pulmonary arterial catheter can alert the anesthesiologist to the possible development of various degrees of cardiogenic shock during the resuscitation. The progress of the resuscitation can be followed by determining mixed venous oxygen content, which will be the best indicator of satisfactory peripheral tissue perfusion. Furthermore, the relationship of pulmonary artery diastolic, pulmonary capillary wedge, and cardiac output determinations will alert the anesthesiologist to the possible development of shock lung, cardiac decompensation, or ischemia.

Rapid blood replacement, however, remains the standard in treatment. It would seem obvious that cold, unreconstituted cells given by gravity will not do the job, but, unfortunately, this event still occurs. The cells should be diluted with 150 to 200 mL of normal saline and pumped under pressure through a warming coil into a 16- or 14-gauge catheter. The ubiquitous use of stopcocks with internal 16-gauge lumina negate the placement of a 14- or 12-gauge IV line. Cold blood should never be administered directly via a central venous line, because the temperature gradient from the cold endocardial to the warmer epicardial surface produces repolarization changes that lead to rhythm problems.

Transfusions of more than 10 units of packed cells will result in thrombocytopenia (platelets $< 100{,}000/mm^3$) in 92% of cases. Factors V and VIII may also fall below the critical 30% level if more than 10 units of packed cells are required. A safe rule is to administer two to three units of fresh frozen plasma and six to eight units of platelet concentrates if diffuse bleeding persists after 10 units of packed cells. If platelet concentrates are not available, whole blood not older than 24 hours will keep the platelet count above $90{,}000/mm^3$.

In the unexpected "crashing" emergencies, type O, Rh-negative screened but uncrossed matched blood can be given, but because some O donors have anti-A and anti-B antibodies, it should always be administered as packed cells. In the packed cells preparation, the plasma antibodies have been centrifuged off. If O Rh-negative whole blood (with anti-A and anti-B antibodies) is used, the patients cannot subsequently receive units of their own type (A, B, or AB), because this infused donor blood would be hemolysed. At a later date, full crossmatching will determine when it becomes safe for a type-specific transfusion.

Full crossmatching requires approximately 45 minutes for incubation processing. I have used 1,000 to 1,500 mL of hetastarch as a temporary expander in addition to high-volume plain Ringer's lactate.

Bicarbonate administration should not be capricious or empirical. The citrate in the blood preservative will metabolize to bicarbonate as tissue perfusion improves and if the body temperature is maintained. Inadvertant swings of the pH into the alkalotic range will shift the oxihemoglobin dissociation curve to the left, reducing tissue oxygen availability. The excess HCO_3 combining with H^+ will form carbonic acid. This dissociates into CO_2, which readily crosses the blood brain barriar and adds to central nervous system (CNS) acidosis with subsequent CNS depression.

The anesthesia technique employed is governed primarily by the hemodynamic data. I favor high-dose narcotic with ancillary pharmacologic intervention to achieve the goals of adequate filling pressures, peripheral perfusion, myocardial oxygenation, and maintenance of urinary output. I have used ketamine as the initial agent for emergency explorations in the severely bleeding patient before full monitoring lines can be established.

SEPTIC SHOCK

Between 70% and 80% of postsurgical septic shock is secondary to gram-negative bacteremia. The primary treatment is antibiotics and the surgical elimination of the source of sepsis. In reanesthetizing such patients, the anesthesiologist is aware that the mortality is at least 47%. Furthermore, young healthy patients develop septic shock infrequently. It is more common in patients with associated diseases; diabetics with possible autonomic dysfunction, cirrotics, cardiorenal patients, and the elderly in general.

The pathophysiology of septic shock is more multifaceted than in hemorrhagic shock, and it is traditionally considered biphasic. In its early phase, the bacterial endotoxin initiates the production of depressive humoral agents that produce profound peripheral dilatation, a drop in afterload, and increased cardiac output. This hyperdynamic state must be maintained to ensure increased peripheral demand. When the cardiac output fails, increased peripheral vascular resistance, acidosis, and the terminal spiral of the hypodynamic phase ensue.

Whereas most cases of hemorrhagic shock can be managed by arterial and central venous pressure monitoring, early pulmonary artery catheterization is imperative in septic shock. Multiple cardiac outputs can be determined and maintained above normal by volume expansion to ensure adequate left ventricular filling pressures and the avoidance of myocardial depressive agents. The choice of fluids will be determined by serial hematocrit values. At hematocrit levels greater than 30%, the increase in viscosity and resistance will diminish peripheral perfusion and oxygen delivery. Red blood cell infusions above this hematocrit level are not beneficial. Vasopressor therapy is appropriate but must be governed by hemodynamics. Vasoconstrictors in general are to be avoided except when the drop in peripheral vascular resistance is so marked as to produce dangerous hypotension in the presence of a normal or above-normal cardiac output. Cardiac inotrops may be necessary if the cardiac output does not respond to increased filling pressures.

The use of steroids has been debatable for 30 years. A combined study of methylprednisolone in septic shock was conducted on 382 patients at 19 centers in the United States and reported by Bone and colleagues.[12] Their results may be summarized as follows. Of those patients who were septic but not in shock at the beginning of therapy, 51% of the steroid group developed shock compared with 37% receiving no steroids. Of those patients already in shock, 65% of patients on steroid therapy had shock reversal compared with 73% receiving no steroids. They further reported no statistical difference between the steroid and placebo groups in overall mortality.

The overall incidence of complications from steroids and their negative impact on the septic state argues against their prophylactic or therapeutic use.

If the syndrome progresses to the second or hypodynamic stage, cardiac output diminishes, peripheral vascular resistance increases, hemodynamics become similar to those in hemorrhagic shock and will direct changes in physiological and fluid therapy.

OBESITY

One area in which the surgeon and the anesthesiologist share a galaxy of trying technical frustrations is in the management of the very obese patient. Patients 45.4 kg above ideal weight or whose weight doubles their ideal weight are by convention morbidly obese. Perhaps 600,000 Americans fall into this category. Minor surgical procedures carry major anesthetic risks in these individuals due to their very precarious cardiopulmonary reserve. Inspite of their morbid habitus, these patients have a high metabolic demand with increased oxygen consumption, carbon dioxide production, expanded blood volume, and increased cardiac output and ventilatory work.

Their embarrassed ventilatory apparatus is not adequate for its demands. The excess fat of the chest wall and abdomen reduce chest wall compliance. In the normal individual as expiration reduces total lung volume and approaches residual volume, a lung volume is reached where dependant alveoli close. This is the so-called closing volume of the lung. In the obese, lung volume is already reduced at the expense of a decrease in functional residual capacity and even residual volume. When the lung volume at the end of a normal tidal expiration is below this closing volume, the collapsed, unventilated, but perfused alveoli will result in a diminution in arterial Po_2. The problems of the lithotomy and Trendelenberg positions are obvious.[3] Intubation and mechanical ventilation with on-line monitoring of oxygenation and Pco_2 are mandatory. The effects of positive end-expiratory pressure, however, are unpredictable and must be evaluated by continuous gas and hemodynamic monitoring.

Routine anesthetic inductions in these subjects with short, rigid, bull necks can be a prelude to disaster. Whenever possible, awake sedated intubations or fiberoptic intubations are often the methods of choice. Hiatus hernias are common in these obese patients; gastric pH is often less than 2.5. Volumes are higher than 25 cc, and the increased abdominal pressure from the obese panniculus predisposes to aspiration. Because of this, many anesthesiologists believe that inhalation inductions are hazardous. The inability to ventilate by bag and mask before or between intubation attempts is the classical catastrophe to be avoided. The traditional thiobarbital relaxant sequence should be used only in those patients with supple, accessable anatomy. The surgeon can anticipate a longer induction time.

Pendulous pyramidal upper arm configurations can make the Riva-Rocci method of blood pressure recording inaccurate or impossible. Automatic blood pressure devices using leg cuffs are only slightly better. I use an intra-arterial line for all except the briefest of cases. It is important to remember that this can be used postoperatively, but preparations must be made for the proper referral of the patient, because not all patient units are equipped or staffed for direct blood pressure monitoring.

The pickwickian syndrome or obesity hypoventilation syndrome (5%–10% of the morbidly obese) can be identified preoperatively by careful history and appropriate laboratory testing. These sleep disturbance problems of hypoxia, apnea, and cardiac arrhythmias may not be cared for equally well on all surgical floors.

Regional techniques can be employed and afford the capability for postoperative pain management. They are almost always used in combination with general anesthesia, and thus far, no specific general agent has proved superior to another. Because the incidence of phlebothrombosis with emboli is twice as common in these patients postoperatively as in the nonobese patient, anticoagulatant therapy is appropriate but may be considered by some anesthesia departments a relative contraindication to the use of epidural catheters for postoperative pain management.

PULMONARY DISEASE

Perineal and lower abdominal procedures do not usually involve the postoperative complications frequently associated with upper abdominal or thoracic procedures. Whereas upper abdominal or thoracic procedures can result in a 60% to 75% decrease in vital capacity within the first 24 hours, lower abdominal procedures decrease the vital capacity by only 30% to 50%, and extremity and perineal procedures per se have minimal effect on changing the preoperative values. Still, the predominant disturbance in lung function should be identified and optimized to assure a safe anesthesia passage and uncomplicated recovery. The anesthesiologist's attention, therefore, is directed to those disturbances that can be improved by preoperative interventions. Simply put, treat infections, secretions, and bronchospasm.[2] A consult to pulmonary therapy or to the internist in this regard should be specifically focused and request more than just a preoperative evaluation of status. I do not usually request spirometery for lower abdominal or perineal procedures. Humidification can make secretions more mobile for coughing and more amenable to tracheal suction. In this regard, the midwinter relative humidity of the ambient air in a typical surgical ward has been found to be as low as 19%.

Asthmatic patients and those with a bronchospastic component of their chronic obstructive pulmonary disease should continue their bronchial dilators up to the morning of surgery. Theophyllin levels may well be requested by the anesthesiologist. Although halothane is favored as the inhalational agent in asthmatic patients, it may produce arrhythmia problems in the presence of theophyllin.

The choice of regional vs. general anesthesia still remains controversial. Provided the patient can tolerate the positioning and does not require continuous tracheal toilet or assisted ventilation, saddle block or low spinal is a reasonable choice for perineal surgery. It is almost axiomatic that when the abdomen is opened, the regional should be of sufficient height for the surgeon to go anywhere in the abdomen. More grief is caused by intravenous (IV) supplementation of an inadequate regional than by the occasional overshoot in dermatone level. A proved clinical rule is that if the patient is using the abdominal musculature for expiration and coughing, abdominal paralysis may cause air trapping and insidious progressive respiratory decompensation. Furthermore, sympathetic blockade rising above the T5 level may aggravate or even precipitate an increase in bronchial tone. Disagreement frequently occurs when the internist or pulmonary consultant documents that the patient should have a regional anesthesia. A well-conducted general anesthetic is more manageable in reversing abdominal paralysis and producing bronchial dilatation. Do not be surprised, therefore, if the anesthesiologist disagrees with the recommendation of the consultant mandating a regional anesthesia. For medicolegal reasons, some anesthesiologists will defer starting such a case until the wording on the consult is made less restrictive regarding the choice of anesthesia.

HYPERTENSION

Primary or essential hypertension is by far the most common hypertensive type encountered. Secondary hypertension due to aldosteronism, renal artery stenosis, pheochromotoma, or renal disease comprises approximately 10% of the hypertensive patients.

The avoidance of excessive swings in blood pressure resulting in cardiac ischemia is the main concern. Preoperative electrocardiogram (ECG) is essential to identify those hypertensive patients with left ventricular hypertrophy, strain, or ischemia. The patient with a hypertrophied less compliant left ventricle will require higher filling pressures to maintain cardiac output and tolerates hypovolemic episodes poorly. Reflex increase in peripheral vascular resistance can be sustained by the hypertrophied ventricle but at the expense of increased work and oxygen demand, which in the presence of associated coronary artery disease can lead to myocardial ischemia. Tachycardia with its resultant decrease in the diastolic filling time is less well tolerated by the hypertrophied heart.

The risks of anesthesia and surgery in the patient with essential hypertension are multifactorial, depending on the status of treatment and the presence of associated cardiac, cerebral, or renal disease, as well as the site and magnitude of the proposed surgery. In the untreated, or inadequately treated hypertensive patient whose diastolic pressure is not higher than 110 mm Hg, elective gynecologic surgery need not be postponed. With close monitoring and treatment of intraoperative and postoperative pressures, these patients are at no greater risk than those with tightly controlled management.[4]

Exaggerated pressor responses to stimuli during anesthesia are the hallmark of the hypertensive patient. Intubation is invariably accompanied by a reflex sympathetic discharge. This anticipated response can be aborted by (1) the use of high dose narcotics, (2) intubation under deep anesthesia by inhalation agents such as halothane, enflurane, or isoflurane, and (3) supplemental beta blockade or direct vasodilators. I have found that automatic blood pressure devices are too slow in response for this phase of the induction and prefer rapid sequence measurements by the Riva-Rocci method. Fentanyl in doses of 10 μg/kg can decrease the response to intubation, but recovery may be inappropriately prolonged for short operations. Alfentanil with its shorter duration of action may be a better choice. If the patient is untreated or inadequately treated, additional beta blockade can be given, preferably with a short-acting agent such as Esmolol.

Persistant arguments in the literature for or against regional techniques would seem to indicate that it is the anesthesiologist's choice. For perineal procedures and for those lower abdominal procedures whose positioning and duration do not require ventilatory assistance, regional epidural or spinal is a frequent choice in my institution.

Preoperative antihypertensive medical regimens should be continued preferably up to the morning of surgery. The issue of diuretics with secondary low potassium values has probably caused more consternation than the myriad of other antihypertensive agents and can be addressed briefly.

LOW POTASSIUM LEVELS

I require potassium levels on preoperative patients who are on diuretic therapy. Total body loss of potassium has long been implicated in clinical muscle weakness, ileus, and diminished cardiac contractility, but a vigorous controversy regarding the arrhythmogenic risk of moderate hypokalemia (i.e., K^+ levels between 2.5 and 3.5 mEq/L persists.

Because the electrophysiologic effect of a decrease in serum potassium level is to diminish cellular threshold potential and increase the slope of diastolic depolarization, the theoretical basis of hypokalemic arrhythmias is well established in the minds of most anesthesiologists, and an arbitrary level for elective surgery has been traditionally 3.5 mEq/L. Equally arbitrary in the minds of many surgeons is the expensive and inconvenient cancellations of cases for moderate hypokalemia 2.7 to 3 mEq/L secondary to diuretic therapy. Replenishment of potassium stores can take days and in itself can be hazardous. Vitez, and co-workers found that the percentage of cardiac arrhythmias in their hypokalemic group (2.6–3.4 mEq/L) was not significantly different from their normal kalemic group (3.5–5.2 mEq/L).[5] In an associated editorial, however, Mcgovern pointed out that these data should not be applied to a larger high-risk population.[6] In the presence of associated ischemia, congestive failure, existing arrhythmias, or digitalis therapy, I would postpone elective surgery if two preoperative potassium values were less than 3.5 mEq/L. Restoration of potassium stores is ideally accomplished by oral potassium, 25 mEq every 6 hours for 1 week. Emergency restoration may be attempted by IV potassium, not to exceed 0.5 mEq/kg/hour and preferably accompanied by 0.5 units of regular insulin/2 gm of dextrose.

CORONARY ARTERY DISEASE

Current statistics indicate that in the United States approximately 10 million people have some form of coronary artery disease. Each year, 150,000 or more of these people will have coronary artery bypass surgery. The incidence of atherosclerosis is most consistently correlated with the life time average concentration of plasma low-density or β-lipoproteins. The incidence of atherosclerosis is low in the premenopausal gynecologic patient because the higher estrogen levels decrease the ratio of low-density β-lipoproteins to high-density α-lipoproteins. With the onset of menopause, the incidence of coronary artery disease approaches and then surpasses that found in men.[7]

The presence and pattern of angina are, of course, diagnostic, but 20% to 30% infarcts on ECGs can be silent. Conversely, a normal resting ECG does not rule out the presence of coronary artery disease. More than 25% of previous myocardial infarctions may not show up on the ECG. The stress testing concomitant with the anesthesia/surgical experience may indicate the presence of coronary artery disease. The ubiquitous report of nonspecific T waves or ST changes or the presence of dysrhythmias should be a signal for a cardiac consultation, specifically asking an opinion as to the presence of an ischemic problem and whether further workup is required. Perioperative ischemic events can lead to infarction, and the reinfarction mortality in these patients may be as high as 50% to 75%.

Although the risks for recurrent myocardial infarctions in the gynecologic surgical patient are not as high as in lengthly thoracic, great vessel, and upper abdominal surgery, there is a concensus on the risk for noncardiac surgery, which can be summarized as follows:

1. Patients with prior myocardial infarctions have an overall reinfarction rate of approximately 7%.
2. With myocardial infarctions within 3 months, the reinfarction rate is 30%.
3. Within 3 to 6 months the rate is 15%.

The implications for the timing of anything but emergent surgery is obvious. Beyond this and in the presence of coronary artery disease per se, the anesthesiologist will be looking for other risk factors and pathophysiology that will determine the management plan.

In chronic coronary artery disease, premature ventricular contractions (PVCs) are the most common dysrhythmia. If the PVCs are frequent, multifocal, or both, this usually means the patient has multivessel disease and poor ventricular function. The presence of Mobitz type 2 block also carries a poor prognosis. The most important prognostic indicator and the one carrying the most significance for intraoperative management is the ejection fraction. Patients with ejection fractions of less than 40% who are to undergo major elective surgery should have full hemodynamic monitoring with Swan-Ganz catheterization and proper postoperative surgical intensive care follow-up. With ejection fractions greater than 40%, for most gynecologic procedures, usually direct arterial monitoring and central venous pressure monitoring is sufficient. The preoperative cardiac consultation, therefore, should be focused on and specifically request studies of left ventricular function. The intraoperative anesthesia manipulation of variations in hemodynamics is beyond the scope of this chapter, but the surgeon and the patient should be aware of trends in perioperative management. Rao and co-workers achieved a reduction in recurrent myocardial infarctions in patients undergoing noncardiac surgery from 7.7 to 1.9%.[8] Implicit in this achievement is the extension of full hemodynamic monitoring for up to 96 hours postoperatively. If valid, this approach has major financial and logistical implications.

SYSTOLIC MURMURS

During preoperative assessment, the anesthesiologist frequently encounters a patient who presents with a history of cardiac symptoms, who may even be taking cardiovascular medications, but no specific cardiac diagnosis is documented. The patient on examination is found to have a systolic murmur. Is the murmur due to mitral insufficiency or aortic stenosis? The intraoperative management may well depend on what condition predominates. In aortic stenosis, the low compliant hypertrophied ventricle squeezes rather than ejects its stroke volume. Systole has to be longer. Early passive diastolic filling is impaired by the rigidity of the chamber. Fast heart rates, therefore, are poorly tolerated. Furthermore, the thick ventricle with its prolonged contractile phase requires a high diastolic pressure for coronary perfusion, and increases in peripheral vascular resistance with vasopressors may be required. With mitral insufficiency, a varying percent of the stroke volume is ejected back into the atrium before the aortic valve opens. A moderately fast heart rate in this condition is beneficial. In contrast to aortic stenosis, increases in peripheral vascular resistance are to be avoided to diminish the amount of regurgitant flow.

Aortic systolic murmurs are a concern to the anesthesiologist because of the management implications between aortic stenosis and idiopathetic hypertrophic subaortic stenosis (IHSS), positive inotrophic agents being indicated in aortic stenosis, but contraindicated in IHSS. Although IHSS is the second most common cause of stenosis in the aortic area, it is not likely to be a problem for the gynecologic patient. Males outnumber females in the most common sporadiac variety of this disease by 4:1.

The night before surgery is a bad time to request of the cardiologist or the internist specifically what conditions we are dealing with. Exact diagnosis may require a more extensive diagnostic workup. If the consult requests nothing more than "cardiac clearance," this is often followed by the pharmacologic history of the patient and the concluding recommendation "okay for surgery." A directed consult will go a long way in refuting any allegations of inadequate workup.

MITRAL VALVE PROLAPSE

Mitral valve prolapse can be expected to be the most common prevelant valve disease in the gynecologic patient. In their report of mitral valve prolapse in the general population, the Framingham Study (9) reported an overall incidence of 5%, with females outnumbering males in all decades, except the ninth.[9] In females, the incidence was 17% in the third decade, with a gradual decline in the incidence to 1.8% in the eighth decade. For reasons not yet clear, it is much more common in those individuals with a thin-chested lordotic ballerina type of habitus. When the patient is symptomatic, the symptoms are most frequently nonspecific and approach those of a benign cardiac neurosis.[10] It is usually detected by a systolic click and a variable systolic murmur in the mitral area. Verification is by echocardiography. No definite association of mitral valve prolapse with coronary artery disease, hypertrophic cardiomyopathy, septal defects, or rheumatic heart disease has been established, and, indeed, it is by far a benign condition. However, clinical reports of an increased frequency of noxious arrhythmias, transient ischemic episodes, and sudden death cannot be disregarded. The prognosis is guarded in young females with abnormal ECGs and/or echocardiographic evidence of redundant leaflets.[11] Furthermore, because mitral valve prolapse is the most common form of isolated mitral regurgitation, the anesthesiologist will be concerned about the hemodynamic management of these cases. The cardiologist or internist can be helpful in determining the appropriateness of echocardiography. Antibiotic prophylaxis against endocarditis is controversial. I believe that the presence of the murmur itself is an indication for such antibiotics.

REFERENCES

1. Katz J, Benumof J, Kadis LB: *Anesthesia and Uncommon Diseases.* Philadelphia, WB Saunders Co, 1981.
2. Stoelting RK, Dierdorf SF: *Anesthesia and Coexisting Disease.* New York, Churchill Livingstone, 1983.
3. Paul DR, Hoyt JL, Boutros AR: Cardiovascular and respiratory changes in response to change of posture in the very obese. *Anesthesiology* 1976; 45:73–77.
4. Goldman L, Caldera DL: Risks of general anesthetic and elective operation in the hypertensive patient. *Anesthesiology* 1979; 50:285–292.
5. Vitez TS, Soper LE, Wong KC, et al: Chronic hypokalemia and intraoperative dysrhythmia. *Anesthesiology* 1985; 63:130–133.
6. McGovern B: Hypokalemia and cardiac arrhythmias. *Anesthesiology* 1985; 63:127–129.
7. Hurst TW, Logue RB: *The Heart,* in *Etiology of Coronary Atherosclerosis,* ed 2. New York, McGraw-Hill Book Co, 1970, pp 909–910.
8. Rao TLK, Jacobs KH, Et-Etr AA: Reinfarction following anesthesia in patients with myocardial infarction. *Anesthesiology* 1983; 59:499–505.
9. Savage DD, Castilli WP, McNamara PM, et al: Mitral valve prolapse in the general population. *Am Heart J* 1983; 106:571–576.
10. Beton DC, Brear SG, Edwards JD, et al: Mitral valve prolapse—an assessment of clinical features associated conditions and prognosis. *Q J Med* 1983; 52:150–164.
11. Wishimura RA, McGon MD, Shub C, et al: Echocardiographically documented mitral valve prolapse. *N Engl J Med* 1985; 313:1305–1309.
12. Bone RC, Fisher CJ, Clemmer TP, et al: A controlled clinical trial of high dose methylprednisolone in the treatment of severe sepsis and septic shock. *N Engl J Med* 1987; 317:653–658.

SUGGESTED READINGS

Hanken AH, Sussman EJ: The physiologic response to surgery and anesthesia, in Goldman DR, Brown FH, Levy WK, et al (eds): *Medical Care of the Surgical Patient.* Philadelphia: JB Lippincott Co, 1982, pp 1–15.

Hirsh RA: An approach to assessing perioperative risk, in Goldman DR, Brown FH, Levy WK, et al (eds): *Medical Care of the Surgical Patient.* Philadelphia, JB Lippincott Co, 1982, pp 31–39.

Johnson JC: Surgery in the elderly, in Goldman DR, Brown FH, Levy WK, et al (eds): *Medical Care of the Surgical Patient.* Philadelphia, JB Lippincott Co, 1982, pp 578–590.

Viljoen JF: Anesthetic considerations in reoperative surgery, in Tomkins RK (ed): *Reoperative Surgery.* Philadelphia, JB Lippincott Co, 1988, pp 9–15.

Chapter 25

Medical/Legal Implications

Saul Lerner, M.D.

Any time that an operation has to be repeated for the same problem, there is a natural assumption on the part of the nonmedical public that the surgeon who performed the first operation did it improperly. Given the present malpractice climate wherein some opportunistic lawyers vigorously advertise free consultation for anyone who believes he or she may have been the victim of such less than perfectly performed surgery, it is inevitable that many of these cases will progress to a lawsuit. What can one do to minimize one's risk in such an atmosphere? If one is to survive in an unfavorable environment, one must accept the fact that the nature of the playing field has changed and mount a defensive strategy to meet the new challenge.

It is impossible to guarantee a perfect result on each case. There are too many extraneous factors beyond the surgeon's control that influence the final result such as poor tissue in an individual patient or lack of compliance on the patient's part. Thus, it is probably inevitable that if a gynecologist is busy enough, he or she will probably be the victim of a lawsuit.

Many surgeons, having informed the patient that surgery will have to be performed to deal with the patient's problem, recognize the patient's apprehensive reaction as inordinate and may tend to overdo it in trying to alleviate that apprehension. In so doing, he or she may leave the patient with the feeling that nothing can go wrong and the result will inevitably be perfect. We all know that we cannot give guarantees of a perfect result. Yet the fact is that many plaintiffs claim that the surgeon guaranteed their problem would be solved by the surgery. The surgeon must go out of his or her way when explaining the operation to the patient to make sure that no guarantee is being offered. The surgeon must honestly explain the possibility of failure and even give honest statistics on failure rates. Certain operations have a higher degree of failure to permanently solve the patient's problem such as repair operations as opposed to ablation of an organ, and recognizing that possibility, the surgeon, in obtaining consent for surgery, must inform the patient of possibilities for failure so that consent will be *informed consent*. But, as a defensive strategy, that would not be enough. The surgeon must take the time to document in the office record that he or she explained the possibility of failure or eventual recurrence of the problem. Most gynecologists are busy and are frequently behind schedule in the office, but if they are unwilling to take the time to do such documentation, they must accept the idea that they are ignoring the reality of the playing field and leaving themselves vulnerable if sued.

Surgery performed to correct such problems as urinary stress incontinence, prolapse of the uterus, fistulas, cystocele, rectocele, or enterocele will generally be successful for a period of time, but there is a definite eventual recurrence rate for each of these. I am not going to discuss each of these separately but will discuss the problem of pregnancy following sterilization (which is generally followed by repeat sterilizing procedure) more in depth since the same principles apply to almost all of the other problems.

It is generally accepted that 2 or 3 sterilization procedures in every 1,000 will fail and the woman will eventually find herself pregnant. It is also generally assumed that in most of the failures the procedure was performed properly. The healing process in the human is unpredictable; fistulous tracts that allow sperm or egg to bypass the manufactured barrier can develop and the patient becomes pregnant—a true natural accident. However, the first reaction of a lay person (i.e., either a patient or a member of a jury) is that the operation was improperly done. Many lawyers know that the resultant pregnancy was not the result of a surgical error, but they are aware of the public perception. Thus, the basis for most lawsuits in this category is not that the operation was improperly done but that the patient was not informed that the operation carries with it a chance of failure. The best defense against the charge that the operation was not properly done is an operative note clearly stating that each tube was traced out to its distal end, the fimbria were seen, and thus the tube was clearly identified before the tubal occlusion was accomplished. Too often the surgeon who is being sued rushes to review the operative note only to find that the resident who dictated the note simply said, "A Fallope ring was applied to each tube." At that point, he or she can only wish that he or she had taken the time to read the note before signing it.

Sometimes, it is impossible during laparoscopic sterilization or minilaparotomy to trace the tube completely to its fimbriated end, but the surgeon is confident that the grasped structure is, indeed, the tube because the round ligament can be traced as a separate structure. What to do? Good medical practice (even if there were no malpractice threat) requires that the patient be informed that there was some uncertainty that the divided structure was tube and that she must not have unprotected intercourse until a hysterogram can be performed 3 months later. Most important, when the operative note is dictated, the plan of management should be clearly stated, and the surgeon should document that he or she so instructed the patient in the record.

Now, let us return to the problem of informed consent. I am repeatedly amazed at how often there is a signed consent form in the medical record, yet the plaintiff claims a lack of informed consent. The general claim is that a clerk thrust a paper at the patient and demanded that it be signed. A good lawyer will note that when one takes his or her car in for repair, a long complicated document must be signed before leaving (without having read the document). There is only one practical precautionary defense against lack of informed consent, and that is proper documentation, reinforced by the surgeon taking the time from an admittedly busy office to explain the nature of the operation, its side effects, its permanence, and its unavoidable inherent failure rate to the patient. Informed consent requires that the patient understand the nature of the act, as in the example of tubal sterilization, that it is not a method of birth control but of terminating the childbearing period. I tell patients that they must not think of the procedure as something that can be reversed if they decide to have another baby since the reversability success rate is only 70%. Since subsequent pregnancy is the cause of most lawsuits in this category, it must be explained to the patient that no matter which technique is used, and, in spite of the fact that the operation is properly performed, about 2 or 3 women in 1,000 will become pregnant because of the body's remarkable capacity to repair itself. Naturally, such explanations must be given in a manner that the surgeon is sure the patient understands what is being said. Survival tactics demand that the surgeon record in his or her notes that he or she explained all of this to the patient. As a further defensive move, I recommend that the surgeon give the patient a booklet on sterilization (e.g., American College of Obstetricians and Gynecologists' booklet), which mentions the inherent failure rate, and record in his notes that such a booklet was given to the patient. The inevitable claim that one hears in court is that "he told me that after this operation I would never be able to get pregnant." Although most hospitals have each patient sign a consent form before surgery, for sterilization procedures, the surgeon should have the patient sign a witnessed form in the office. Such a consent form must explicitly include information about the permanence of the procedure and the lack of guarantee.

Not all second operations are done because of recurrence of the original problem. On occasion a patient will require a second operation very soon after the first operation to deal with an unexpected complication such as postoperative hemorrhage, intestinal obstruction, or evisceration. Once again the nonmedically trained person suspects that the original operation was not properly done, and such a situation lends itself to exploitation by an opportunistic lawyer. It is most important to have careful documentation of the surgeons preoperative assessment of the case. Keep in mind that the claim frequently made in the ensuing lawsuit is that the diagnosis of the complication should have been made earlier in the course of events, and this would have prevented the serious sequelae that followed. When the patient is not doing as well as should have been expected postoperatively, that is the time for the surgeon to seek consultation—not a corridor consultation but an official one documented in the record. Granted that such consultation may not be necessary for management of the patient's problem, it is of great help in mounting a defense in a subsequent lawsuit (or, better still, in discouraging a stalking lawyer).

Frequently, when such emergency surgery has to be performed, the patient may not be alert and in command of all of her senses. Under such circumstances, the husband or parent should be asked to substitute for the patient and grant consent for the surgery. Again, it must be informed consent. Sometimes the husband or other close relative is not immediately available and the situation is urgent, requiring haste in getting the patient to the operating room. In that case, a surgical colleague (or even a medical one) should be asked for a consultation to agree that the surgery is both necessary and urgent.

Many times the lawsuit, when filed, will also be directed against the hospital. It would be wise under certain circumstances when it is reasonable to anticipate such a possibility to alert the administrator on call so that he or she can set in motion such risk management moves that are indicated.

All surgeons have had the experience of being in the midst of an operation and making an unanticipated discovery requiring removal of another organ or doing something other than what was told to the patient before surgery. Even though the surgeon is fully competent to handle this new development, he or she should seek supportive consultation with a colleague as an extension of the consent process. Naturally, the existance of such a consultation should be recorded in the surgeon's operative note but also the consultation report should be written separately in the record signed by the consultant.

The most common malpractice claim against gynecologists concerns failure to diagnose breast cancer early enough, but that is beyond the scope of this book on repeat gynecologic operations and will not be discussed. The next most common problems concern alleged failure to sterilize properly and ectopic pregnancy. Most suits related to ectopic pregnancy involve delayed diagnosis, but a certain number involve repeat ectopic pregnancy in the same tube. Most gynecologists prefer to conserve organs whenever possible, and many operations are done in which the pregnancy is removed from the tube by one means or another and the tube reconstructed. There is some disagreement on the wisdom of this approach, since it leaves a scar in the tube that could trap the fertilized egg on its journey through the tube to the uterus, setting up another ectopic pregnancy. I will not discuss the merits of the different surgical techniques employed to reduce the possibility, but I will point out that this possibility should be properly disclosured to the patient before surgery. Although there still are some true emergencies with ruptured ectopic pregnancy requiring rapid course of action to deal with hemorrhage threatening the patient's life, most ectopic pregnancies are diagnosed early using a combination of quantitative human chorionic gonadotropins, ultrasound, and/or laparoscopy, leaving plenty of time for discussion of her problem with the patient. The various approaches to her problem with their advantages and disadvantages, should be explained to the patient. The possibility of repeat ectopic pregnancy should be presented to the patient fairly, and she should be allowed to select the procedure of her choice, conservation of the tube or excision. The gynecologist can certainly recommend his or her choice to the patient as long as it is done fairly. Consent to surgery must be informed consent. This means explaining alternatives, side effects, possible complications, and possible failure rates to the patient. The wise surgeon not only explains all of these, but also documents in the chart that he or she has done each of them.

Index

R

S